Statistical Methods in Spatial Epidemiology

WILEY SERIES IN PROBABILITY AND STATISTICS

Established by WALTER A. SHEWHART and SAMUEL S. WILKS

A complete list of the titles in this series appears at the end of this volume

Statistical Methods in Spatial Epidemiology

ANDREW B. LAWSON
University of Aberdeen, UK

JOHN WILEY & SONS, LTD
Chichester • New York • Weinheim • Brisbane • Singapore • Toronto

Telephone (+44) 1243 779777

Email (for orders and customer service enquiries): cs-books@wiley.co.uk
Visit our Home Page on www.wileyeurope.com or www.wiley.com

Reprinted December 2001, June 2004, January 2005

Other Wiley Editorial Offices

John Wiley & Sons Inc., 111 River Street, Hoboken, NJ 07030, USA

Jossey-Bass, 989 Market Street, San Francisco, CA 94103-1741, USA

Wiley-VCH Verlag GmbH, Boschstr. 12, D-69469 Weinheim, Germany

John Wiley & Sons Australia Ltd, 33 Park Road, Milton, Queensland 4064, Australia

John Wiley & Sons (Asia) Pte Ltd, 2 Clementi Loop #02-01, Jin Xing Distripark, Singapore 129809

John Wiley & Sons Canada Ltd, 22 Worcester Road, Etobicoke, Ontario, Canada M9W 1L1

Library of Congress Cataloging-in-Publication Data

Lawson, A. B. (Andrew B.)
Statistical methods in spatial epidemiology / A.B. Lawson.
p. cm.—(Wiley series in probability and statistics)
Includes bibliographical references and index.
ISBN 0-471-97572-9 (alk. paper)
1. Medical geography—Statistical methods. 2. Epidemiology—Statistical methods. I. Title. II. Series.

RA792 .L39 2001
614.4′2′0727—dc21 00-043389

British Library Cataloguing in Publication Data

A catalogue record for this book is available from the British Library

ISBN 0-471-97572-9

Typeset in 10/12pt Times by T&T Productions Ltd, London.
Printed and bound in Great Britain by Antony Rowe Ltd, Chippenham, Wiltshire.
This book is printed on acid-free paper responsibly manufactured from sustainable forestry in which at least two trees are planted for each one used for paper production.

Contents

Preface

The development of statistical methods in spatial epidemiology has had a chequered career. One of the earliest examples of the analysis of geographical locations of disease in relation to a putative health hazard was John Snow's analysis of cholera cases in relation to the location of the Broad Street water pump in London (Snow, 1854). However, until recently, developments in statistical methods in this area have been sporadic. While medical geography developed in the 1960s (Howe, 1963), only a number of papers on space-time clustering (Mantel, 1967; Knox, 1964) appeared in the statistical literature. More recently, developments of methods in spatial statistics, image processing, and in particular Bayesian methods and computation, have seen parallel developments in methods for spatial epidemiology (see Marshall (1991b) for a review). It is notable that methods for the analysis of case locations around a source of hazard (such as Snow's cholera map) have only recently been developed (Diggle, 1989; Lawson, 1989). The current increased level of interest in statistical methods in spatial epidemiology is a reflection, in part, of the increased concern in society for environmental issues and their relation to the health of individuals. Hence, the 'detection' of pollution sources or sources of health hazard can be seen as the backdrop to many studies in environmental epidemiology (Diggle, 1993). The correct allocation of resources for health care in different areas by health services is also greatly enhanced by the development of statistical methods which allow more accurate depiction of 'true' disease incidence and its relation to explanatory variables. Previous work in this area has been reviewed by Lawson and Cressie (2000), and Marshall (1991b) and Elliott *et al.* (1992a) discuss the general epidemiological issues surrounding spatial epidemiological problems.

It is the purpose of this book to provide an overview of the main statistical methods currently available in the field of spatial epidemiology. Inevitably, some selectivity in choice of methods reviewed will be apparent, but it is hoped that our coverage will encompass the most important areas of development. One area which we do not examine in detail is that of space-time analysis of epidemiological data, although the modelling of infectious disease data is considered in Chapter 11.

As this book is mainly a review of recent research work, its target audience is largely confined to those with some statistical knowledge and is appropriate for third level degree and postgraduate students in statistics, or epidemiology with a strong statistical background.

A considerable number of people have directly or indirectly contributed to the production of this book. First, I acknowledge the support of Sharon Clutton and Helen Ramsey at Wiley and Tony Johnson of Statistics in Medicine for their support from Budapest onwards. Fundamental influences in the development of my ideas in spatial epidemiology have been Richard Cormack and Peter Diggle. I also acknowledge the encouragement of Noel Cressie, who has supported my work through visits to Iowa State and Ohio State Universities, and important collaborations with Martin Kulldorff, Annibale Biggeri, Dankmar Boehning, Peter Schlattmann, Emmanuel Lesaffre, Jean-Francois Viel, Adrian Baddeley, Niels Becker and Andrew Cliff.

Andrew B. Lawson
Aberdeen, March 2000

Part I

The Nature of Spatial Epidemiology

CHAPTER 1

Definitions, Terminology and Data Sets

Spatial epidemiology concerns the analysis of the spatial/geographical distribution of the incidence of disease. In its simplest form the subject concerns the use and interpretation of *maps* of the locations of disease cases, and the associated issues relating to map production and the statistical analysis of mapped data must apply within this subject. In addition, the nature of *disease* maps ensures that many epidemiological concepts also play an important role the analysis. In essence, these two different aspects of the subject have their own impact on the methodology which has developed to deal with the many issues which arise in this area.

First, since mapped data are spatial in nature, the application of *spatial* statistical methods forms a core part of the subject area. The reason for this lies in the fact that the study of any data which are georeferenced (i.e. have a spatial/geographical location associated with them) may have properties which relate to the location of individual data items and also the surrounding data. For example, Figure 1.1 shows the total number of deaths from respiratory cancer found in 26 small areas (census tracts) in central Scotland over the period 1976–1983. This map displays a number of features which commonly arise when the geographical distribution of disease is examined. On this map the numbers (counts) of cases within each area are displayed. In some areas of the map the counts are similar to those found in the immediately surrounding areas (e.g. in the south and southeast of the map counts of 4 and 6 are recorded, while in the northwest of the map, lower counts are found in many areas). This similarity in the count data in groups of tracts is unlikely to have arisen from the allocation of a random sample of counts from a common statistical distribution. The counts may display some form of correlation in their levels based on their location, i.e. counts close to each other in space are similar. This form of correlation does not arise from the usual statistical models assumed to apply to independent observations found in, for example, clinical medical studies or other conventional statistical application areas. Hence, methods which apply to the analysis of these data must be able to address the possibility of such correlation existing in the mapped data under study. Another feature of this example, which commonly arises in the study of spatial epidemiology, is the irregular nature of the regions within which the counts are observed, i.e. the census tracts have irregular geographical boundaries. This may arise as a feature of the

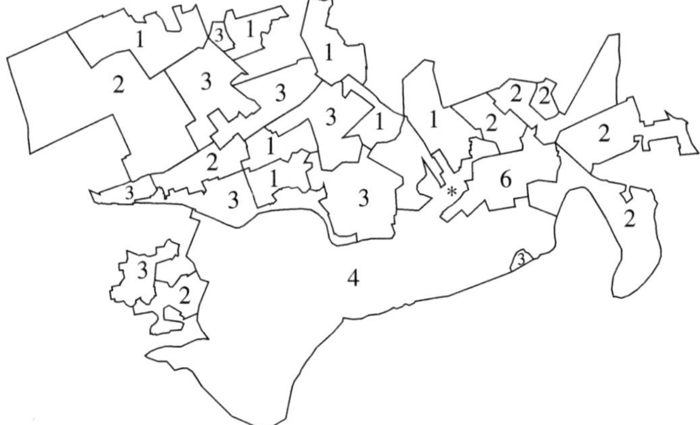

Figure 1.1 Falkirk: central Scotland respiratory cancer counts in 26 census enumeration districts over a fixed time period. $*$ Putative health hazard.

whole study region (*study window*) or may be found associated with tracts themselves. In some countries, notably in North America, small areas are often regular in shape and size and this feature simplifies the resulting analysis. However, in many other areas irregular region geometries are common. Finally, in some studies, the spatial distribution of cases or counts of disease are to be related to other locations on the map. For example, in Figure 1.1 the location of a potential (*putative*) environmental health hazard is also mapped (a metal-processing plant), and the focus of the study may be to assess the relationship of the disease incidence on the map to that location, perhaps to make inferences about the environmental risk in its vicinity.

The second feature which uniquely defines the study of spatial epidemiology is that the mapped data are often *discrete*. Unlike other areas of spatial statistical analysis, which are often focused on continuous data, e.g. geostatistical methods, the data found in spatial epidemiology often take the form of point locations (the address locations of cases of disease) or counts of disease within regions such as census tracts or, at larger scale, counties or municipalities. Hence, the mapped data often consist of cartesian coordinates in the form of a grid reference or longitude/latitude of an address of a case, or a count of cases within a region with the associated location of that region (either as a point location of a centroid or as a set of boundary line segments defining the region). Given this form of data format, it is not surprising that models which have been developed for applications within this area are derived from stochastic point process theory (for case locations) and associated discrete probability distributions (for counts within arbitrary regions).

Finally, the epidemiological nature of these discrete spatial data leads to the derivation of models and methods which are related to conventional epidemiological studies. For example, the case control study, where individual cases are matched to control individuals based on specific criteria, has parallels in spatial epidemiology where spatial control *distributions* are used to provide a locational control for cases. This is akin to the estimation of background hazard in survival studies. One fundamental epidemiological issue which arises in these studies is the incorporation of the local population which is at risk of contracting the disease in question. As we must control for the spatial variation in the underlying population, then we must be able to obtain good estimates of the population from which the cases or counts arise. This estimation often leads to the derivation of *expected* rates in the region count case and further to the estimation of the ratio of count to expected count/rate or the *relative risk*, in each area. Relative risk is a fundamental epidemiological concept (Clayton and Hills, 1993) in non-spatial epidemiological studies.

1.1 MAP HYPOTHESES AND MODELLING APPROACHES

In any spatial epidemiological analysis, there will usually be a study focus which specifies the nature and style of the methods to be used. This focus will usually consist of a hypothesis or hypotheses about the nature of the spatial distribution of the disease which is to be examined, and it is convenient to categorise these hypotheses into three broad classes: *disease mapping*, *ecological analysis* and *disease clustering*. Usually, the distribution of cases of disease, whether in the form of counts or case address locations, can be thought to follow an underlying model, and the observed data may contain extra noise in the form of random variation around the model of interest. Often, the model will include aspects of the *null* (hypothesis) spatial distribution of the cases, which captures the 'normal' variation which is expected, and also aspects of the *alternative* spatial distribution. In much of spatial epidemiology, the focus of attention is on identifying features of the spatial distribution which are not captured by the null hypothesis distribution. This is mainly related to *excess spatial aggregation* of cases in areas of the map. That is, once the normal variation is allowed for, the residual spatial incidence *above* the normal incidence is the focus. Seldom is there any need to examine areas of lower aggregation than would be normally expected. Note that 'normal' variation is usually assumed to be defined by the underlying population distribution of the study region/window and cases are thought to arise in relation to the local variation in that distribution.

The first class, that of *disease mapping*, concerns the use of models to describe the overall disease distribution on the map. In disease mapping, often the object is simply to 'clean' the map of disease of the extra noise to uncover the underlying structure. In that situation, the null hypothesis could be that the case distribution arises from an *unspecified* or partly specified null spatial distribution (which includes the population spatial distribution) and the object is to remove the extra noise/variation. In this sense disease mapping is close in spirit to image processing where *segmentation* usually describes the process of allocating pixels or groups of pixels to classes.

The second class, that of *ecological analysis*, concerns the analysis of the relation between the spatial distribution of disease incidence and measured explanatory factors. This is usually carried out at an aggregated spatial level, and usually concerns regional incidence compared to explanatory factors measured at regional or other levels of aggregation (Greenberg *et al.*, 1996). This contrasts with studies which use measurements made on individual subjects. However, many of the issues concerning interpretation of ecological studies are concerned with *change* in aggregation level and not aggregated data per se. For example, the *ecological fallacy* concerns making inference about individuals from analyses carried out at a higher scale, e.g. regional or country-wide level. Equally, the *atomistic fallacy* concerns making inferences about average characteristics from individual measurements. In what follows we assume a relatively wide definition of ecological, more in the sense of ecology itself, that any study which seeks to describe/explain the spatial distribution of disease based on the inclusion of explanatory variables. Two classic studies of this kind are presented by Cook and Pocock (1983), who examined the relation of cardiovascular incidence in the UK to a variety of variables (including water hardness, climate, location, socio-economic and genetic factors and air pollution), and Donnelly (1995), who examined the respiratory health of school children and volatile organic compounds in the out-door atmosphere. Note that this general definition can include the situation where case address locations are related to a pollution hazard via explanatory variables such as distance and direction from the hazard. In that case individual data is related to explanatory variables.

The final class, that of *disease clustering*, concerns the analysis of 'unusual' aggregations of disease, i.e. assessing whether there are any areas of elevated incidence of disease within a map. This type of analysis could take a variety of forms. First, the analysis could include the assessment of a complete map to ascertain whether the map is *clustered.* This is often termed *general clustering*. In this case, the null hypothesis would be that the disease map represents normal variation in incidence given the population distribution. The alternative hypothesis would include some specified clustering mechanism for the disease cases. This mechanism could be descriptive or include some notion of how the clusters form (e.g. clusters can form if infectious diseases are examined, and the contact rate of individuals can be modelled). General clustering is often treated as a form of *autocorrelation* and models for such effects are often employed. This form of clustering can be termed *non-specific* as it does not seek to determine where clusters are found but instead simply seeks to determine whether the pattern is clustered.

Second, *specific* cluster studies attempt to ascertain the locations of any clusters if they exist on the map. These clusters could have known (fixed) locations and the incidence of disease around these locations may be assessed for its relation to the location(s). Studies of putative pollution hazards fall within this category. This is often termed *focused* clustering. If the locations of clusters are unknown *a priori*, then the locations must also be estimated from the data; this is termed *non-focused* clustering. Often, ecological regression methods can be used in focused clustering studies. whereas, for non-focused studies special methods must be constructed which allow the estimation of cluster locations and their form.

In all the above areas of study, fundamental to the methods employed is the inclusion of spatial location in the analysis and so spatial statistical methods are often employed to model the observed data, that epidemiological considerations should be employed in any study of the distribution of disease incidence, in that the concept of normal variation of disease (i.e. that generated from the population at risk from the disease)

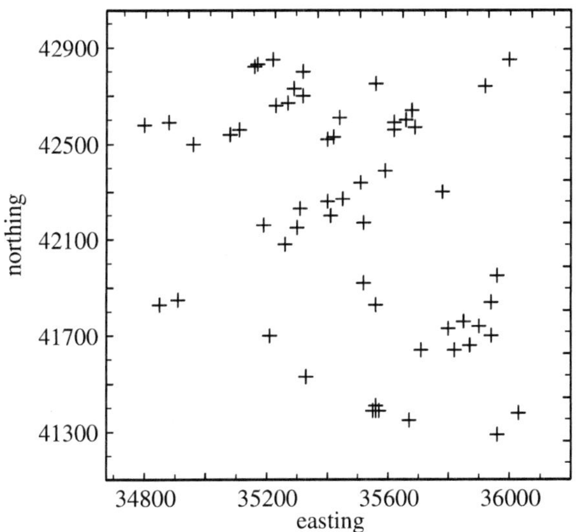

Figure 1.2 The locations of larynx cancer cases in an area of central Lancashire, UK, for the period 1974–1983.

must be catered for in any model of incidence, and that methods used should be appropriate to the analysis of georeferenced discrete data.

1.2 DEFINITIONS AND DATA EXAMPLES

In this section, some basic definitions and concepts are introduced which are used throughout this book. In addition, a number of data examples make their first appearance and these will be referred to at various stages throughout the work.

In what follows we will mainly be concerned with data which are available within a single period of time. Hence, we do not provide notation for space-time problems here. Where such notation is appropriate, we provide it locally.

We define 'epidemiology' as the study of the occurrence of disease in relation to explanatory factors. A strict dictionary definition of the term implies the study of 'epidemic diseases'. However, in this work we mainly restrict attention to *fixed* time period studies and do not directly examine the dynamic behaviour of disease incidence. This area has recently been reviewed in Mollison (1995). Some discussion of epidemic models appear in Chapter 11. Here the term 'spatial epidemiology' is defined to mean the study of the occurrence of disease in spatial locations and its explanatory factors. Usually, the disease to be examined occurs within a *map* and the data are expressed as a point location (case event) or are aggregated as a count of disease within a subregion of the map. Two examples of such data are provided in Figures 1.2 and 1.3. These two data types lead to different modelling approaches, and we make specific the following definitions as a basis for further discussion.

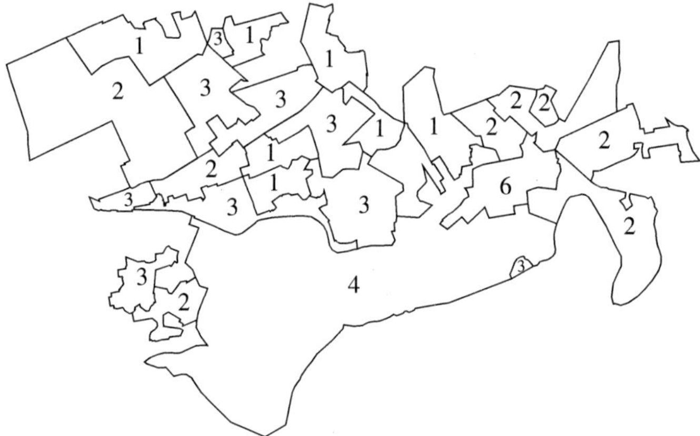

Figure 1.3 Respiratory cancer counts within census tracts (enumeration districts) of Falkirk, central Scotland, for the period 1978–1983.

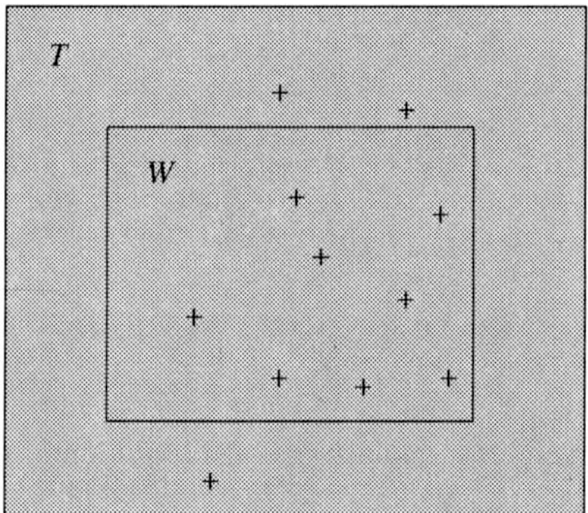

Figure 1.4 A notional study area (W) and a guard area (T).

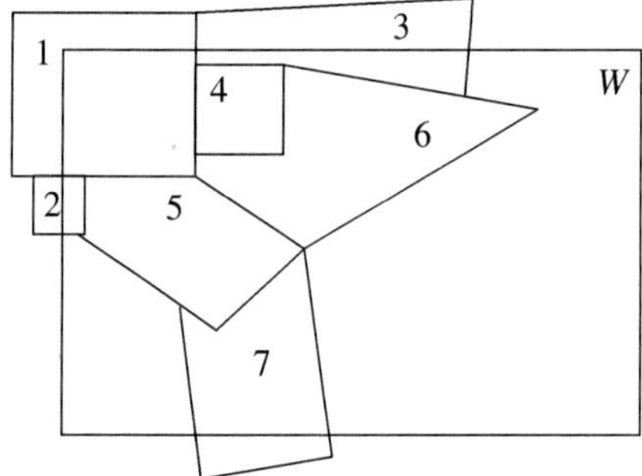

Figure 1.5 A study region within which counts are observed in subregions (tracts).

1.2.1 Case Event Data

We define the study window (W), within which m disease case events occur at locations $\boldsymbol{x}_i$, $i = 1, \ldots, m$. The area of W is denoted by $|W|$, Lebesgue measure on $\mathbb{R}^2$. Figure 1.4 displays these definitions.

1.2.2 Count Data

We define the study window (W) as above, within which m *arbitrarily bounded* subregions, wholly or in part, lie. The count in m subregion tracts is denoted n_i, $i = 1, \ldots, m$. In Figure 1.5, only regions 4, 5 and 6 are wholly within the window. Regions 1, 2, 3 and 7 are cut by the window boundary. The effect of this region truncation will be discussed in detail later. However, it should be noted that, *usually*, the count available (n_i) is from the complete region and *not* from the truncated region which appears in the study window.

Usually, the m subregions are politically defined administrative regions and are often tracts defined for the purposes of population censuses. We adopt the term 'census tract' to denote an arbitrarily defined region. In addition, the counts in census tracts are just an aggregation of case event data counted within the bounding tract boundaries. Hence, the data in Figure 1.5 could be derived from the data in Figure 1.4 by counting case events in census tract subregions of the window.

The object of analysis of case event or count data can define the type of summary measures used to describe the data. Usually, as a basic summary measure it is common to compute a local measure of relative risk, or to use a local measure of relative risk as the dependent variable in a more substantial analysis. Here, relative risk is taken to mean the measure of excess risk found in relation to that supported purely by the local population, which is 'at risk'. This population is sometimes called the 'at-risk' population or background. Relative risk is derived or computed from the relation of observed incidence to that which would be expected based on the 'at-risk' background. It is common practice within epidemiology to derive such risk estimates. In the case of spatial epidemiology, it is common, when tract count data are available, to compute a standardised mortality (or morbidity) ratio (SMR), which is simply the ratio of the observed count within a tract to the expected count based on the 'at-risk' background. A ratio greater than 1.0 would suggest an excess of risk within the tract. These SMRs are often the basis for atlases of disease risk (see, for example, Pickle *et al.*, 1999).

1.3 FURTHER DEFINITIONS

Some further definitions are required in relation to data which arise in such studies.

1.3.1 Control Events and Processes

Often, an additional process or realisation of disease events is used to provide an estimate of the 'background' incidence of disease in an area. Define $\boldsymbol{x}_{cj}$, $j = 1, \ldots, m_c$,

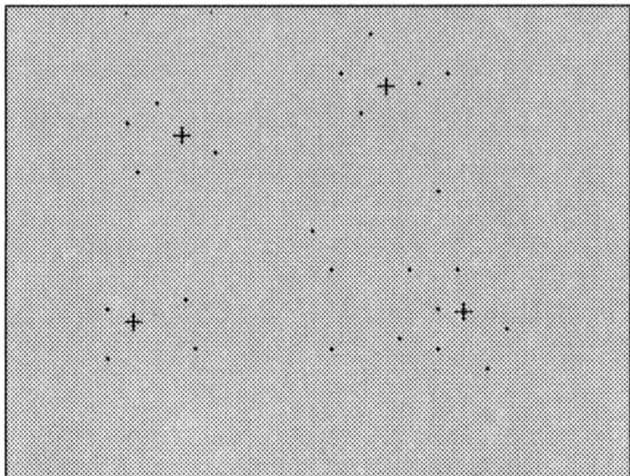

Figure 1.6 Pictorial representation of clustering definitions; $\cdot$, offspring $\{x\}$; $+$, centre, $\{y_c\}$.

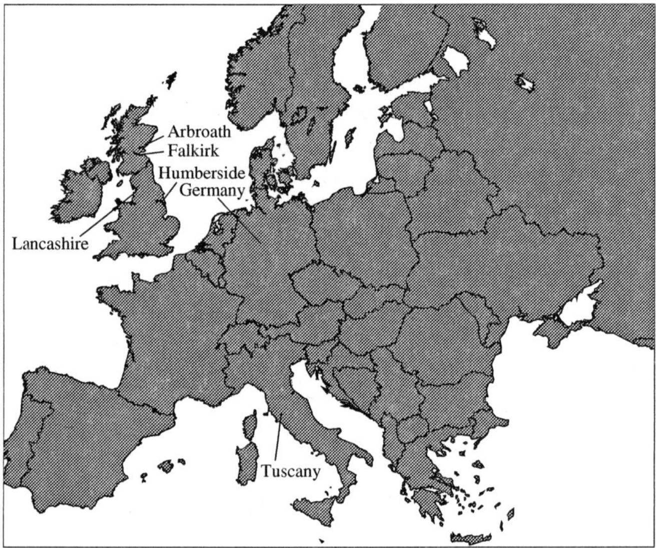

Figure 1.7 European location map.

to be these m_c control event locations. The use of such data will be detailed in a later section.

1.3.2 Census Tract Information

The census tract count of a control disease is defined to be n_c.

Instead of using a control disease to represent 'background', the 'expected' incidence of disease can be used. This is usually based on known rates of disease in the population (Inskip *et al.*, 1983). Denote this expected incidence as e_i, $i = 1, \ldots, m$. The total population of a tract is p_i, while the extent of the tract is defined as a_i. The tract centroid, however defined, is denoted by $\boldsymbol{x}_{n_i}$.

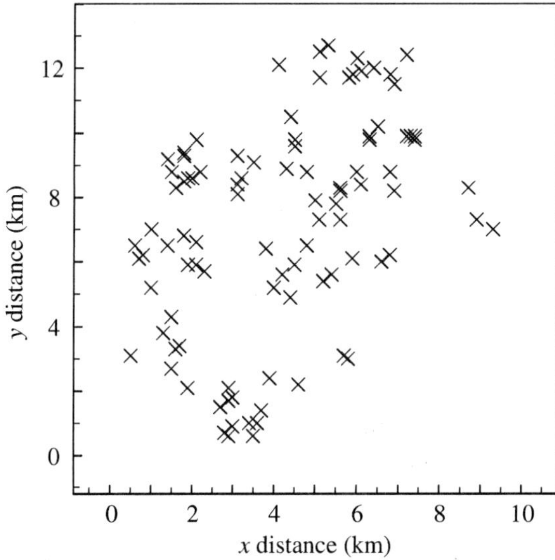

Figure 1.8 Arbroath: respiratory cancer case event map.

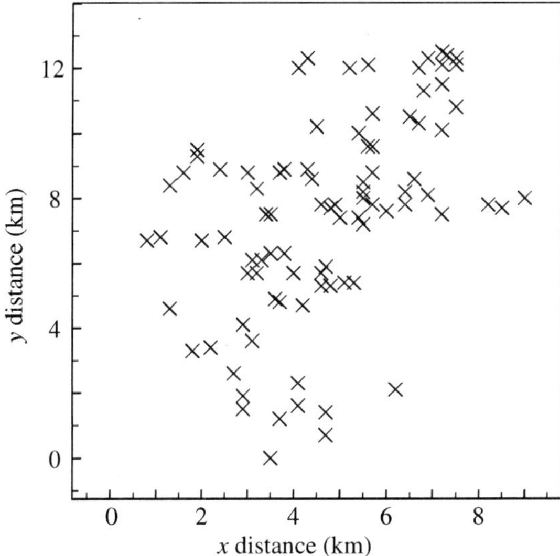

Figure 1.9 Arbroath: gastric and oesophageal cancer case event map.

For models involving explanatory variables measured at tract level, we define F as an $m \times p$ matrix whose columns represent p explanatory variables, and α as a $p \times 1$ vector of parameters. (For case event models the row dimension of F will usually be m also.)

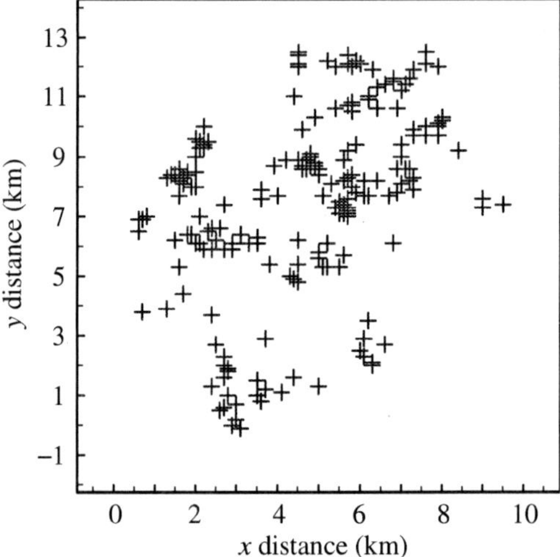

Figure 1.10 Arbroath: bronchitis case event map.

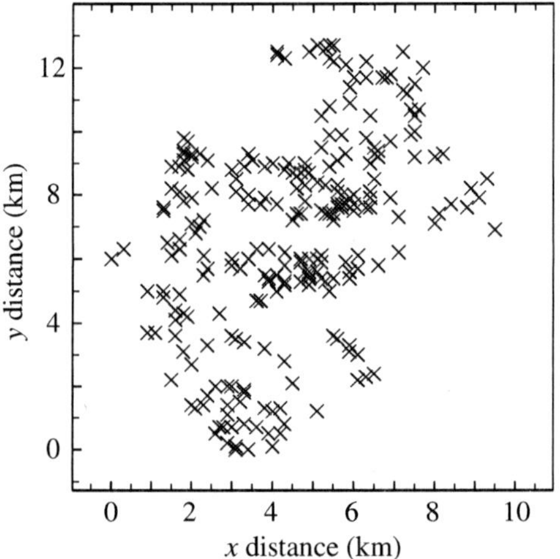

Figure 1.11 Arbroath: control disease (lower-body cancers) case event map.

1.3.3 Clustering Definitions

In cases where clustering is studied, a number of additional definitions are required. First, cluster centre locations are defined as $\boldsymbol{y}_j$, $j = 1, \ldots, k$, where k is the number of centres in a suitably defined window. The term 'parent' is used here synonymously with cluster centre. This does not imply any genetic linkage with the observed data. The observed data belonging to a cluster are sometimes referred to as offspring. Again, there is no genetic linkage implied by this term. In addition, the offspring (or tract

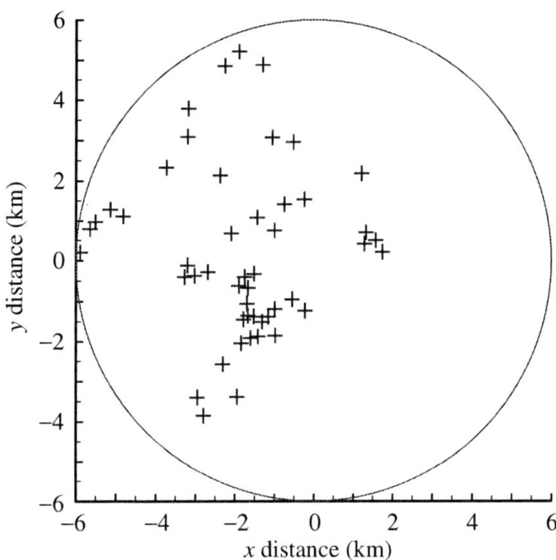

Figure 1.12 Armadale: 49 respiratory cancer death certificate addresses, within circular window.

count) associated with a particular parent, $\mathbf{y}_i$ say, have an integer label, z_i, denoting their associated parent. These definitions are displayed in Figure 1.6.

1.4 SOME DATA EXAMPLES

In the following discussion a number of data examples will be examined. These are used to motivate discussion of certain modelling issues and to provide insight into the nature of the data which arise in this area. The examples are chosen to represent different approaches to the study of the spatial distribution of disease. The data sets are available as a link from a website: http://www.maths.abdn.ac.uk/maths/department/staff/pages/lawson_a.html.

In Chapters 10 and 11 additional data sets are introduced which are only referenced in those chapters.

1.4.1 Case Event Examples

The following examples have been analysed previously and represent different aspects of analysis.

Arbroath: Multiple Disease Study

Arbroath is a small town on the east coast of Scotland. A retrospective study of the health status in that town was initiated following concerns over airborne emissions from a centrally located steel foundry. For the period 1966–1976, the address locations

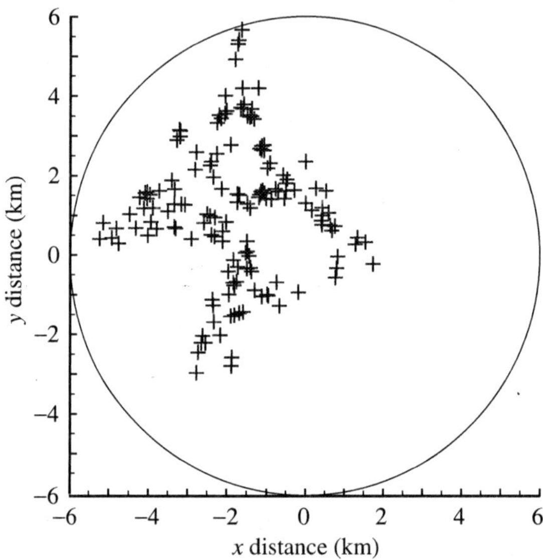

Figure 1.13 Armadale: realisation of CHD death certificate addresses, within circular window.

of death certificates for a range of diseases were recorded. The diseases chosen were thought to be related to air pollution risk. These included respiratory cancer, gastric and oesophageal cancer, and bronchitis. To provide a representation of the background 'at-risk' population at case event locations, a realisation of a 'control' disease was also recorded. The control disease was a composite of lower-body cancers (prostate, penis, breast, testes, cervix, uterus, colon and rectum). These diseases are thought to be largely unaffected by air pollution.

Figure 1.7 displays the location map and Figures 1.8, 1.9, 1.10 and 1.11 display the case event maps of the three case diseases and the control disease.

Armadale: Respiratory Cancer Data

This data set was first analysed by Lloyd (1982) and consists of 49 respiratory cancer death certificate addresses for the period 1968–1974 for the small town of Armadale, central Scotland. This town is located in an industrial area close to Falkirk (see location map 1.7). A standardised mortality ratio of 150 for each of the years of the period was recorded and this unusual excess of deaths was dubbed the Armadale Epidemic. Accompanying the case locations are a realisation of coronary heart disease (CHD) death certificate locations which have been used as a control disease realisation (Lawson and Williams, 1994). A circular study window was used so that directional sampling bias would be minimised. The case and control realisations are displayed in Figures 1.12 and 1.13.

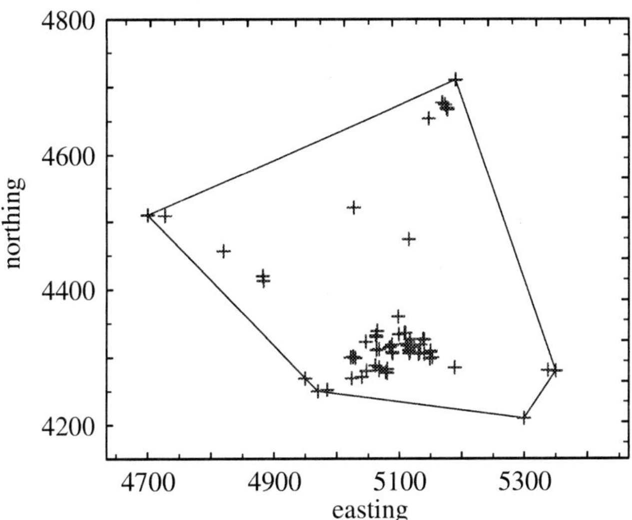

Figure 1.14 Humberside: leukaemia and lymphoma case event map (1974–1986). Reproduced from Lawson and Cressie (2000) with permission from Elsevier Science.

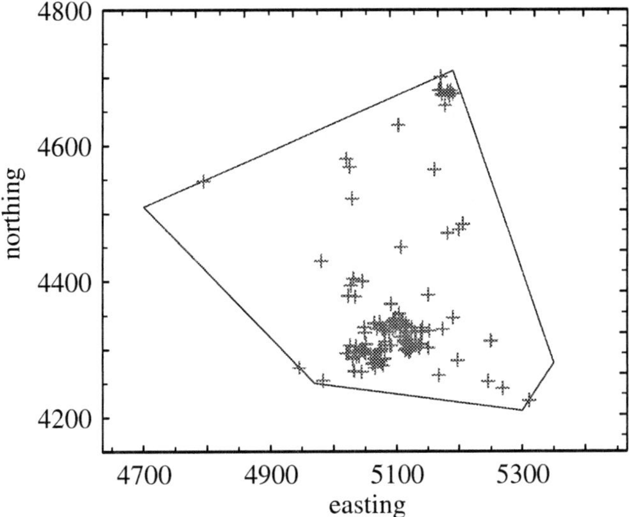

Figure 1.15 Humberside: leukaemia and lymphoma control event map (1974–1986).

Humberside: Leukaemia and Lymphoma Data

This data set was first analysed by Cuzick and Edwards (1990) and consists of a realisation of case events of childhood leukaemia and lymphoma in the north Humberside region of England for the period 1974–1986. As a 'control' for the population 'at risk' in the area, the authors obtained a large sample of births from the birth register for

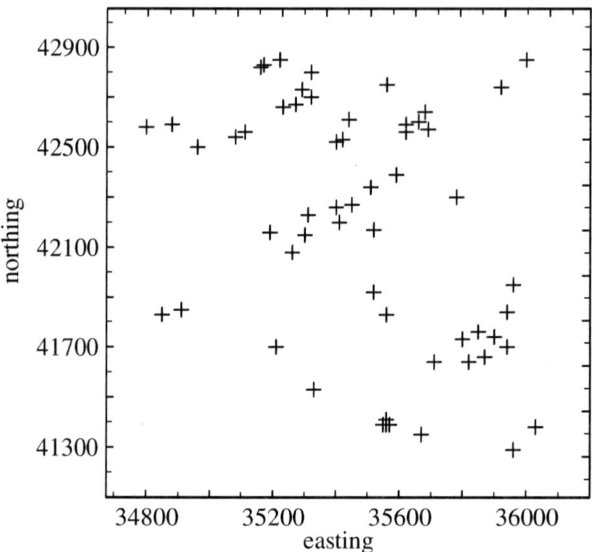

Figure 1.16 Lancashire: larynx cancer case event map (1974–1983).

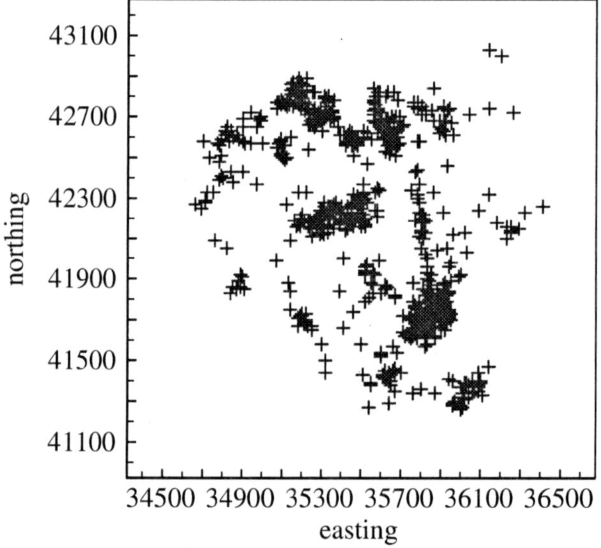

Figure 1.17 Lancashire: respiratory cancer control event map (1974–1983).

the region and period. This provides a spatial 'childhood' control but not a disease-specific control. Figures 1.14 and 1.15 display the case event and control maps for this example. The original purpose of the example was to examine the clustering tendency of the case events.

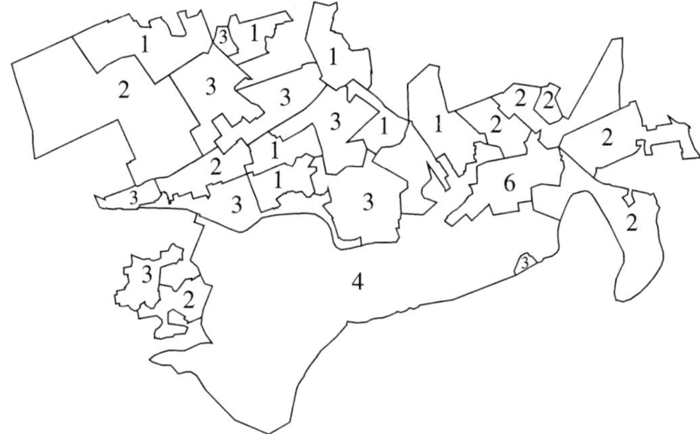

Figure 1.18 Falkirk: map of respiratory cancer enumeration district counts (1978–1983).

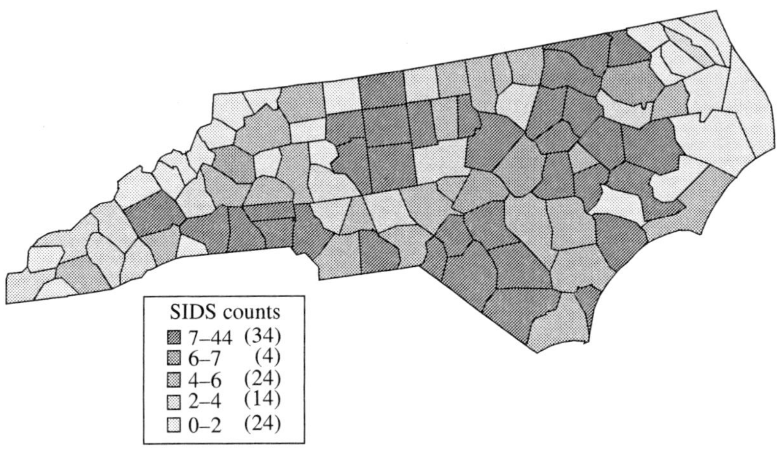

Figure 1.19 Thematic map of counts of sudden infant deaths (SIDs) in North Carolina for the period 1974–1978.

Lancashire: Larynx Cancer

The incidence of cancer of the larynx in a part of Lancashire, England, has been studied by Diggle (1990). This example consists of a realisation of 58 larynx cancer case events in the period 1974–1983. A control event realisation of 192 cases of respiratory cancer in the same period was also available. Figures 1.16 and 1.17 display the case and control maps. The object of the original analysis was to assess evidence for the existence of an environmental air pollution source in the area of the map (an incinerator; location: (35 450, 41 400)). While respiratory cancer may represent the 'at-risk' population for larynx cancer, its distribution is also affected by air pollution and hence the comparison of these two diseases is a relative risk comparison only. Discussion

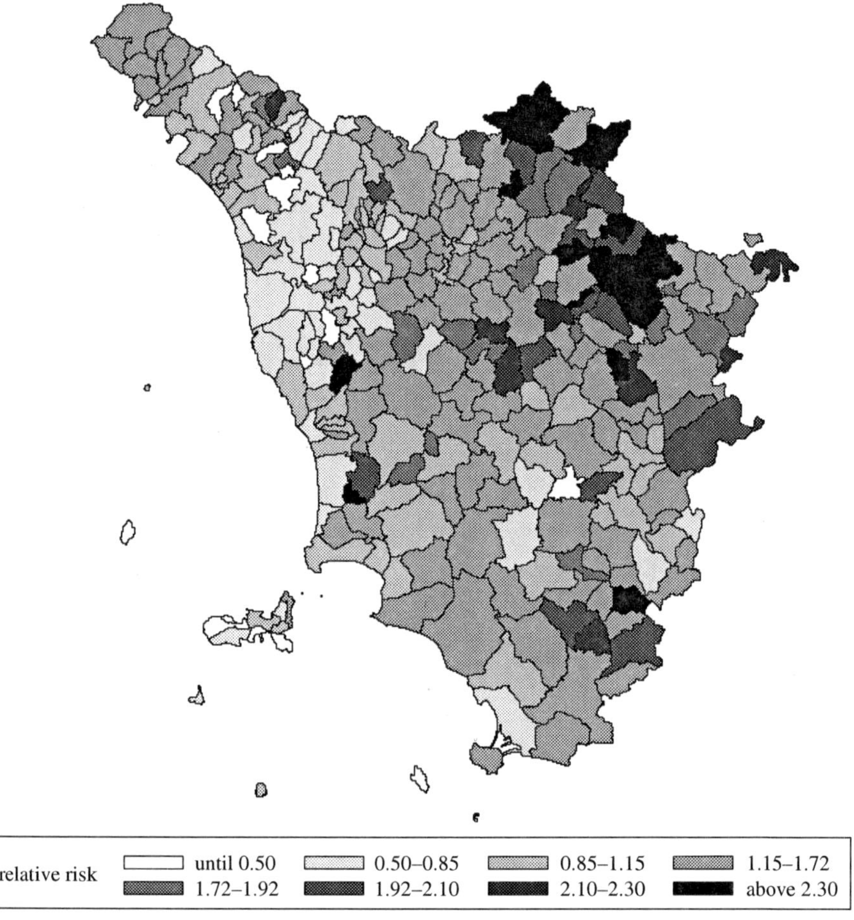

Figure 1.20 Tuscany: gastric cancer morbidity 1980–1989. Standardised mortality ratios.

of the choice of control disease or other sources of standardisation is postponed to a later section.

1.4.2 Count Data Examples

In this work we also examine a number of examples of count data maps where the disease of interest has been collected within small areas. These small areas vary from census enumeration districts (Falkirk) to districts (North Carolina), municipalities (Tuscany) and Landkreise (Germany).

Falkirk: Respiratory Cancer Mortality

In this example, counts of respiratory cancer in 26 census enumeration districts for the period of 1978–1983 in central Falkirk, a large town in central Scotland, are

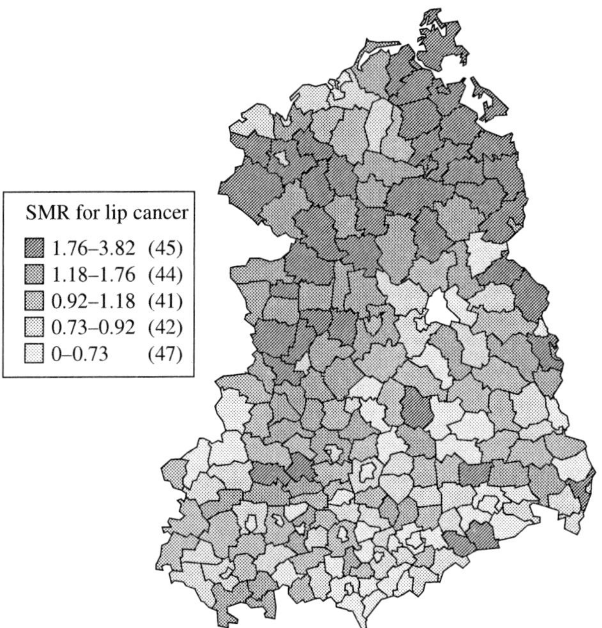

Figure 1.21 Thematic map of SMRs for lip cancer in Eastern Germany for the period 1980–1989.

given. These data form a small part of a larger study of respiratory cancer incidence in this urban area. The enumeration district map with associated counts is displayed in Figure 1.18. Total expected rates based on Scottish national rates for 18 age × sex groups are also available.

North Carolina: Sudden Infant Mortality

The incidence of sudden infant death (SID) in North Carolina, USA, has been studied by Cressie and Chan (1989) and Lawson (1997), amongst others. The counts of infant death in the 100 counties for the period of 1974–1978 have been collected and total births for the counties are also available. Figure 1.19 displays the county map and death counts.

Tuscany: Gastric Cancer Morbidity

The incidence of gastric cancer in the Tuscany region of Italy is of particular interest due to large variations in incidence between the northeastern areas and the south and west. Figure 1.20 displays the standardised mortality ratios as a choropleth map for the period 1980–1989.

Lip Cancer in Eastern Germany

This data set consists of age–sex standardised counts for lip cancer in administrative regions in Eastern Germany for the period 1980–1989. A set of counts for the regions (Landkreise) is provided, and the standardised mortality ratio map is displayed (Figure 1.21).

CHAPTER 2

Scales of Measurement and Data Availability

It has long been recognised that analysis of spatial data should be carried out at appropriate scales. Examples of such discussion extend back to the 1960s in geography (Schumm and Lichty, 1965). It is clear that not only are certain scales *appropriate* for examination of particular spatial structures, but also that *changes of scale* will change the structural features of the data themselves. For example, the occurrence of four cases of a rare disease in a suburban street (street level), in its isolation, could be regarded as a 'cluster' of disease, by some definition. However, when the incidence is aggregated with that from a large number of streets (which could have negligible incidence), then the total incidence for the area may not be detectable as representing a 'cluster'. Essentially, the effect of arbitrary aggregation was to change the *scale* of analysis and effectively produced a smoothing of the incidence surface. The duality of smoothing and scale change occurs wherever case events are aggregated into tract counts. In that case, the locational information held in the case events is 'blurred' by the scale change to tract level. This loss of information was noted by Diggle (1993) and Lawson (1993c), and both authors have stressed the importance of using methods appropriate to the observation scale when this is available.

The related aspect of appropriate scales of analysis relates to 'a scale at which phenomena occur', and it is this sense of scale which geographers have addressed. This is also of great relevance to any statistical analysis as (1) within any window, phenomena of interest may occur at different scales, (2) the scales of spatial variation may be required to be estimated, and (3) there may be regions within the window which are associated with certain spatial scales. Examples of all three situations are plentiful. For (1), a localised pollution hazard may increase incidence of disease around a source, but not elsewhere. For (2), the size of disease clusters can vary, due to spatial variation in aetiological factors. For (3), the boundaries between urbanised and rural areas can occur in study regions and the effect may yield considerably different spatial variation in these regions. The appropriate spatial scale of analysis can be defined, on an increasing measure, for a variety of types of study and these scales are detailed in the following sections.

2.1 SMALL SCALE

The analysis of an individual disease cluster or group of clusters, whether related to a known source of hazard or not, usually requires the examination of areas of size 0.5–10 km^2. Often the exact scale of operation of the process or processes affecting the clustering is unknown, and hence a reasonably large study window is used, large enough to encompass the scale of the clustering effect. At this small scale it is also possible to analyse spatial 'ecological' problems, i.e. the study of the relation of disease to explanatory variables (Cuzick and Elliott, 1992). Indeed, the analysis of the relation between a cluster of data events and a putative hazard could be regarded as a special case of this type of analysis. Usually, the object of spatial ecological analysis is to assess the *general* relations between data and covariates (see, for example, Donnelly *et al.* (1994), Cressie and Chan (1989) and Marshall (1991a) for a review).

2.2 LARGE SCALE

At larger spatial scales, the aggregative effects of scale lead to different analysis objectives. The analysis of variation in incidence of disease within regions of a country could be to provide a disease map of the country or to carry out large-scale ecological analysis. Disease mapping has as its objective the provision of a 'clean' map of disease incidence, with all random effects removed, so that an accurate estimate of the underlying rate in different areas is provided. In this sense, the objective is a type of smoothing, and methods related to smoothing are typically employed.

The screening of large areas of a country for 'anomalies' in incidence (or 'clusters') (Besag *et al.*, 1991a) has as its objective the isolation of 'areas of raised incidence'. These studies are related to disease mapping, in that a 'clean' disease map can be used to assess such 'areas of raised incidence'. Such cluster detection can be based on case event data (Openshaw *et al.*, 1987). Disease mapping on the other hand is usually based on regional count data. Large-scale ecological analysis can also be based on either data type. Cook and Pocock (1983) give an example of the analysis of regional variation in heart disease, within the United Kingdom, based on regional explanatory variables.

2.3 RATE DEPENDENCE

While the scale change criteria in Sections 2.1 and 2.2 apply to a given disease, a suitable scale for analysis will depend on the normal rate of occurrence of that disease. For example, with very rare diseases it may require a continental scale to analyse even a case event map. Indeed cluster patterns may even have scale cycles. This should be considered when making choices of scale for analysis.

2.4 DATA QUALITY AND THE ECOLOGICAL FALLACY

A number of issues arise in the use of case event and count data and their interpretations. As mentioned above, count data are formed, usually, as an aggregation of case event data. In that sense, count data are an approximation to case event data. However, there are significant advantages and disadvantages associated with both data types.

Case event data are usually available as the street address of a case of disease recorded as having occurred within a fixed time period. While this is an exact location, its relation to the disease aetiology may be uncertain. For example, if the event is a *morbidity* event (e.g. the address at diagnosis), it may be that (a) the disease was not contracted at that address, (b) the case has subsequently moved. If the event is a *mortality* event (e.g. the address on a death certificate), it may be that the disease was contracted while at another address. In both cases, the exact location may not be appropriate. For example, the case may be someone who has a work-related disease. Therefore, the home address may be of little importance. Alternatively, a pollution source may have been influential in causing cases of bronchitis amongst people travelling daily to work. Hence, home address could be, at least, an approximation to the 'at-risk' environment.

However, case event locations, when properly validated (Lawson and Williams, 1994), can provide detailed spatial information, which would be lost when counts are used. This information could be very important in detailed assessment of environmental gradients. The conflicting results which can occur when data are aggregated to counts are evidenced by Diggle (1990) and Elliott *et al.* (1992b). Two disadvantages of case event data are that (1) the exact addresses are not always readily available due to possible confidentiality problems, and (2) often inferences about individuals at locations are functions of a smoothed regional 'at-risk' population surface which is interpolated to the case address. Hence, regional average characteristics are being ascribed to a particular location and a particular individual. This is an example of the ecological fallacy, which affects many studies in this area (Rothman, 1986).

On the other hand, count data, by the fact that they are aggregated, can avoid some of the problems of case events but introduce some new problems. Aggregation increases the 'local' sample size and avoids the need to use 'exact' addresses which may not be truly exact for the reasons specified above. Census tract data are more closely matched to the underlying population in tracts, and are usually readily available from central government agencies, with little confidentiality problems associated. However, the smoothing involved in counts does yield an invariance at regional level, and disjunction between individual risk and location. There is no relation which maps the number of cases in a region to locations within the region and, usually, region-wide explanatory factors are only available. Hence, there is another level of ecological fallacy in operation with count data: that is the problem of ascribing each item in the count to a location and to ascribe a relevant value of explanatory factor at that location. This additional problem is somewhat balanced by the gain in sample size.

In general, if case event data are available, then this level of resolution should be analysed. If only aggregated data are available, then methods suitable for counts should be employed, although case event models should be used, given that these underlie the counting process. It is not usually recommended that spatial information be lost by aggregation of case events into counts.

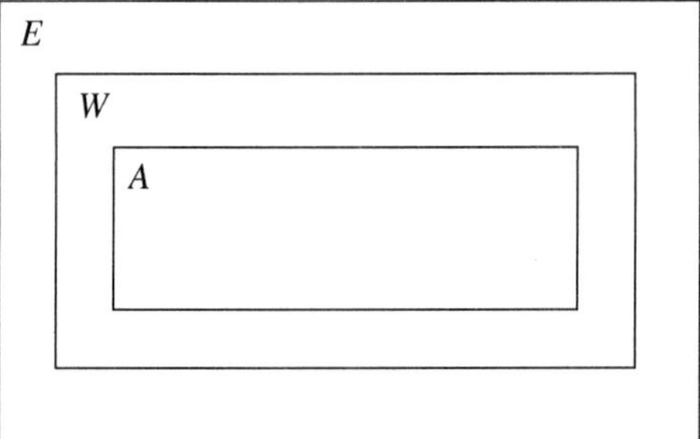

Figure 2.1 Representation of a study region (W) and associated external and internal guard areas.

2.5 EDGE EFFECTS

In most mapping exercises where statistical data are to be represented, edge effects are present and may need to be accommodated in the analysis. When data are spatially autocorrelated, then observations made within a study window will relate to unobserved data outside the window. This is a form of spatial censoring (Baddeley and Gill, 1997). Even when data are not autocorrelated, a method used to estimate the smoothed surface representation of the data will have greater variability at the edges due to the fact that such smoothing operators use neighbouring data observations to compute estimates and at edges these neighbourhoods are censored. Also, if only data *within* the window are used to estimate edge values, then a bias will appear in this edge estimation.

The main areas where edge effects play an important role in disease mapping are in the assessment of specific clustering of disease cases, in the assessment of large-scale autocorrelation and in the analysis of count data where the estimation of rates of disease in small areas depends on values observed in neighbouring areas. A number of methods can be used to make allowance for such edge effects. First, it is possible to employ a guard area around the map, which provides extra data support at the edges, but is not included in the main study area. The guard area could be internal to the study region or an external addition to the region. Figure 2.1 displays a study region within an external guard area ($E : \forall \boldsymbol{x} \in E$), an internal guard area ($W : \forall\, \boldsymbol{x} \in W$) and an internal area A. The study region was defined as $\forall\, \boldsymbol{x} \in T \cup A$. Internal guard areas are commonly used in the analysis of point process data, and a number of methods have been proposed for the incorporation of such areas in the analysis of such data (Ripley, 1988). For case event data, this implies that any events falling within the predefined internal guard area are given different weights from those within A. Weighing schemes for guard areas are discussed by Cressie (1993) and Ripley (1988). These vary from simple binary schemes to those employing proportions of nearest-neighbour circles intersecting the window boundary.

External guard areas are less commonly used, but in the case of stationary Poisson point processes within study windows of regular geometry, it is possible to employ a wrapping method called toroidal edge correction, which does not require additional data outside the study window. Instead, the window is wrapped on a torus so that opposite edges of the window become neighbours. Hence, data close to the edges of the study window act as external additional data for the opposite edge of the window. This form of correction is *not* usually available for disease mapping as it is to be expected that either non-stationarity in mean or covariance is likely to be encountered and often the study window is highly irregular. This implies that any external guard area must be provided from additional observations outside the study window.

Further consideration of edge-effect problems is deferred until Chapter 5, where an example of the effect of different edge compensation schemes is considered.

CHAPTER 3

Geographical Representation and Mapping

It is often the case that the results of the analyses of georeferenced health data are presented in the form of a map. In addition, the map depicting these results is often the basis from which decisions concerning health status of an area, or epidemiological hypotheses are generated. Unfortunately, the construction of such a visual form of representation can lead to additional stages of processing of the statistical data, and so interpretational problems can arise from the use of such maps. The production of large-scale atlases of mortality or morbidity for countries has as its focus the presentation of visual information about the spatial distribution of disease incidence, often without presentation of the associated statistical data. Often, these atlases use colour schemes to represent different classes of incidence, and the viewer must interpret the map based on the scheme chosen. Without the availability of concomitant statistical information, this task could be prone to bias.

In this chapter, a review of issues related to map production and representation of statistical information is provided. As many of these issues are cartographic or lie in the area of visual cognition, it appears before discussion of the main statistical issues in the book. Some issues do depend on the nature of statistical processing of georeferenced data, but these can be discussed at a general or generic level.

3.1 INTRODUCTION AND DEFINITIONS

Initially, consideration is given to issues relating to the map construction for statistical data, in general. In a later section we consider the use of georeferenced health data. The topic of *statistical mapping* requires some definition before considering its many facets. Here, the concept of a *map* is first defined, and then the area of statistical disease map construction and related interpretational issues will be discussed.

3.2 MAPS AND MAPPING

A map can be defined as '*a collection of spatially defined objects*' (MacEachren, 1995; Monmonier, 1996). As such a map is simply a display of the spatial properties of an

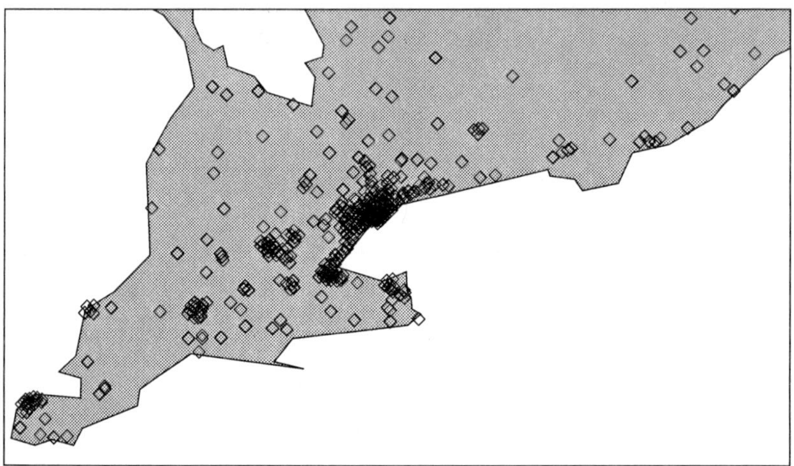

Figure 3.1 Canada, Toronto area: urban centres (diamonds depict centre locations).

object set. This usually implies a two-dimensional display of the cartesian or polar coordinate locations of objects and also their attributes, e.g. a street map displays the locations of streets and houses on these streets (if the *resolution* of the map is high enough). In addition, the houses may have attributes which relate to the population of each household. Hence, a variety of maps could be constructed even from this simple example. We could have a simple street map, a more detailed house map and a map of household attributes at the highest resolution. The display of such varied information in a graphical form has been the concern of *cartography* for a considerable time (MacEachren, 1995). Many of the concerns of those within statistics about the representation of data in graphical forms have also been explored within geography for mapped displays. The psychological/visual perceptual implications of chosen mapping methods has been studied extensively (Monmonier, 1996, Chapters 3–6), and these issues also apply to the construction of maps of statistical information. Walter (1993) and Pickle and Hermann (1995) have examined visualisation issues related to medical mapping. The stages of map construction can each be associated with some form of processing of spatial information and hence can be of concern to anyone wishing to use such methods of presentation.

The main stages are

(1) choice of scale,

(2) choice of symbolisation or representational processing,

(3) further processing required to construct a suitable map.

In stage (1), a suitable scale for the map must be chosen. Any choice of scale, however, inevitably leads to a process of *averaging* of spatial information from higher levels of resolution. For instance, a map of urban centres in the vicinity of a large city (Figure 3.1, Toronto area) will usually have such areas represented as sets of

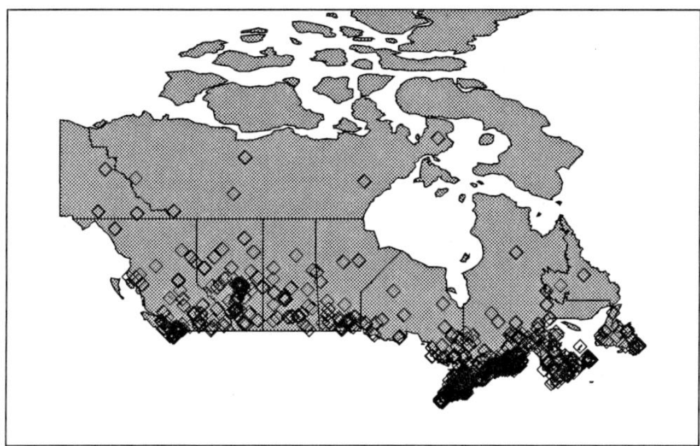

Figure 3.2 Canada: zoomed map of urban areas.

geometric symbols depicting locations, but if a larger country scale was to be used (Figure 3.2, Canada), within which the urban centres were but a small part, then the centres would be replaced by alternative symbols, otherwise a large loss of information occurs. Hence, in this case, the scale change has resulted in averaging of the spatial information. Stage (2) is also represented in the street map example. At the detailed scale, linear features represent the streets while at the country scale, the whole city is represented by a dot. This represents a change in symbolic representation as well as a scale change. This can have both a visual perceptual effect for the map user and is an averaging of spatial information. Stage (3), that of further processing, can occur when information on the spatial structure of the objects and/or attributes is not available in the form required by the representational system. For example, often we want to, or need to, compute a map representation from a set of sampling points which are predefined, whereas we need to have measurements at the intersections of a fixed grid which do not correspond to the sampling points. This arises in many statistical mapping problems and leads to the use of *interpolation* or *smoothing* of data. Another example of further processing is the use of *transformations* of the mapped data to represent some feature of the spatial structure. Map projections (Monmonier, 1996, Chapter 2) are a classic example of transformation. Schulman *et al.* (1988) give an example of using projection and transformation in a medical statistical application.

Hence, in two of the three stages of map production, some form of statistical processing of the spatial information usually occurs. This applies in most forms of mapping exercise and hence it can be claimed that map construction is, for a large part, a statistical processing task.

3.2.1 Statistical Maps and Mapping

The three stages of map production discussed above map easily onto the data types which are often the basic ingredients for mapped representation. Within the subject of spatial statistics a spectrum of spatial information and data formats are found.

This spectrum ranges from the locations of points or objects (point and object processes) to the measurements made on random variates at specific spatial locations (random fields). In the former case, the subject area of stochastic geometry concerns the probabilistic modelling of the locations of objects (Stoyan *et al.*, 1987). In the latter case, the subjects of geostatistics and image processing deal with observations made on random fields (Cressie, 1993). Image processing characteristically studies random fields observed on a grid mesh of regular sampling points (pixels), and its task is usually restricted to the processing of the pixel data to obtain the underlying 'ground truth' or noise-free image. Hence, this form of processing is not closely akin to mapping as there is usually no need for interpolation or scale averaging. On the other hand, the subject of geostatistics, does involve smoothing and interpolation and can involve the estimation of areas or blocks of information which are averages of underlying sampling point data. In addition, the analysis of object processes often involves the averaging and scale change from locational data to localised intensity data, i.e. the locations of objects are converted into a continuous surface describing the local density/intensity of objects. Both of these data types then, lead to scale change and interpolation/smoothing operations which are integral to the mapping process.

In applications in disease mapping, some of each data type may be encountered. Maps of case events are object maps, while covariates which are measured at spatial sampling sites can be regarded as geostatistical data. Count data observed within *fixed* arbitrary administrative regions are 'averages' of an object process.

3.2.2 Object Process Mapping

An object process map is a presentation of the spatial locations of objects, usually in two dimensions. Define $\boldsymbol{x}_i$, $i = 1, \ldots, m$, to be the locations of the objects within a spatial window W. Usually, objects are mapped at a specified point (the associated point) which can be uniquely identified for each object. For example, a process of circles could have the circle centres as associated points. Hence, to construct a map of such a process it suffices to plot the locations of such points and then to construct circles with given radii. For this example, the locations of the circles could follow a stochastic process and also the circle radii could be the realisation of a random variable. A simpler example of this idea is the point process, which has a point location as its observation unit and the realisation of point locations are the objects. For example, the address locations of cases of a disease form a point process and a map of all addresses of disease within W would be a mapping of the process. Figure 1.8 depicts a case address map for respiratory cancer in a small Scottish town for the period 1966–1976.

Often, it is important to transform an object map by converting the object locations into a continuous surface representation of the objects. This kind of transformation can be achieved by computing the local density of objects. Density estimation (Silverman, 1986) can be used to provide such local densities and the resulting density surface can be mapped over the study window. Usually, such a surface is displayed as a contour plot or, in three dimensions, as a surface perspective view. The contour plot is often preferred, as some spatial information is hidden in perspective views. To

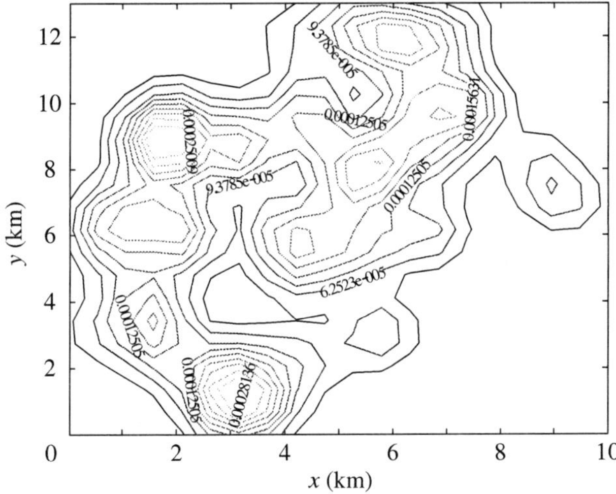

Figure 3.3 Contour plot of respiratory cancer density using 10 contour levels.

demonstrate how scale and symbolisation affect such mapping, the contour plot of a density estimate of the case event data in Figure 1.1 has been drawn for two different contour densities (10 and 5 heights) in Figures 3.3 and 3.4. Note that the arbitrary choice of fewer contours effectively produces a smoother surface and can change the perception of the object map. In addition, the derivation of these contour maps has proceeded through a number of stages which may affect the final visualisation. First, the process of density estimation involves the production of estimates in a grid mesh (interpolation) and the choice of a smoothing constant (bandwidth) which controls the smoothness of the gridded data. Then a graphical package has constructed contours using a further interpolation/smoothing step.

3.2.3 Geostatistical Mapping

Geostatistical data differ from the above in that a network of sites are usually used to sample or measure some spatially distributed variate. For example, the early geostatistical work related to estimation of geological structures in mining applications where concentrations of particular minerals were sampled at fixed locations (Wackernagel, 1995; Cressie, 1993). In principle, the basic mapping considerations apply in this case also: for visualisation, the data can be displayed as an object map with each sample site becoming the location of an object representing the measurement at that site. For example, a circle of radius equal to the magnitude of measurement could depict the distribution. Other display forms are available, such as needle plots, where the length of vertical lines drawn at the sites are scaled to represent the measurement magnitude (Ripley, 1981). Often, a surface interpolated from the measured data is to be constructed. This surface also requires an interpolation or smoothing step to provide a gridded data set, which can be subsequently contoured. Such interpolation

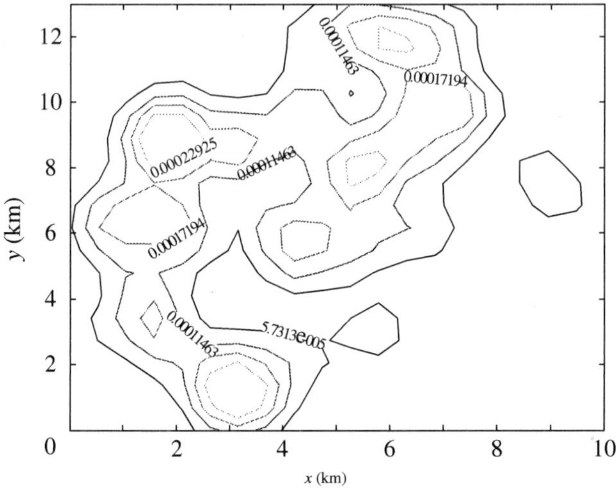

Figure 3.4 Contour plot of respiratory cancer density using 5 levels.

can be achieved by a wide range of smoothing techniques. The method of *kriging* was developed within geostatistics to provide such processing.

Other notable forms of smoothing available for such data are: *non-parametric regression* or *kernel smoothing* (Härdle, 1991), and *thin plate splines* (Green and Silverman, 1994, Chapter 7)). A wide variety of mathematical interpolation methods are also available, e.g. finite-element methods (Lancaster and Salkauskas, 1986).

3.3 STATISTICAL ACCURACY

Any step of map production which requires statistical estimation will have associated with it a measure of the reliability or variability of that estimation. Hence, any map of estimated values (such as interpolated or smoothed data) should have a variance estimate available at the estimation points. The variance estimate can also be represented as a surface, or a pointwise confidence interval for the estimated surface can be produced. The visualisation of such surfaces can cause some problems as there are no simple clear methods of displaying multiple surfaces without losing spatial information. If areas of the estimated surface which exceed limits of variability are of interest, then it may be possible to construct a Monte Carlo p-value surface (Gelman *et al.*, 1995). This idea has been exploited by Kelsall and Diggle (1995b) in the depiction of excesses of disease risk for georeferenced health data.

3.4 AGGREGATION

It is important to consider the interconnection between some mapping concepts and the related statistical issue of aggregation. The effect of aggregation of data into spatially larger areas has a variety of effects on the subsequent interpretation. First, aggregation is a scale change. That is, by accumulating observations into larger spatial units, this changes the scale of analysis. In addition, aggregation acts as a smoothing operation. That is, by accumulation of data, detailed variation in the data will be lost and will not be retrievable. A classic example of this is the arbitrary regionalisation of case events into census tracts in medical small-area studies. In that case the detailed spatial variation of cases is lost within the census tract count (for discussion, see, for example, Lawson (1993c)). This type of averaging of spatial effects is inherent in scale changes, and it is important that any spatial structural effects observed in data at one scale are scale labelled, i.e. the scale at which the effect is found is permanently associated with the effect. For example, clustering of disease data in space may occur on a case event map, but when aggregated into census tract counts this effect may disappear. Hence, the clusters are only apparent at a scale below the count aggregation level.

3.5 MAPPING ISSUES RELATED TO AGGREGATED DATA

The visual representation of aggregated count data has been the focus of study for some time. Often, the ready availability of aggregated count data for diseases has led to the widespread use of visualisation to depict spatial distributions. Often, the purpose of mapping count data is to display the spatial variation of disease so that interpretation of disease variation can be made. Variation of interest to, say, public health workers, could be the identification of 'clusters' of high incidence of disease or the isolation/identification of areas of similar incidence. In the first case, some public health intervention may result from the identification. In the second case, allocation of public health resources to 'like' areas may be the focus.

Once statistical processing of the aggregated data has been performed, the resulting map of disease risk (usually relative risk) is often used as the basis of interpretation. Unfortunately, the interpretation of such maps without recourse to additional statistical information relating to estimates and their variability can be extremely difficult. This is akin, in the simpler clinical trials field, to computing the means of a parameter of interest in two dose groups in a trial, and basing judgement of group differences on a visual display of the means. Certainly, this kind of analysis would not pass Federal Drug Administration guidelines.

The main problem with the use of such maps for these purposes is that the map is a visualisation tool, but is being used for an inferential task without recourse to statistical inference procedures. Hence, it is extremely important to present such georeferenced data with all relevant statistical information. At the minimum, any map of relative risk for a disease should be accompanied with information pertaining to estimates of rates within each region as well as estimates of variability within each region. At the other extreme it could be recommended that such maps be only used as a presentational aid, and not as a fundamental decision-making tool.

Some issues relating to disease map interpretation have been studied within cognitive science (Pickle and Hermann, 1995; Mungiole *et al.*, 1999; Lewandowsky

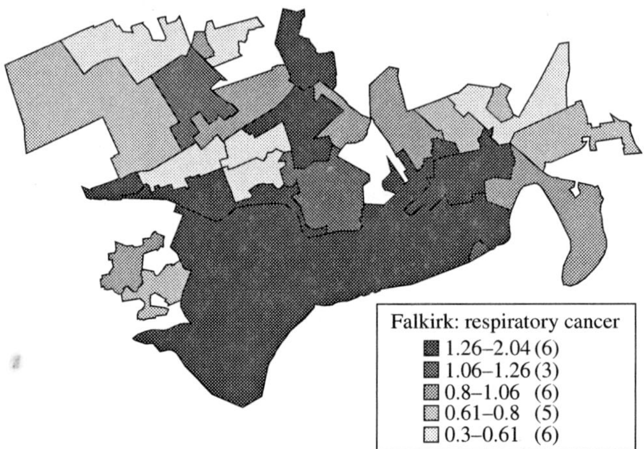

Figure 3.5 Respiratory cancer relative risk (SMR) thematic map: Falkirk, central Scotland. Reproduced from Lawson and Cressie (2000) with permission from Elsevier Science.

et al., 1993). In these studies, certain aspects of map presentation have been examined in relation to the ability of map observers to detect 'clusters' of disease and in their ability to assess given areas of risk. In most of these studies, estimation of observer variability was attempted, but no comparison of observer ability in recovering 'true' features were made. These studies have mainly focused on the construction of thematic maps, i.e. the use of colour schemes or shading to represent the relative risk within regions of the map. See Figure 3.5 for an example.

In these studies, it has been established that

(i) monochrome thematic maps yield lowest observer variability in detection of areas of risk,

(ii) two-colour map schemes have higher variability, but are *preferred* by observer focus groups (of end-users),

(iii) dot density maps tend to emphasise small clusters and yield higher variability in identification of risk areas,

(iv) observer focus groups prefer double-coloured maps over monochrome maps or contoured risk surfaces,

(v) these studies also support the use of coloured monochrome maps over greyscale maps.

These results support the use of monochrome colour thematic maps for the presentation of disease incidence. In addition, it has been found that the use of particular colours can reduce interpretational variability. Red monochrome maps appear to be favoured for identification of risk areas. However, it should be noted that although cognitive research has shown that monochrome maps are to be preferred, many observers within focus groups 'prefer' multiple-colour maps (Pickle *et al.*, 1999). Hence, if atlases of disease risk are produced based on focus group recommendations, then these may be suboptimally designed for interpretational purposes. In addition, if an end-user is given a choice of which map to use, they are likely to choose a map which is suboptimal for the purposes of interpretation. This further supports the contention that maps should be used as wallpaper (as observer preference may be for pleasant colour schemes) and not for inferential purposes.

3.6 CONCLUSIONS

In conclusion, it would appear that, in general, the use of map displays should be minimised and only used when ancillary statistical information is available. Any map which may be used for interpretation should be as simple as possible and report statistical information closely without undue extra processing. For case event data, the simplest form of representation of relative risk is a contoured risk surface. While this form of display is not favoured by end-users of thematic maps, it would appear that if the contouring algorithm does not distort the inferential results, then this must be the recommended method of display. To reduce the potential bias in interpretation of such surfaces, it is probably better to portray the surface as a probability (p-value) surface which displays the associated variability directly, rather than presenting the estimated relative risk surface itself.

For aggregated count data, the use of monochrome thematic mapping is likely to yield the least user variability; however, there remains considerable arbitrary choice of grouping of colour classes. Although users may prefer coloured maps there is some justification for the use of greyscale maps in that tonal quality can bias interpretation. The use of class boundaries defined by percentiles of the observed distribution or other cut points which produce internally standardised relative schemes should be avoided in favour of reporting of grouped rates.

In general, the use of maps of relative risk should be limited to an aid to presentation of statistical results rather than a basic inferential tool.

CHAPTER 4

Basic Models

In the study of the spatial distribution of disease, it is recognised that there are basic models which are usually assumed to apply, at least as a starting point, in the analysis of case event or count data. As counts within regions are usually derived from case events which have been aggregated into the regions of interest, then it is useful to consider first the basic models for case event data. In what follows a key role is played by the Poisson process, related point process models and the Poisson distribution, which is often used as a starting point for analysis of count data. Both these basic models lead to straightforward likelihood-based modelling and inference, when the appropriate assumptions are met by the data under consideration. However, the fundamental assumptions of these models are often not completely met in applications, and in these situations, more complex models must be invoked. These models often consist of random effects which can describe *unobserved* features of the data and for estimation under these models a Bayesian approach is often required. In fact in situations where spatial (auto)correlation is to be directly modelled within a data set, then the inclusion of such a feature within a prior distribution is a natural approach to modelling. In the next sections, we consider the role of sampling related to the use of likelihood-based inference compared to a full Bayesian approach to modelling.

4.1 SAMPLING CONSIDERATIONS

Fundamental to the method of analysis of data in spatial epidemiology is the consideration of how the data have been observed or sampled and the effect of the method of data collection on the further analysis of the data. Here we will mainly be concerned with the impact of sampling on the spatial domain of observation. While there are many issues connected with the validation and collection of epidemiological data (Elliott *et al.*, 1992a), it is the specific statistical issues relating to sampling of spatial epidemiological data that are of concern here.

The main spatial sampling methods are described by Ripley (1981), Cressie (1993) and Thomson (1992). Specialised methods of sampling for spatial epidemiological data have not developed greatly. This is largely due to the fact that most available data are in the form of complete enumeration of events within a fixed window. Hence, the data usually form a *realisation* (a completely mapped occurrence), rather than a subsample of a larger population. This is true for data obtainable routinely from registry offices or government statistical offices. The 'completeness' of the data may be questioned on the basis of registration error or problems of misdiagnosis of disease. However, if little is known about the *spatial* effects of such errors, then it is reasonable to approach the statistical analysis of such data on the basis of a complete realisation.

In studies where complete enumeration within a specified window is not possible, then subsampling considerations could become important. For example, if a study were based on the notification of respiratory disease incidence to a selection of general practitioners within a fixed time period, then the study window could be variable and only a subsample of the spatial window may be sampled at any fixed time. Another example arises when spatially segregated small areas are sampled for specific disease incidence (see Nejjari *et al.* (1993): the Paquid study). In this case the subsampling mechanism must be taken into consideration in the subsequent analysis. This would involve the estimation of between and within subsample characteristics.

4.2 LIKELIHOOD-BASED AND BAYESIAN APPROACHES

Define the probability density of a vector random variable $\boldsymbol{x}$, which depends on a parameter vector $\boldsymbol{\theta}$, as $P(\boldsymbol{x} \mid \theta)$. Often, when a realisation of $\boldsymbol{x}$ is observed, we assume that a likelihood can be defined for the parameter vector. In frequentist inference, decisions concerning the true values of parameters are based on the likelihood itself. In the Bayesian paradigm, parameter values are assumed to be governed by prior distributions and inference must be based on a posterior distribution which incorporates both likelihood and prior distributions. In spatial epidemiology similar considerations apply, in that models based on likelihood can be derived and inference based on this alone, or models admitting prior distributions for parameters can be examined within a Bayesian framework. In the next sections we examine both approaches in the construction of basic models for disease incidence.

4.3 POINT EVENT MODELS

Point event data consist of address locations of cases of disease. Hence, the data represent, or can be considered as, a point map of disease events. Usually, a complete realisation of cases within a spatial and temporal window is observed. At the lowest level of data structure, the data are simply represented as a point process, and appropriate models for such data can be employed. The effects of scale are also important in this regard. For example, the exact locations of cases may be known only within a census tract, and not at street address level. This would allow the use of count models (Section 4.4). However, if the observational *scale* was very large relative to the census tract resolution level (say, for example, 1000 times), then observations in tracts could be regarded as point process realisations. This is most valid for rare diseases, where the probability of any *multiple* occurrence in a tract is negligible. Point process theory relies on the notion of orderliness, which has as its basic tenet that multiple coincident events cannot occur, i.e. for a infinitesimal region around $\boldsymbol{x}$, $\mathrm{d}\boldsymbol{x}$ say, then

$$P_r\{N(\mathrm{d}\boldsymbol{x}) \succ 1\} = o(|\mathrm{d}\boldsymbol{x}|) \quad \text{as} \quad |\mathrm{d}\boldsymbol{x}| \to \mathbf{0}$$

(see, for example, Daley and Vere-Jones (1988, p. 28) and Cox and Isham (1980)).

The 'exact' address location of a case is used in such modelling as the basic data unit. However, the use of this data unit can lead to problems in epidemiological interpretation or inference (see Section 2.4). For example, a case address is often used to represent residential exposure to risk, particularly environmental pollution hazard. However, individual exposure could occur at a workplace, related to residence, at school, during shopping trips, or at regular weekend visits. Hence, the residential address may both be too precise, and spatially inaccurate as a surrogate for exposure. In the case where genetic or viral aetiology is to be considered, then some consideration of address locations may identify clusters of disease which have epidemiological 'significance'. However, in either case purely residential exposure is difficult to ascertain: both genetic and viral clusters may invalidate point process model assumptions, and in the case of viral causes then residence may not be a reliable surrogate for exposure, for the reasons sited above.

Given the above caveats, it is useful to consider basic statistical models for case event data and their possible extensions to accommodate, at least, some of the above problems. We assume a study window W, within which are observed m cases at address locations $\{\boldsymbol{x}_i\}$, $i = 1, \ldots, m$. Figure 1.2 is an example of a case event map within a rectangular study window. To put in context the development of models in this area, we briefly review basic point process models and their application.

4.3.1 Point Process Models and Applications

The development of applications of models for spatial point processes has gone through various phases. Many early developments took place in ecological applications and, in particular, forest science (Matérn, 1986). In these applications, it was often the case that relatively large realisations of points were observed (e.g. plant communities or forests), mainly in a homogeneous environment. This led to the analysis of models for events on homogeneous environments, and to special methods for 'sparsely sampled' problems, which are found particularly in ecological examples. These methods, which relate to spatial subsampling of complete realisations of points, are necessitated by the expense in cost or time of mapping large realisations of events. In applications examined here, sparse sampling is not usually required and is not discussed further.

In these early studies a number of basic models for point processes were applied. Among these models the three most important in applications were complete spatial randomness (CSR), spatial cluster processes, and spatial inhibition processes. Diggle (1983), Ripley (1981) and Cressie (1993) provide reviews of this work. These models were particularly applicable to ecological examples because (1) under a homogeneous environment CSR is a tenable null hypothesis, and (2) simple first-order stationary alternative models such as cluster/inhibition processes could be applied. In addition, given the computational resources available in the 1970s and early 1980s, simple global summary measures were computable for these models (e.g. $K(t)$ functions).

For applications in spatial epidemiology these basic models must be modified. The reasons for this are

(1) case events occur within a population which is heterogeneous in its propensity to contract a disease (its 'at-risk' structure), and its spatial distribution;

(2) environmental gradients and other spatially dependent covariables are often included in models and the first-order stationarity assumption made in many earlier point process studies is usually inappropriate;

(3) the case events are not 'fixed' at particular locations, and also have case historical information which affects their 'at-risk' status.

In many published analyses, the final consideration has been ignored in favour of evaluation of case events using simple point process models. If spatial location is the *only* available information, then such modelling is justified, but is likely to have value limited to early-stage exploratory analysis.

4.3.2 The Basic Poisson Process Model

Here we modify the basic point process models to accommodate the above extensions to model spatial epidemiological data. First, it is reasonable to assume that at a residential location $\boldsymbol{x}$ the probability of observing a case is independent of such a probability at other locations. This will at least hold true conditionally, given knowledge of a spectrum of ancillary information (covariates and other spatial structure information). This model assumption essentially regards individuals as having an independent probability of becoming a case. In addition to conditional independence of case events, it is possible to include both heterogeneous background and non-stationarity or long-range spatial trend components in our models by adopting a special type of Poisson process model. A heterogeneous Poisson process (HEPP) model is a simple extension of the homogeneous Poisson process where first-order intensity λ is allowed to be spatially dependent ($\lambda(\boldsymbol{x})$).

For this case, the expected number of events in an area T, say, is now

$$E\{n(T)\} = \int_T \lambda(\boldsymbol{u})\,\mathrm{d}\boldsymbol{u}. \tag{4.1}$$

The definition of $\lambda(\boldsymbol{x})$ is quite flexible and allows the inclusion of a modulating function which can represent the heterogeneous (population) background, and also covariate information. In addition, any realisation of m events in T has likelihood:

$$\prod_{i=1}^{m} \lambda(\boldsymbol{x}_i)\mathrm{e}^{-\int_T \lambda(\boldsymbol{u})\,\mathrm{d}\boldsymbol{u}}. \tag{4.2}$$

Table 4.1 Some link types for HEPP models.

$m(F(x)\alpha)$	link
$F(x)\alpha$	multiplicative-identity
$\exp(F(x)\alpha)$	multiplicative-log
$1 + F(x)\alpha$	additive-identity
$1 + \exp(F(x)\alpha)$	additive-log

This is the unconditional likelihood for a realisation of m events in T. The number of events (m) is Poisson distributed with parameter ρ. A basic theoretical discussion of non-stationary point process models can be found in Chapters 3 and 6 of Cox and Isham (1980), and examples of applications in temporal examples can be found in Snyder (1975) and spatial examples in Cressie (1993). It is also important to note that the likelihood (4.2) can be simplified by conditioning on the realised value of m. This may be useful when we are only concerned with the *spatial* structure of events and not the overall intensity (which is characterised by the realised value of m). This conditioning leads to the likelihood:

$$\prod_{i=1}^{m} \lambda(\boldsymbol{x}_i)\left\{\int_T \lambda(\boldsymbol{u})\,\mathrm{d}\boldsymbol{u}\right\}^{-m}. \tag{4.3}$$

Note that if a constant intensity parameter (ρ) is included in the parametrisation of $\lambda(\boldsymbol{x})$, then this factors out of (4.3), and greater parsimony is a result.

The inclusion of population background in the above models is usually achieved by defining an extra modulating component in $\lambda(\boldsymbol{x})$. A basic formulation for the modulated intensity is

$$\lambda(\boldsymbol{x}) = g(\boldsymbol{x})m(F(\boldsymbol{x})\alpha), \tag{4.4}$$

where $g(\boldsymbol{x})$ is a function of the 'at-risk' population distribution, and $F(\cdot)$ is an $m \times p$ (spatially dependent) design matrix of spatial and non-spatial covariates, α is a $p \times 1$ vector of parameters. The function $F(\boldsymbol{x})$ represents the design matrix evaluated at the location $\boldsymbol{x}$. The function $m(\cdot)$ is usually included to provide a flexible link between the background population-induced intensity and covariates included in the design matrix F. Breslow and Day (1987, Chapter 5) discuss a variety of specifications for $m(\cdot)$ in the context of cohort survival studies. Some possibilities are defined in Table 4.1.

Note that a scaling parameter can be included in the specification of F, which allows the covariate contribution to be scaled separately from the background intensity.

The link functions defined in Table 4.1 represent a range of possible effects which may be thought relevant in the relation of disease incidence to background rate. The multiplicative models represented by the first two entries require that $g(\boldsymbol{x})$ is directly related to any change in disease incidence, and further that the change is proportional to the background rate. For some applications, this specification may not be realistic. In some cases where the disease concerned can be regarded as adding to the background propensity, then the last two links may be more appropriate. In fact the additive–log link has a number of significant advantages in applications where it is important to maintain background risk where there is negligible excess risk predicted and the log component ensures positivity. This type of link has been applied in the analysis of putative sources of health hazard (see Chapter 7). It is not always clear *a priori*, however, which of these links is appropriate in any given situation, and in that case it may be appropriate to examine a range or family of link functions to determine the best specification. Breslow and Day (1987, pp. 160–161) discuss the use of general risk functions which have additive and multiplicative risks as special cases. It may be appropriate to consider such a range of models in any particular application.

The basic additive and multiplicative models for case event data were independently proposed by Lawson (1989) and Diggle (1989) in applications to analyses of putative sources of health hazard.

In the original definition of $\lambda(\boldsymbol{x})$, the background $g(\boldsymbol{x})$ function appears in the likelihood, and hence must be estimable at the case event locations $\{\boldsymbol{x}_i\}$. This implies that the 'at-risk' population must be able to be interpolated to the case locations, if not already available and measured at these sites. This assumption has implications for the epidemiological interpretation of this model.

First, the assumption of a continuous $g(\boldsymbol{x})$ background over a study region may require re-specification if areas of no population occur within the study window. Although this consideration relates to the method of estimation of $g(\boldsymbol{x})$, detailed discussion of which is postponed to Section 4.3.2, the issue is related to the 'ecological fallacy'. The ecological fallacy can occur 'when a suspected risk factor and disease are associated at the population level, but not at the individual subject level' (Greenberg *et al.*, 1996). This can also apply to the use of a population background function $g(\boldsymbol{x})$ used to describe the probability of an individual case at $\boldsymbol{x}$. In general, the problem can be interpreted as the attribution of *average* characteristics to an individual within a region. Evidently, individuals rarely display such 'average' characteristics, but randomly varying ideographic features.

The idea of attribution of such 'random' effects to groups or individuals is the subject of *frailty* models (Clayton, 1991), and in principle the inclusion of such effects requires the addition of a random component in $\lambda(\boldsymbol{x})$.

The $g(x)$ Estimation Problem

The function $g(\boldsymbol{x})$, as defined here, is a spatially continuous function representing the propensity of the local population towards contraction of the given case disease. This is termed the 'at-risk' structure of the population. As this function appears within the intensity (4.4), it must be included in any analysis of this intensity function. Hence, either (1) $g(\boldsymbol{x})$ must be estimated and this estimate must also be capable of interpolation to a variety of spatial locations (including the observed case locations $\{\boldsymbol{x}_i\}$); or (2) $g(\boldsymbol{x})$ must be removed from the problem. In the first case, $g(\boldsymbol{x})$ can be estimated prior to analysis of parameters in $m(\cdot)$, in which case inference concerning these latter parameters would be made conditional on the estimated value of $g(\boldsymbol{x})$, $\hat{g}(\boldsymbol{x})$ say. This could lead to a type of profile likelihood analysis. An alternative approach could be to include $g(\boldsymbol{x})$ estimation within a general procedure which explores the interaction between $g(\boldsymbol{x})$ estimation and $m(\cdot)$ estimation. The disadvantage of the profile approach is that it could lead to estimates of α which are sensitive to the value and variability of $\hat{g}(\boldsymbol{x})$. Methods for the estimation of $\hat{g}(\boldsymbol{x})$ were first proposed by Diggle (1989) and Lawson (1989) independently, and are also found in Diggle (1990). These developments were in the analysis of small-area health data around putative sources of health hazard, but the methods have wide applicability in situations where the 'at-risk' population related to a realisation of case events has to be estimated.

The second approach to the function $g(\boldsymbol{x})$, that of removal from the problem, can be accomplished in a variety of ways. First, it might be possible to integrate $g(\boldsymbol{x})$ out of the intensity and use the resulting integrated intensity ($\lambda^*(\boldsymbol{x})$) in further analysis. An alternative approach, which is only available when another case event map is used to estimate $g(\boldsymbol{x})$, is to condition on the realisation of case/control marks on the two disease map locations. This leads to a binary logistic regression and $g(\boldsymbol{x})$ is factored out of the analysis. The advantage of this approach is that it does not require any knowledge of, or manipulation of, the $g(\boldsymbol{x})$ function. The disadvantage is that it is limited to situations where two disease maps are available.

Methods for the estimation of $g(\boldsymbol{x})$ require that data be available which describe the 'at-risk' structure of the population. Traditionally, when examining counts of disease within small areas, use is frequently made of a standardised rate for each region, which is calculated from known regional or national rates for the case disease. This is usually scaled by the population structure of the region to allow for local effects. This standardisation is readily available at census tract level in many countries. However, it is often only available at an aggregate level and hence at a level of aggregation *above* that of case event data. Instead of using such data, it is possible to use a surrogate measure which is available at the case event resolution level. It has been proposed that a mapped realisation of another disease could be used to represent the 'at-risk' population structure which must be controlled for in the analysis of case disease data. This additional disease map is used as a spatial 'control' for the case disease and in principle should be matched closely to the population affected by the case disease, but unaffected by the case effects under study. For instance, in a study of clustering of a cancer (case disease) it may be thought appropriate to use coronary heart disease (CHD) as a control disease. If the cancer affects similar ages and sexes in the population, then any excess clustering in the cancer will be apparent *above* the local variation in CHD. This approach to estimating the 'at-risk' structure was adopted by Diggle (1989, 1990), Lawson (1989) and Lawson and Williams (1994). In the original work, a two-dimensional kernel density estimate was used to interpolate the control disease to the case data points. Subsequent inference was made conditional on the value of $\hat{g}(\boldsymbol{x})$ found optimally by cross-validation of the kernel bandwidth smoothing parameter. However, there are drawbacks to the use of such control diseases which limit their usefulness as a general panacea in this case. First, the problem of false accuracy of the residential address of the control could lead to misinterpretation. For example, a control disease could be related to factors which are not strongly related to the spatial address structure of the case disease. Hence, in this case the only argument for the use of such a control is the aggregate relevance of the spatial expression. In addition, the idea that such controls can be interpolated to case data points is also an assumption which should be verified.

An alternative approach is to use aggregated standardised disease rates from a higher level than the case disease. This has the advantage of being directly related to the disease of interest and already an average. However, the degree of smoothing of this aggregate may crucially affect the resulting parameter estimation in $m(\cdot)$, as noted by Lawson and Williams (1994). Those authors also suggested a mixed-level hybrid model, which does not require such arbitrary smoothing. This is discussed in Section 4.3.3.

Finally, Diggle and Rowlingson (1994) have suggested an approach which 'factors out' the $g(\boldsymbol{x})$ function from the analysis. This conditional approach directly models the probability of a location being a case rather than a control, given the joint realisation of cases and controls. This leads to a different joint likelihood for the case and control data, but conditions the analysis on the observed pattern.

Given the joint intensity of cases and controls is $g(\boldsymbol{x}) + g(\boldsymbol{x})m(F\alpha)$, define the probability of a case at $\boldsymbol{x}$ as

$$P(\boldsymbol{x}) = \frac{g(\boldsymbol{x})m(F\alpha)}{g(\boldsymbol{x}) + g(\boldsymbol{x})m(F\alpha)} = \frac{m(F\alpha)}{1 + m(F\alpha)}, \tag{4.5}$$

then the conditional likelihood of a joint realisation of cases and controls is given by

$$L = \prod_{i=1}^{m} \left\{ \frac{m(F_i\alpha)}{1 + m(F_i\alpha)} \right\} \prod_{j=m+1}^{m+n} \left\{ 1 - \frac{m(F_j\alpha)}{1 + m(F_j\alpha)} \right\}, \tag{4.6}$$

where there are m cases and n controls.

While there are many benefits to this approach, not least of which is the fact that $g(\boldsymbol{x})$ does not require to be estimated and window boundaries no longer need be considered, it remains limited by the fact that it requires the use of a control point map, which, as noted above, has a number of significant drawbacks. If, in addition, only aggregate level standardised rates are available, then it cannot be used.

Matched Case Control Modelling

In most of the models considered above, the 'at-risk' population background was assumed to be represented by a continuous function $g(\boldsymbol{x})$. In that case the use of control diseases or other expected rate estimators does not allow the inclusion of information about individuals who are matched to the case on selected criteria but who have not expressed the disease. Such matching is fundamental to matched case control studies in epidemiology and the usefulness of such individual controls is clear. It is possible to define a conditional probability of a particular location, x_{j0} being a case, given the occurrence of the case-control location pair x_{j0} and x_{j1}. This probability is

$$p_{jo} = \frac{m(F(x_{j0})\alpha)}{m(F(x_{j0})\alpha) + m(F(x_{j1})\alpha)}.$$

It is possible to construct a likelihood based on this derivation, and also to extend the derivation to multiple matched controls (Diggle *et al.*, 2000). In Chapter 7 this approach is discussed further.

4.3.3 Hybrid Models and Regionalisation

The models of the previous section dealt with the situation where case events are modelled directly with the 'at-risk' background estimated or conditioned out of the analysis. However, it is sometimes the case that the *only* available information pertaining to the population of the study window is based on census tract level data which is at a higher aggregation level than the case event data. While it is possible in this case to regard such information as pertaining to a fixed region point (such as a region centre, however defined), it is possible to define a different model for this situation which directly uses the aggregated information *without* the requirement of interpolation or smoothing. Here we define the probability of a case event at $\boldsymbol{x}$ as

$$P(\boldsymbol{x}) = \lambda(\boldsymbol{x}) \Big/ \sum_{j=1}^{p} \lambda^*(\boldsymbol{x}_{nj}), \tag{4.7}$$

where p is the number of census tracts and $\boldsymbol{x}_{nj}$ is the location of the jth tract centre.

In addition,

$$\lambda^*(\boldsymbol{x}_{nj}) = g_j \int_{a_j} m(F\{\boldsymbol{u}\}\alpha)\, \mathrm{d}\boldsymbol{u}/|a_j|,$$

where $|a_j|$ is the area of the jth tract and g_j is the background population hazard function for the jth tract. The resulting likelihood is given by

$$L = \prod_{i=1}^{m} \lambda(\boldsymbol{x}_i) \left[\sum_{j=1}^{p} \lambda^*(\boldsymbol{x}_{nj})\right]^{-m}. \tag{4.8}$$

Note that if it can be assumed that a regional average spatial intensity is appropriate, then the intensity can be rewritten as $\lambda^*(\boldsymbol{x}_j) = g_j m(F(j)\alpha)$, which further simplifies the analysis. Lawson and Williams (1994) developed this analysis for an application in putative hazard source analysis, but this method can be used in a range of applications where only an aggregated background is available.

4.3.4 Bayesian Models and Random Effects

The models described in preceding sections are all available under the frequentist approach to inference, and can all be fitted via conventional maximum-likelihood methods. However, in many epidemiological problems it is natural to regard some or all of the model parameters as random variates which are governed by a probability distribution. This can apply to any parameters which are included within the α vector, and this can then lead to a conventional Bayesian analysis of hierarchical models (Gelman *et al.*, 1995). The prior probability distributions specified for the α vector can themselves contain hyperparameters, and subjective prior beliefs could be incorporated.

However, there are some unique features of spatial epidemiological problems where it is natural to model data via prior distributions, and indeed is difficult to avoid such a formulation. Random effects can take a variety of forms in spatial epidemiological data. A short list of possible effects is given below.

(i) Population strata (age $\times$ sex) random effects (uncorrelated heterogeneity).

(ii) Population strata (age $\times$ sex) random effects (spatially correlated heterogeneity).

(iii) Individual case event random effects (uncorrelated heterogeneity).

(iv) Individual case event random effects (spatially correlated heterogeneity).

(v) Region-specific random effects (uncorrelated heterogeneity).

(vi) Region-specific random effects (spatially correlated heterogeneity).

(vii) Random-object effects (e.g. cluster centres).

(viii) Background $g(\boldsymbol{x})$ smoothing random effects.

The above list represents an abbreviated view of the possible role of random effects in spatial epidemiological data. The effects which are peculiar to spatial problems are *spatially correlated heterogeneity* and *random-object effects*. These two topics represent two separate areas of spatial statistics: the analysis of spatial correlation and stochastic geometry. Many studies have focused on how to incorporate spatial autocorrelation in spatial data. For Gaussian observations sampled at fixed spatial sites, the methods of kriging and universal kriging have been developed. Cressie (1993, Chapters 1–5) gives a detailed discussion of the work in this area of geostatistics. An alternative, though closely related approach, is the use of simultaneous autoregressive (SAR) or conditional autoregressive (CAR) models for the observations (Cressie, 1993, Section 6.2). For images where regular arrays or lattices of observations (pixels) are available, then Markov random field models have been developed (Besag, 1974, 1986; Besag and Green, 1993). One common feature of all these models is that the spatial correlation structure is incorporated within the prior distribution for the parameter(s) of interest. This can be applied to strata, parameter or region-specific random effects and examples of this can be found in Cressie and Chan (1989), Clayton and Bernardinelli (1992), Lawson (1994b), Clayton and Kaldor (1987), Donnelly *et al.* (1994), Breslow and Clayton (1993), Lawson *et al.* (1996a) and Besag *et al.* (1991b). Uncorrelated heterogeneity can also be incorporated via a simpler prior distribution structure. Examples of the application of these random effects can be found in Marshall (1991a), Clayton and Kaldor (1987), Besag *et al.* (1991b), Manton *et al.* (1981) and Tsutakawa (1988). Marshall (1991b) and Lawson and Waller (1996) provide reviews of these areas in specific applications.

Among the non-spatial random effects which could be thought appropriate in analysis of spatial epidemiological data, those specifically related to cases themselves are perhaps the most important. The idea of attribution of random effects to groups or individuals is the subject of frailty models (Clayton, 1991), and in principal the inclusion of such effects requires the addition of a random component in the specification of $\lambda(\boldsymbol{x})$. For an individual random effect, it is possible to define

$$\lambda(\boldsymbol{x}_i) = g(\boldsymbol{x}_i)\xi_i m(F\alpha), \tag{4.9}$$

where ξ_i is the random effect for the ith individual. For non-spatial applications, Clayton (1991) recommended the use of a gamma distribution for the prior distribution of ξ.

The random-object effects noted above can arise when spatial epidemiological data are related to the spatial distribution of another random process. A classic example of this type of effect is the idea that data cluster around, usually unknown, cluster centres. These centres have associated with them sets of case events. The clusters may be of a variety of predefined shapes but the locations of the centres are unknown and are to be estimated as part of the modelling problem. In this case, the cluster centres will have a prior spatial distribution often defined as spatially uniform or Markov inhibited (Lawson, 1996a). Hence, the centres can be regarded as random objects which have to be recovered from the case events. In this way, such analysis is directly related to high level object recognition tasks in image processing (Baddeley and Lieshout, 1993). Such methods are not limited to cluster detection and can be applied to any situation where small-area health data are thought to be related to an unobserved spatial feature. The aim in such analysis may be to recover the location of the spatial feature. A hypothetical example may be the release of a chemical pathogen in a subsurface area which is spatially continuous. In this case the resulting health gradients observed in the human population could lead to reconstruction of the deposition sites/areas of maximum exposure of the chemical. Of course, where the location of the health hazard source is *known*, then methods related to putative pollution source analysis are appropriate (see Chapter 7, and Lawson *et al.* (1999a) for a review).

The background estimation problem discussed in Section 4.3.2 can also be approached via the use of prior distributions. The problem of estimation of the continuous $g(\boldsymbol{x})$ surface from either a control disease event map or from standardised tract disease rates involves the process of smoothing. This smoothing, whether based on density estimation or non-parametric regression, is controlled by a bandwidth smoothing parameter (h). In early studies kernel smoothing has been applied to either data type (Diggle, 1990; Lawson, 1992, 1995; Lawson and Williams, 1994). However, in those studies subsequent inference concerning parameters in $m(\cdot)$ was made conditional on the fixed value of h separately estimated from a control or externally standardised rates. Even if h is assessed via 'optimal' methods such as cross-validation, the variability in this estimate has not been included in the analysis. In addition, the contribution of the case disease distribution to the estimation of the background is not considered.

It is possible, however, to regard the smoothing constant as having arisen from a distribution of possible constants, and hence a prior distribution can be specified for this parameter. The exploration of the joint posterior distribution of h and the other parameters can be facilitated by constructing special iterative simulation methods such as Markov chain Monte Carlo (MCMC) samplers (see Appendix B; see also Lawson and Clark (1999a)).

4.3.5 MAP Estimation, Empirical Bayes and Full Bayesian Analysis

For the Bayesian models discussed in Section 4.3.4, there are a variety of approaches to the examination of posterior information provided by the sample found. A full Bayesian analysis evaluates the full posterior distribution of parameters and associated summary measures, if required. This approach provides general information on parameter variability and between-parameter correlation. In this section a brief description of estimation methods relating to Bayesian models is provided. A fuller discussion of these methods is postponed to Chapter 5 (Sections 5.2 and 5.2.4).

It is also possible to avoid this full exploration by attempting to find the *modal* values of the posterior distribution of parameters, and this approach is akin to maximum likelihood estimation in the non-Bayesian approach. Maximum *a posteriori* (MAP) estimation is an example of this approach, and is often used in spatial problems, such as image analysis (Besag, 1986; Ripley, 1988). This form of analysis is sometimes known as empirical Bayes (EB) as it uses conventional frequentist estimation in the posterior distribution, although more recently this term has become associated with the approximation of features of the posterior after estimation of parameters from empirical data (see, for example, Bernardo and Smith (1994, p. 373)). Examples of the application of such estimators to case event data are few, although in principle, it is straightforward to specify a suitable model. For example, assume (4.9) but with $m(\cdot) = 1$, and $\xi_i \sim G(\alpha, \upsilon)$, then the posterior distribution is proportional to

$$\prod_{i=1}^{m} \xi_i g(\boldsymbol{x}_i) \mathrm{e}^{-\xi_i \int g(u)\,\mathrm{d}u} p(\xi_i),$$

where $p(\cdot)$ is the prior distribution for the random effect. In this case EB methods would lead to the estimation of α and υ, and the substitution of these estimates in a functional of the posterior distribution, such as an expectation.

Examples of the use of EB estimators for census tract data are more numerous. In the case of counts observed in census tracts, a number of authors have proposed estimators of tract relative risk based on different random-effect assumptions. For example, if observed counts are defined as n_i with expected count e_i and relative risk θ_i, then, with $n_i \sim \text{Poisson}(e_i\theta_i)$ and $\theta_i \sim G(\alpha, \upsilon)$, the posterior distribution of θ_i is

$G(e_i + \alpha, n_i + \upsilon)$ conditional on n_i. The posterior expectation of θ_i reduces to

$$\frac{n_i + \upsilon}{e_i + \alpha}.$$

Note that the crude relative risk estimator, the standardised mortality/morbidity ratio (SMR) is just n_i/e_i and this is the maximum likelihood estimator for the ordinary saturated Poisson model.

Hence, a full Bayesian analysis of this model would require sampling $\boldsymbol{\theta}$ from the above conditional gamma distribution, whereas an EB approach could estimate $\boldsymbol{\theta}$ from the conditional expectation with suitable estimates of α and υ substituted. Further discussion of this example is postponed to Section 5.2 and Chapter 8.

4.3.6 Bivariate/Multivariate Models

In the analysis of case event data it is often found that, rather than a single disease being of sole concern, a range of diseases are studied within a window area. This kind of study can arise, for instance, when a local area is thought to suffer from an environmental problem (such as an, as-yet, unidentified, putative form of pollution) and a range of diseases are studied to assess the health status of the local area (Lenihan, 1985). In general, where it is required to study the spatial distribution of a number of diseases, then there is a requirement to consider a bivariate or multivariate distribution of disease case events.

In principle, it is straightforward to extend the case event models defined above to describe multiple disease realisations. For any given study window W, define the intensity of the kth disease as $\lambda_k(\boldsymbol{x})$, where $k = 1, \ldots, n_d$. The kth intensity is the realisation of a spatial stochastic process on $\mathbb{R}$, and conditional on the realisation of the n_d intensities, then the kth disease is distributed independently as a modulated heterogeneous Poisson process with intensity $\lambda_k(\boldsymbol{x})$. Notice that this definition allows the formalisation of a *conditional independence* model for the case events from the disease types which has considerable generality. Under this specification complete independence of the diseases (i.e. no spatial cross-correlation) can be assumed, while it is also possible to specify prior correlation between disease occurrences via the definition of the spatial stochastic processes which generate the intensities. One obvious possibility is that the realisation of the log of the intensities at spatial locations is multivariate normal with specified covariance matrix and the intensity cross-correlation represents a multivariate extension of this model.

Specifically, assume that the case events are described by $\lambda_k(\boldsymbol{x})$ given above and that the 'at-risk' population background for each disease can be represented by the function $g_k(\boldsymbol{x})$. The total intensity of disease at $\boldsymbol{x}$ is now $\sum_{k=1}^{n_d} \lambda_k(\boldsymbol{x})$. The case intensity includes the background intensity and it can be defined as

$$\lambda_k(\boldsymbol{x}) = g_k(\boldsymbol{x}) m(F_k \alpha_k).$$

It is now possible to make probabilistic statements concerning the spatial distribution of case events. First, the probability of any case at location $\boldsymbol{x}$ is given by the corresponding Poisson process probability:

$$\lambda_{\mathrm{T}}(\boldsymbol{x}) \exp\left\{-\int_W \lambda_{\mathrm{T}}(\boldsymbol{u})\,\mathrm{d}\boldsymbol{u}\right\},$$

where

$$\lambda_{\mathrm{T}}(\boldsymbol{x}) = \sum_{k=1}^{n_d} \lambda_k(\boldsymbol{x}).$$

In addition, given a case at $\boldsymbol{x}$, the probability that the case is of the lth disease is given by

$$\lambda_l(\boldsymbol{x}) \Big/ \sum_{k=1}^{n_d} \lambda_k(\boldsymbol{x}).$$

Hence, the probability of a case of the lth disease at $\boldsymbol{x}$ is given by

$$\lambda_l(\boldsymbol{x}) \exp\left\{-\int_W \lambda_{\mathrm{T}}(\boldsymbol{u})\,\mathrm{d}\boldsymbol{u}\right\}.$$

It is therefore possible to derive a likelihood for a realisation of n_d disease events within W. It can also be shown that such a likelihood factors into independent components for each disease type as the log-likelihood can be written:

$$l_{\mathrm{cr}} = \sum_{k=1}^{n_d}\left\{\sum_{\phi_k} \log \lambda_k(\boldsymbol{x}_{\phi_k}) - \int_W \lambda_k(\boldsymbol{u})\,\mathrm{d}\boldsymbol{u}\right\},$$

where ϕ_k is the set of all cases of the kth distance.

This is the fundamental model governing multiple disease incidence and can be regarded as equivalent to the competing risk models of survival analysis (Lawson and Williams, 2000). The above model is capable of describing the joint distribution of case event diseases within a study window. This model includes the background functions $g_k(\cdot)$, and it is important to decide how to incorporate such functions into any analysis. A number of options are available. First, it is possible to estimate each function separately from some external data, such as standardised rates for the area, or from the spatial distribution of a 'control' disease. Further, when a control disease is used it is sometimes also possible to factor out the background functions as in the single disease case (see, for example, Section 4.3.2). However, in general, it is not possible to condition-out the background $g_k(\boldsymbol{x})$ functions, when there are multiple disease occurrences. In the special case where a control disease is used to represent the background for each disease, then it is possible to condition-out the control, but only when a common control disease is assumed for all diseases (i.e. $g_1(\boldsymbol{x}) = g_2(\boldsymbol{x}) = \cdots = g_{n_d}(\boldsymbol{x})$). This may be appropriate when a common factor, such as an environmental pollution agent, affects a particular population profile.

To see this an alternative formulation can be derived. First, define the total intensity of cases and controls of the jth disease at $\boldsymbol{x}$ as $g_j(\boldsymbol{x}) + \lambda_j(\boldsymbol{x})$. Then the conditional probability of a case of the jth disease, given a case has occurred at $\boldsymbol{x}$, is given by

$$\frac{\lambda_j(\boldsymbol{x})}{\sum_{k=1}^{n_d}\{g_k(\boldsymbol{x})+\lambda_k(\boldsymbol{x})\}}=\frac{g_j(\boldsymbol{x})m(F_j\alpha_j)}{\sum_{k=1}^{n_d}\{g_k(\boldsymbol{x})[1+m(F_k\alpha_k)]\}}.$$

If a common $g(\boldsymbol{x})$ function can be assumed, then the binary logistic model can be applied. Define a disease indicator variable d which takes the value j when referring to the jth disease, and also a case/control indicator variable c which equals 1 when an event is a case and 0 when a control. Then

$$\Pr(c=1\mid d=j)=\frac{m(F_j\alpha_j)}{n_d+\sum_{k=1}^{n_d}m(F_k\alpha_k)}$$

and

$$\Pr(c=0\mid d=j)=\frac{1}{n_d+\sum_{k=1}^{n_d}m(F_k\alpha_k)},$$

and the conditional likelihood becomes

$$\prod_{k=1}^{n_d}\left\{\prod_{l=1}^{n_k}\frac{m(F_{jl}\alpha_j)}{n_d+\sum_{k=1}^{n_d}m(F_{kl}\alpha_k)}\right\}\left\{\prod_{t=1}^{c_k}\frac{1}{n_d+\sum_{k=1}^{n_d}m(F_{kt}\alpha_k)}\right\},\qquad(4.10)$$

where l denotes the case event index and t denotes the control event index, and F_{jl} refers to the lth case event in the jth disease set. However, the likelihood does not factor into independent components in this case.

The models described here provide a general framework within which it is possible to assess multiple disease incidence without resort to multiple comparison methods (Haybrittle *et al.*, 1995), which can lead to interpretational problems (Lawson and Waller, 1996). The methods can also be extended to include prior weighting of evidence (Lawson and Williams, 2000).

4.3.7 Hidden Structure and Mixture Models

The idea that the structure of a disease map should have a single general model structure has been assumed in the previous discussion. That is the model had single components governing the *overall* spatial structure of the disease. An attractive alternative to this approach is to assume that a number of components underlie the structure. This approach is sometimes called the *hidden structure* method (Quian and Titterington, 1991), and can provide a rich class of methods for characterisation of structure. In the disease mapping context, these methods could be used to isolate some general underlying factors or characteristic groupings in the disease map. Hence, these methods may provide answers to questions relating to the discrimination/classification of tracts into disease groups. While general Markov mesh models could be adapted to apply here, there has been little development of such applications in disease mapping. Section 4.4.4 describes some examples of mixture models developed for count data.

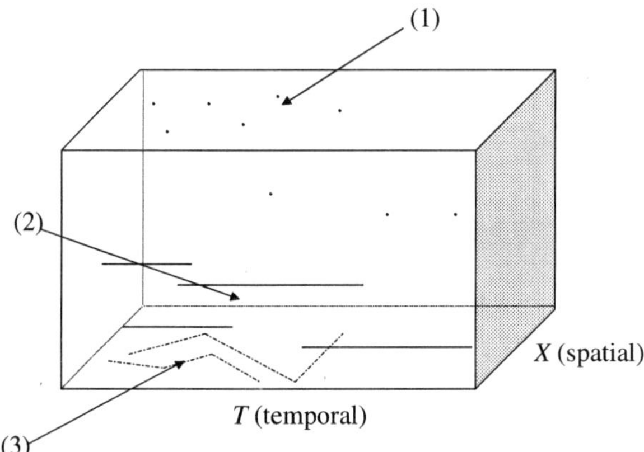

Figure 4.1 Typical forms of space-time process found in epidemiology.

4.3.8 Space-Time Extensions

In principle, it is straightforward to extend the basic Poisson process intensity model (Chapter 4) to incorporate temporal effects. By inclusion of such terms, the possible number of effects which could be modelled are increased considerably, as not only are spatial and temporal main effects possible, but spatio-temporal interaction is also possible.

Before considering detail of models to be derived, it is useful to consider how spatio-temporal data on case event incidence can arise. Cox and Isham (1980, p. 160) provide a useful pictorial summary of different possible patterns of spatio-temporal incidence. Figure 4.1 displays some types of incidence typically found in spatio-temporal disease incidence studies.

Three main types of spatio-temporal data are described in Figure 4.1. First, case events may occur within a spatial domain and their time of diagnosis or notification/registration may be recorded. In this case, the case event realisation takes the form of spatio-temporal point process, and inference can be focused on point process models. The second situation that may arise is that further time-dependent features of the individual case may be known or recorded. This may be dates of remission or recurrence of the disease in question. In this case a type of spatio-longitudinal analysis may be appropriate. The third situation displayed is where movement of the individuals is monitored within a spatial region, while the individual remains infected. Each of these situations could be further extended by variants of the basic patterns. For example, it may be possible to monitor a variety of disease episodes on individuals where the disease types differ, and this could lead to multiple disease (competing risk) models with a spatial component. Yet another possibility is the observation of multiple types of disease, with times of event diagnosis known. This is similar to type (1) in Figure 4.1, but the points are marked with disease-type labels. This could lead to multivariate or marked spatio-temporal point process models. Further, another possible extension to any of these situations would be the inclusion of individual case histories in the analysis.

In this section, we consider the simplest situation: that of single disease case events recorded in space-time. For this case, we initially assume, as before, that individual response to disease is independent and hence a modulated Poisson process model may be appropriate for the description of individual response, but unobserved factors could lead to apparent correlation or clustering in the data, and we assume that these effects can be modelled via suitable prior distributions where appropriate. A first-order intensity $\lambda(\boldsymbol{x}, t)$ can be defined for a general spatio-temporal Poisson process model which leads to a likelihood for individual response to disease risk. Define

$$\lambda(\boldsymbol{x}, t) = g(\boldsymbol{x}, t) m_x(F_x \alpha_x) m_t(F_t \alpha_t) m_{xt}(F_{xt} \alpha_{xt}), \tag{4.11}$$

where $g(\boldsymbol{x}, t)$ is a function dependent on space and time, which represents the 'at-risk' population locally at $\boldsymbol{x}$ and at time t. The functions $m_x(\cdot)$, $m_t(\cdot)$ and $m_{xt}(\cdot)$ represent the link functions of spatial, temporal and spatio-temporal design matrices (F_x, F_t, F_{xt}). These matrices can include variables measured at specific locations only, specific times only and measured conjointly in space-time. Note that in principle there is no difference in subsequent development as

$$E\{n(\boldsymbol{x}, \Delta t)\} = \int_W \int_{\Delta t} \lambda(\boldsymbol{u}, v) \, \mathrm{d}\boldsymbol{u} \, \mathrm{d}v$$

and where time of disease occurrence is known, then the sample realisation is $\{\boldsymbol{x}_i, t_i\}$, $i = 1, \ldots, m$. Hence, the corresponding likelihood for observations within a time window $(0, T_*]$ is given by

$$L = \prod_{i=1}^{m} \lambda(\boldsymbol{x}_i, t_i) \exp\left\{ - \int_W \int_0^{T_*} \lambda(\boldsymbol{u}, v) \, \mathrm{d}\boldsymbol{u} \, \mathrm{d}v \right\}. \tag{4.12}$$

Although in principle the addition of temporal effects does not change the basic modelling approach, many new considerations arise when time effects are included. For example, different approaches are usually adopted when types of temporal censoring arise in a problem. For instance, if we observed cases at locations and noted the duration of illness for each case, then we would have a type (2) space-time realisation and hence some cases could be censoring, in that they will not have been observed to have completed their illness before the end of the study period. Here there are obvious connections with the methods of longitudinal data analysis which focus on the temporal progression of effects. Spatial censoring can also occur due to the inability to fully observe the complete time sequence of disease. That is, some events could occur outside the spatial window during the time period studied but will be unobserved. This type of spatio-temporal censoring has been addressed in a hypothesis-testing context (Lawson and Viel, 1995; Diggle *et al.*, 1995).

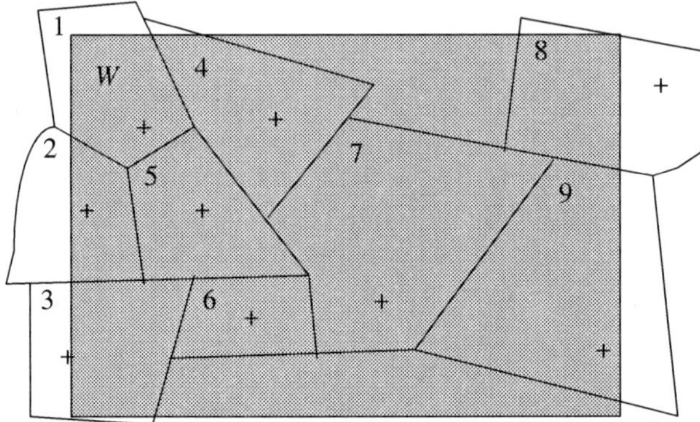

Figure 4.2 An idealised study window (W) with nine associated regions. A '+' denotes the centroid of the region.

4.4 COUNT MODELS

When observations are made on arbitrary regions, such as census tracts or administrative districts, then the locational information inherent in case event data is no longer available. Denote the jth tract as a_j, the Borel open set on $\mathbb{R}^2$. Then n_j, the count in a_j, is defined

$$n_j = \sum_{\forall \boldsymbol{x}_i} 1\{\boldsymbol{x}_i \cup a_j\}. \tag{4.13}$$

Often, the counts in such regions are the only available data which describe the spatial distribution of case events. This form of data is often routinely available from government statistical offices, and due, in part, to this ready availability has been the subject of considerable methodological development in recent years.

The basic models for count data can be derived from the case event example. We assume that we observe a map of arbitrarily defined tracts and that we observe m tracts and the complete count realisation within these m tracts. Some complications arise from how the study window is defined. Figure 4.2 describes the most common sampling situation, where a study window is defined and all the tract areas which lie, at least in part, within the window are mapped.

The fact that some regions will intersect the window adds a sampling step to the study. It must be decided how to choose tracts for inclusion. If whole tract counts are only available, as would usually be the case, then a choice must be made as to which boundary tracts (i.e. those that intersect the boundary) should be included. Such a choice has been studied in stereology, where the methods of *minus*, *plus* and *associated point* sampling have been developed (Baddeley, 1993). Minus sampling only accepts into a sample those tracts which lie wholly inside the study window (Figure 4.2, regions 5–7), whereas plus sampling includes all tracts which lie in part in the window. Associated-point sampling only includes all tracts whose associated point lies within the study window. The associated point of census tracts is any uniquely defined point associated with the tract. The tract centroid, however defined, would be an obvious choice in this situation (Figure 4.2, regions 1, 2, 4–7 and 9). The reason for the distinction between these methods is that it is known that certain methods lead to biases in the choice of tract based on tract size. For example, plus sampling is biased towards larger regions, while minus sampling tends to favour small regions. Of the three methods, only associated-point sampling leads to size-unbiased tract choice.

If any of the above methods are used and only whole tracts are to be examined, then the implication for study design is clear: for tract-based studies, the study window will be the external tract perimeter of all chosen boundary tracts, and *not* the original study window. Hence, in the following we assume that a sample of tracts has been selected and that its outer perimeter defines the study region, i.e.

$$W \equiv \bigcup_{j=1}^{m} a_j.$$

4.4.1 Standard Models

We assume that given m tracts, the count n_j within each tract is observed for a fixed time period. Based on the assumptions used to define the case event Poisson process model, it is possible to derive basic model results for counts in tracts. Assuming an underlying modulated heterogeneous Poisson process model for case events, then it is known that for such a process, counts of events within disjoint subregions of the process are independent and the expected count in the jth tract is

$$E\{n_j\} = \int_{a_j} \lambda(\boldsymbol{u})\,\mathrm{d}\boldsymbol{u}. \tag{4.14}$$

In addition, it is also the case that the counts in these regions are Poisson distributed with expectation given by (4.14). This model implies that within a realisation of counts in m regions, the tract counts are independent Poisson distributed with expectation and variance equal to (4.14). Define the integral in (4.14) as λ_j for brevity. The likelihood of m tract counts is then

$$L = \prod_{j=1}^{m} \left\{ \frac{\lambda_j^{n_j} \mathrm{e}^{-\lambda_j}}{n_j!} \right\}, \tag{4.15}$$

and log-likelihood (bar a constant involving only the data) is

$$l = \sum_{j=1}^{m} n_j \log(\lambda_j) - \sum_{j=1}^{m} \lambda_j. \tag{4.16}$$

This also implies that, conditional on $n_{\mathrm{T}} = \sum_{j=1}^{m} n_j$, the total sum of the tract counts (the window or region total), the counts in tracts have a multinomial distribution with likelihood given by

$$L_{\text{cond}} = \prod_{j=1}^{m} \left(\frac{\lambda_j}{\sum_{j=1}^{m} \lambda_j} \right)^{n_j}. \tag{4.17}$$

These likelihoods (4.15), (4.17) mirror the unconditional and conditional likelihoods found for the case event situation. In principle, it is possible to use these models as a basis for the analysis of count data found in arbitrary regions. Given the general availability of software for fitting discrete data likelihoods such as the Poisson (e.g. GLIM, S-Plus, Minitab), it is surprising that many examples of count data analysis employ approximations to the likelihoods. The integration over arbitrary regions of space is largely eschewed by most examples of analyses in this area, the favoured method being to assume that λ_j is a constant within tracts (see, for example, Chapter 5). This assumption can lead to considerable problems, as the parameters related to spatially continuous covariates included in the analysis could have considerable bias in their estimated values.

The Parametrisation of λ_j

As in the case event situation, the function λ_j can be parametrised to describe both the background 'at-risk' population and additional functions describing the spatial variation of the count intensity and relation of the counts to covariates such as measurements made on the spatial distribution of pollution within the study window. The inclusion of individual covariates is not possible due to the aggregation of the individual case data to tract count level. A basic parametrisation could be

$$E\{n_j\} = \lambda_j = m_1(F_j\alpha) \int_{a_j} g(\boldsymbol{u}) m_2(F^*(\boldsymbol{u})\alpha^*) \, \mathrm{d}\boldsymbol{u}, \tag{4.18}$$

where $m_1(\cdot)$ is a (link) function of tract level covariates, F is an $m \times p$ matrix of tract level covariates, α is the corresponding $p \times 1$ parameter vector, $m_2(\cdot)$ is a link function to spatially dependent covariates, $F^*(\boldsymbol{u})$ is an $m \times q$ matrix of spatially dependent covariates, and α^* is the corresponding $q \times 1$ parameter vector.

As a basic model for tract counts this serves as a starting point to consider extension, both in terms of approximations and in terms of inclusion of more sophisticated random-effect terms which can describe unobserved heterogeneity and clustering of the data.

Often, the basic model in (4.18) has to be modified to accommodate the level of aggregation of available covariates or external referencing of the case disease. For example, it may be that only tract level data are available from which to estimate the $g(\boldsymbol{u})$ function. This can occur when population-based rates, computed from national or regional incidence of the case disease, are used to estimate the tract-specific 'expected count' for the disease. Typically, this expected count is then used to estimate the $g(\boldsymbol{u})$ function for the tract of interest. This could be achieved by smoothing and interpolation or the function could be regarded as constant throughout that tract. In the latter case it is often assumed that the $g(\boldsymbol{u})$ function can be removed from the integral in (4.18) and, in doing so, remove any ancillary spatial information relating to the tract from the resulting g_j function. However, this ignores tract geometry and size or shape differences between tracts.

The estimation of the $g(\boldsymbol{u})$ function can also be achieved by interpolation either from an already aggregated level of observation, or from non-parametric regression methods from lower levels of aggregation. For example, it may be that a control disease realisation is available, and so density/intensity estimation could be used to provide estimates of the $g(\boldsymbol{u})$ function at a variety of locations within any tract of interest. However, interpolation of such aggregated data could lead to multiple stages of smoothing and this can affect subsequent inference significantly (Lawson and Williams, 1994).

An alternative approach to this problem is to extend the conditional logistic approach of Section 4.3.2 to include the situation where counts of the case disease and the control disease are available within each tract. Define the count of the control disease in the jth tract as n_{cj}. Using this definition it is possible to derive conditional probabilities for the realisation of n_j cases and n_{cj} controls in each of the m tracts. By conditional arguments, it is possible to derive the probability of n_j cases in the jth tract as

$$\left\{\frac{\lambda_j}{\sum_{k=1}^{m}\int_{a_k}[g(\boldsymbol{u})+\lambda(\boldsymbol{u})]\,\mathrm{d}\boldsymbol{u}}\right\}^{n_j}$$

and the probability of n_{cj} controls in the jth tract is

$$\left\{\frac{g_j}{\sum_{k=1}^{m}\int_{a_k}[g(\boldsymbol{u})+\lambda(\boldsymbol{u})]\,\mathrm{d}\boldsymbol{u}}\right\}^{n_{cj}},$$

where

$$g_j = \int_{a_j} g(\boldsymbol{u})\,\mathrm{d}\boldsymbol{u}.$$

These expressions can be included within a standard likelihood which, bar a constant only depending on the data, is of the form:

$$L = \prod_{j=1}^{m}\left\{\frac{\lambda_j}{\sum_{k=1}^{m}\int_{a_k}[g(\boldsymbol{u})+\lambda(\boldsymbol{u})]\,\mathrm{d}\boldsymbol{u}}\right\}^{n_j}\left\{\frac{g_j}{\sum_{k=1}^{m}\int_{a_k}[g(\boldsymbol{u})+\lambda(\boldsymbol{u})]\,\mathrm{d}\boldsymbol{u}}\right\}^{n_{cj}}. \tag{4.19}$$

This model reduces to a simpler form when both $g(\boldsymbol{u})$ and $m(F(\boldsymbol{u}))$ can be regarded as constant within tracts. In that case, substituting g_j and m_j as constant functions we have

$$L = \prod_{j=1}^{m}\left\{\frac{g_j m_j |a_j|}{\sum_{k=1}^{m} g_k |a_k|\{1+m_k\}}\right\}^{n_j}\left\{\frac{g_j |a_j|}{\sum_{k=1}^{m} g_k |a_k|\{1+m_k\}}\right\}^{n_{cj}}.$$

Of course, as noted above, there would have to be substantive reasons for this approximation in any particular case study which employed this general modelling approach.

4.4.2 Approximations

The extreme form of approximation of the model (4.18) is found by considering all explanatory and background functions to be constant within tracts. This can be called the *decoupling* approximation, and has been discussed by various authors. By making this approximation, analysis via standard discrete generalised linear models (GLMs) is possible. However, this leads to a number of problems related to the discretisation of variates and the replacement of the point estimate of an integral over an area by a point estimate unrelated to that integral. Essentially, to correctly estimate the expected count in any tract j, the point estimate of $E\{n_j\}$ must represent the integral of a continuous function across the whole study area. Hence, the value of the point estimate in any tract is related to that in any other as it is the integral of a continuous function over all tracts.

The most common approximation of this kind is the assumption that

$$E\{n_j\} = \rho g_j m(F_j \alpha), \tag{4.20}$$

where ρ is an overall disease risk parameter, not dependent on the specific tract, and all other parameters are constant within each tract. Often, g_j is estimated from some known rate for the disease by standardising on national or regional rates for the population groups in the tract. This leads to the use of expected deaths (e_j) as an estimate of the background 'at-risk' function g_j. This approach is commonly employed in a wide range of applications of disease mapping. Of course, without consideration of the spatial tract structure or compensation by inclusion of random effects for each tract, then this approximation could yield considerable bias in parameter estimation and hence subsequent inference. Diggle (1993), and others (Lawson and Cressie, 2000), discuss the implications of such an ecological bias.

4.4.3 Random-Effect Extensions

As discussed in Section 4.3.4, it is possible to extend the models described for count data by inclusion of various types of random effects which can make some allowance for unobserved heterogeneity in the observed counts. The rationale for inclusion of such effects will vary depending on the nature and purpose of the study. For example, it is possible to include random effects for each tract at the tract level to allow for, or compensate for, the effect of assuming that covariates are constant within tracts. Alternatively, although we assume that individual responses to disease risk are independent and, given the Poisson count model, have linked and equal expectation and variance, these assumptions may not appear valid in observed data. This can be due to the existence of variates which are unmeasured in the study but which can produce *apparent* heterogeneity or lack of independence in the observations. In addition, the data may naturally cluster in space and this effect is not explicitly modelled in the above formulation, and hence could produce *real* heterogeneity due to model misspecification.

All of the above effects can be incorporated in the specification of models for count data as they were for case event data, except that individual effects or frailties are not relevant. Hence, the list of types of effect in Section 4.3.4 can apply to counts equally, as in the case event situation. Discussion of specific random-effect models is postponed to Section 5. However, it should be noted that a large literature has arisen in the application of random-effect models to count data.

4.4.4 Hidden Structure and Mixture Models

As in the case event situation it is possible to consider hidden structure or mixture models for count data.

The application of simpler mixture models, has been developed by Schlattman and Böhning (1993) and Ayutha and Böhning (1995). These models describe hidden structure in the *marginal* intensity of the counts and have not been applied in the case event situation. The counts are assumed to be independent Poisson distributed with expectation $E(n_i) = e_i \sum_{j=1}^{k} w_j \lambda_j$, where it is assumed that $\sum_{j=1}^{k} w_j = 1$ and the w_j are a set of weights (probabilities), and the λ_j are a set of intensity components. Here the relative risk is a mixture of components where all elements of the mixture are unknown (including the number of components k). The authors use likelihood and expectation-maximisation (EM) algorithms for estimation. The methods have been extended to include covariates (Schlattmann *et al.*, 1996).

A more elaborate mixture formulation has been proposed by Knorr-Held and Rasser (2000) where the expected count in the ith tract is defined as $E(n_i) = e_i\lambda_j$, where there are $j = 1, \ldots, k$ cluster-partitioned relative risks. This model implies a discrete non-overlapping partition of the relative risk surface and may be useful where discontinuities in risk are found. There is no allowance for probabilistic allocation of tracts to clusters under this approach. There does not seem to be great *a priori* epidemiological justification for division of large-scale risk maps into risk categories that are step functions.

A similar specification underlies the development of models where it is assumed that $n_i \sim \text{Poisson}(\sum_{j=1}^{k} w_{ij}\lambda_j)$, where the weights have spatial correlation prior distributions (Carmen Fernandez, personal communication, 2000). In this case a weight vector is attached to each tract and so differential membership can be accommodated.

4.4.5 Space-Time Extensions

As in the case event situation, the basic Poisson model can be extended to accommodate space-time extensions. The spatio-temporal model described by (4.11) can be applied to count data by specification within the usual integration scheme. That is, we can derive the expected count over a given time period and spatial area by integration of the spatio-temporal intensity specified by (4.11) suitably parametrised for the study in hand.

However, as noted above, in many studies of tract counts, this is eschewed in favour of the assumption of constant within-region and within-time period rate parametrisation (Bernardinelli *et al.*, 1995b; Waller *et al.*, 1997; Heisterkamp *et al.*, 2000; Knorr-Held and Besag, 1998; Knorr-Held, 2000; Boehning *et al.*, 2000; Pickle, 2000; Sun *et al.*, 2000; Zhu and Carlin, 2000). In many examples it is realistic to consider that individual responses to risk are continuously varying in time and could be a continuous function of spatial location. Counts recorded in tracts which represent the sum of all cases could also be viewed in this way. The level of counts in tracts could have both a purely spatial component, of whatever degree of complexity, and a purely temporal component reflecting changes in temporal disease trends. In addition, there could also be an extra effect due to the added interaction of temporal and spatial effects. This interaction occurs when a particular spatial pattern becomes correlated with particular temporal patterns. For example, the incidence of childhood leukaemia may form into spatial aggregations and these aggregations or clusters are represented by areas of elevated disease incidence within a study window. In addition, it may be found that when the time of occurrence of the cases is taken into consideration, the clustering of the disease in space becomes particularly marked. This interaction, or space-time correlation as it is known, can arise amongst count data as well as case event data, and has been separately studied for a considerable time (Knox, 1964; Mantel, 1967). The existence of spatial aggregations and spatio-temporal interaction are both of great significance within spatial epidemiology. Purely temporal effects have little importance in the interpretation of spatial patterns *unless* they interact with the spatial structure. A fuller discussion of issues relating to aggregation and interaction is postponed to Chapters 8 and 10, which focus in detail on particular application areas.

CHAPTER 5

Exploratory Approaches, Parametric Estimation and Inference

In many studies of the incidence of disease, it is appropriate to consider whether models of the disease process are to be employed, whether any pre- or post-exploratory analysis is to be pursued, and also if non-parametric alternatives to these approaches are appropriate. In this section we assume that the main process of model examination follows a sequence of stages.

First, exploratory analysis of the data may be pursued to examine some underlying structure which could be present, or to generate hypotheses concerning the example. The nature of this exploration will depend crucially on the nature and purpose of the study to be undertaken. Often, this exploration is non-parametric in nature, in that the methods used do not rely on the specification of a model. Clearly, it is appropriate to undertake exploratory analysis when only limited knowledge exists concerning the study window of concern. However, some problems can arise when analyses are made *a posteriori*, that is, when knowledge of a particular spatial feature leads an investigator to test for the structure or even the existence of such a feature. Examples of these problems often arise in the analysis of small-area health data around putative sources of hazard, such as incinerators or nuclear power stations. Often, in these examples some adverse health effect ascribed to the putative source is reported by local residents, and following this, a study is focused on the health in the local area (Lenihan, 1985; COMARE, 1988). In these cases, knowledge of a putative source exists and therefore inferences made concerning such a source could lead to *a posteriori* inference problems. Indeed, any hypotheses concerning the existence of a putative source of pollution fall in this category. However, analyses of the *spatial structure* of disease incidence within the study window does not, per se, lead to such problems. In addition, if prior knowledge of a *raised* incidence of disease within the study window exists this does not relate directly to *any* specific hypothesis concerning the spatial structure within the window, including any hypotheses concerning the existence of a putative source.

While hypothesis testing itself is sometimes regarded as an exploratory tool, here, it is assumed that exploratory tools are those which can be used with little or no prior knowledge of the underlying spatial structure. Section 5.4 provides discussion of the role of hypotheses testing in the analysis of spatial epidemiological data.

The second stage of analysis can be regarded as a model-fitting stage. Usually, we want to fit parsimonious models for the spatial structure of the data observed within the window. This allows a flexible approach to assessing spatial effects without limiting the analysis to a restricted set of hypothesis tests. Whether it is appropriate to employ fully parametrised models, or approaches which are essentially non-parametric, is often dictated by the level of prior information provided by the study and the data themselves. For example, in many applications of spatial statistics the asymptotic distribution of estimators is not known and resort must be made to Monte Carlo testing (see Appendix A.2). Hence, even when fully parametric models are employed, the methods used to assess the significance of model fits are, at least in part, non-parametric. At this stage it is usual to pursue parameter estimation and to assess the reliability of estimators and the overall goodness-of-fit of the model.

Following the model-fitting stage it is usual to examine residual diagnostics to assess the pointwise goodness-of-fit. In addition, it is also possible at this stage to assess the overall goodness-of-fit via functions of residuals. The use of simulation envelopes in this area is one which is pursued here as a general method of pointwise model assessment, regardless of whether Bayesian or likelihood models are applied to the study data. Appendix A.3 discusses the use of such envelopes in detail. Gelman *et al.* (1995) propose the use of these envelopes in general Bayesian modelling. It is also possible, at this stage, to apply exploratory tools to assess the structures found in residual fields, although we do not pursue this here.

Finally, it may be appropriate to re-examine the model-fitting process as a result of the examination of residuals and goodness-of-fit of the model. In fact, the iterative examination of model fits and residuals in a continuous process of model improvement can be advocated in this application area. A common example of this process arises when a model assuming independence of observations is fitted and following this the residual diagnostics suggest that spatial autocorrelation remains in the observations. It may then be appropriate to include such autocorrelation in a subsequent model fit.

5.1 EXPLORATORY METHODS

The use of exploratory methods in the analysis of disease incidence has a considerable history. Ever since a map of disease locations was first constructed, visual exploration has been pursued. The construction of a map of locations of disease incidence allows the visual exploration of the spatial distribution of a disease. The construction of the map of cholera cases around the Broad Street pump in London by John Snow in 1854 must rank as one of the first published attempts to use spatial information in an epidemiological or public health study. The map of disease incidence is a fundamental *visual* tool for the analysis disease, and as such can be useful. However, care must be taken in the interpretation of such maps, both from the visual/perceptual viewpoint and from understanding how the map represents or seeks to represent the disease information. In addition to the mapping and perceptual process, the choice of what to map is often a statistical task, in that the map often represents an 'average' of the observed data. John Snow represented the address locations of cases of disease on a street map of the Broad Street pump area. The intention of the map construction was to provide some visual evidence for a link between the disease incidence and possible sources of water-borne infections. Hence, this forms an early example of the analysis of a putative source of health hazard. The interpretation of the map was based on the density of cases around the Broad Street pump, and how these cases decreased with distance from the pump. One factor which is not represented on this map is the changes in population density with distance from the pump. While maps of disease incidence can be used without such information, it is usually important to incorporate such information in the analysis. Otherwise, raised incidence of disease could be spuriously thought important when it simply represents increases in the 'at-risk' population.

5.1.1 Cartographic Issues

Esteve *et al.* (1994) have discussed some issues related to cartographic representation of disease incidence data. The representation of spatial data has been a concern of geographers for a considerable time and many cartographic texts have arisen dealing with map construction and the visual perception of mapped information (MacEachren, 1995; Monmonier, 1996). Within epidemiology there has been a considerable development of the publication of disease atlases, which have as their focus the presentation of large domain maps, usually country- or continent-wide (Pickle *et al.*, 1999), and many developments of mapping methods have been related to these developments.

Here, as our concern is with statistical issues related to mapping, we focus only briefly on the main concerns of map representation. First, the purpose and audience of the putative map should have some impact on the design of visual information in mapped form. For example, a map of case event data presented to health researchers or planners, may lead to a search for disease 'clusters'. Clustering of objects on maps is often readily picked out by eye (Ripley, 1981). Equally, if counts within census tracts are depicted, then a similar potential audience may look for areas of high incidence. Hence, the interpretation of mapped data can be largely based on the visual/perceptual properties of a map. Because visual perception is linked to classification of objects or ideas within each individual, then the use of particular visual effects can have dramatic perceptual effects. For example, if all census tracts on a map which have a high incidence of a disease (say, above a threshold value) are coloured fluorescent purple and all those below threshold are depicted by a cold colour then the perceptual incidence of disease is raised by the colour of the map! This generalises to choropleth maps, where arbitrary choices of colour shading must be used to represent different incidence levels of disease. The use of colouring has considerable potential in the perceptual distortion of visual information (see Section 3.5).

The map presentation issue discussed above is really the last stage in a process of visual representation of statistical information. Before this stage there often lies a graphical processing stage which allows the information to be represented in a visual form. This stage could consist of statistical processing, e.g. smoothing or interpolation, as well as strictly graphical processing. The first stage is usually statistical in that it concerns issues of how to estimate parameters related to the data. For example, for tract counts this might be the estimation of the relative risk of disease in each tract, the second stage would be representation of these relative risks over a mapped area (e.g. interpolation onto a grid mesh). The final stage would be the choice of symbolic representation of different levels of relative risk on the map. In any map production, at least two of these stages are always met, and often the intermediate stage occurs implicitly within a graphical package. For example, it is often desirable to represent the local intensity of case events on a map by an intensity function which can be estimated non-parametrically using a two-dimensional density estimation procedure (Diggle, 1985b). Once this density estimate is available, it can be computed at a variety of locations within the domain of interest (the study window). For the purpose of visual representation of the estimate, a set of estimates is computed usually on a grid mesh and some method is chosen to represent the continuous intensity surface over the area. If a contour or surface drawing procedure is used, then it may itself employ interpolation and smoothing stages, *in addition* to those used to compute the density estimate at each location. Counts within tracts represent averages and as such can be regarded as continuously defined over the study window. That is, it is possible to interpolate counts to provide estimates at locations other than where the count is 'located'. Often, counts are ascribed to tract centroids, however defined, and these are treated as points in subsequent analysis. Hence, similar considerations apply to this case as in the case event situation except that a different smoothing procedure would be used (e.g. non-parametric regression).

To avoid extra stages of interpolation it is usually best to use simple known smoothing operations and to avoid graphical packages with unknown interpolation procedures. For example, the INTERP command in S-Plus uses the high-dimensional Akima interpolator (Ripley, 1981). The IMSL library (Visual Numerics) provides a number of interpolators, including Akima. If little can be done about the choice of representational package, then at least it is important to note that a number of stages are always involved in the processing of mapped data, even after the major statistical estimation issues are resolved.

5.1.2 Case Event Mapping

Maps of case events have limited use without association with the background 'at-risk' population distribution. It is commonplace in the analysis of tract counts to examine the spatial distribution of disease counts *with* the distribution of the 'at-risk' population incorporated in the analysis. In the case event situation, it is also possible to represent the background 'at-risk' population within a map of case event distribution. Bithell (1990) first suggested the idea of mapping case event intensity with the background

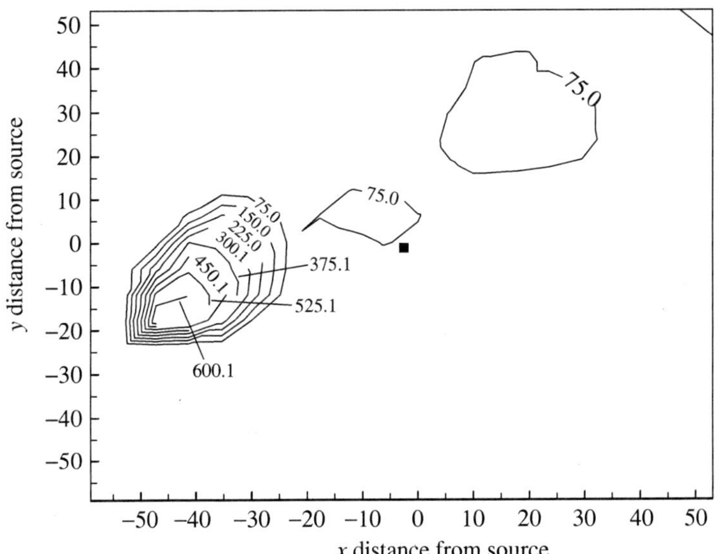

Figure 5.1 Ratio extraction surface for the Armadale example, using CHD control smoothed using a two-dimensional kernel estimator with smoothing constant estimated via cross-validation. Reproduced with permission from Lawson and Williams (1994).

'extracted' from the cases. Essentially, the idea is that the first-order intensity can be defined as $\lambda(\boldsymbol{x}) = g(\boldsymbol{x})\lambda^*(\boldsymbol{x})$, where $g(\boldsymbol{x})$ represents the 'at-risk' background population, and $\lambda^*(\boldsymbol{x})$ represents a modulating function related to residual disease incidence, i.e. any incidence locally differing from that 'expected' from $g(\boldsymbol{x})$. As the case events represent both the population variation *and* the residual disease incidence, then $\lambda(\boldsymbol{x})$ can be estimated from the complete case event map realisation by, for example, a two-dimensional density/intensity estimate. Call this estimate $\hat{\lambda}(\boldsymbol{x})$. The background function $g(\boldsymbol{x})$ can also be estimated separately as $\hat{g}(\boldsymbol{x})$. Methods of $g(\boldsymbol{x})$ estimation are discussed in Section 4.3.2. It is then possible to form the ratio:

$$\frac{\hat{\lambda}(\boldsymbol{x})}{\hat{g}(\boldsymbol{x})}, \qquad \forall\, \boldsymbol{x} \in W. \tag{5.1}$$

This ratio provides an estimate of the difference in risk between the observed case intensity and that expected from the background and hence can be used to provide information about areas with different risks. In particular, the results of this computation can be mapped, and these maps are often examined for areas of excess risk. Figure 5.1 displays the ratio extraction process applied to the Armadale example with CHD control used as the background estimator.

The process of mapping of ratio estimates has been called 'extraction mapping' by Lawson and Williams (1993), who developed the idea by using an alternative extraction method based on non-parametric regression. The issue arises in the estimation of (5.1), of whether it is better to use separate estimation of numerator and denominator,

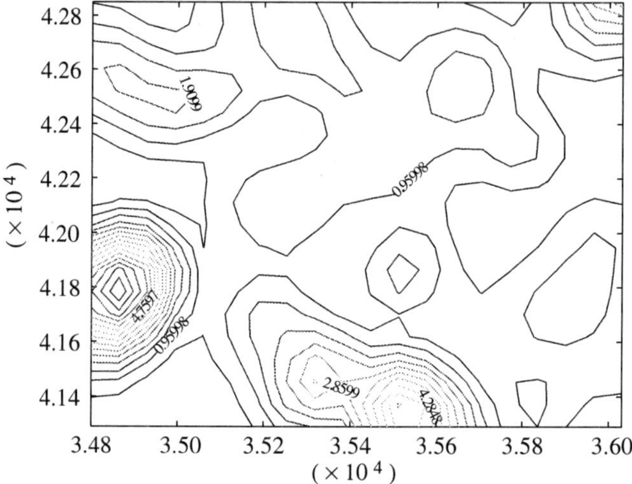

Figure 5.2 Lancashire larynx cancer example: extraction surface using the respiratory cancer control estimated by two-dimensional kernel density estimation. The smoothing constants were estimated using cross-validation criteria.

or to apply a common smoothing operation to both. Kelsall and Diggle (1995a, 1995b) have shown that, in the cross-validation method used, which minimises the integrated squared error of the log density ratio estimate, a common smoothing constant is preferable. Their result applies to densities estimated from two-point processes and hence applies when a control disease map is used to estimate $g(\boldsymbol{x})$. The application of this to situations where $g(\boldsymbol{x})$ is estimated from other sources has not been investigated. Specifically, define

$$\hat{f}_h(\boldsymbol{x}) = n^{-1} \sum_{i=1}^{n} h^{-2} K\{h^{-1}(\boldsymbol{x} - \boldsymbol{x}_i)\},$$

which is a bivariate kernel density estimate of a density f, where $K(\cdot)$ is a bivariate kernel function and h a smoothing parameter. It is possible to regard the ratio of intensities $R(\boldsymbol{x}) = \lambda(\boldsymbol{x})/g(\boldsymbol{x})$ as being represented by a ratio of densities as, if the intensities govern independent Poisson processes, $r(\boldsymbol{x}) = \log R(\boldsymbol{x}) = \log\{f(\boldsymbol{x})/d(\boldsymbol{x})\} + r_0$, where f and d are densities. The constant r_0 is the log ratio of integrated intensities and, due to the conditioning inherent in the method, this does not need to be further considered. By estimating f and d using the bivariate kernel above, and also the ratio $\hat{r}_h(\boldsymbol{x}) = \log\{\hat{f}_h(\boldsymbol{x})/\hat{d}_h(\boldsymbol{x})\}$, it is possible to construct a cross-validation criterion which can be minimised to find the optimal h.

This criterion is

$$\mathrm{CV}(h) = -\int_W \{\hat{r}_h(\boldsymbol{x})\}^2\,\mathrm{d}\boldsymbol{x} - 2m^{-1} \sum_{i=1}^{m} \frac{\hat{r}_h^{-i}(\boldsymbol{x}_i)}{\hat{f}_h^{-i}(\boldsymbol{x}_i)} + 2m_{\mathrm{c}}^{-1} \sum_{j=1}^{m_{\mathrm{c}}} \frac{\hat{r}_h^{-j}(\boldsymbol{x}_{\mathrm{c}i})}{\hat{d}_h^{-i}(\boldsymbol{x}_{\mathrm{c}i})}, \tag{5.2}$$

where m and m_c are the number of cases and controls respectively and, the superscript $-i$ means that the all the sample except the ith item is used. The same applies to superscript $-j$.

The resulting surface of $\hat{r}(\boldsymbol{x})$ can be used for visual inspection within an exploratory analysis. Of course, the previous comments concerning the display of such surfaces also apply here, and in fact to reduce the chance of perceptual misrepresentation, it is useful to obtain some measure of the reliability of the estimated surface. This can be achieved by computing pointwise tolerance intervals. Under the usual null hypothesis, that the cases are just a realisation of a Poisson process with intensity $g(\boldsymbol{x})$, then in the case/control situation, this implies that the cases and controls come from the same distribution. In that case, it is possible to randomly reassign the case/control labels to the joint data set and to compute a Monte Carlo p-value surface from $\hat{r}(\boldsymbol{x})$ computed from s realisations of the label reassignments. In the case where it is inappropriate to compute $g(\boldsymbol{x})$ from a control disease, it is still possible to generate pointwise tolerance intervals. However, in this case it is not possible to condition the joint distribution of cases and controls. Instead, s realisations of the m case events would have to be generated from the distribution with density $\hat{g}(\boldsymbol{x})/\int_W \hat{g}(\boldsymbol{u})\,\mathrm{d}\boldsymbol{u}$. This can be achieved by standard rejection sampling methods (Ripley, 1987, pp. 60–63).

Alternative exploratory methods exist where particular effects are to be assessed or examined. For example, it is possible to examine particular distance effects, such as the distance of cases from known locations (e.g. putative hazard sources) or the overall marginal distribution of local intensity of cases compared to controls. In the first case, if it is possible to regard the intensity of cases as based on a simple distance function from the nearest known location, then, assuming the intensity decline is monotone with increasing distance, certain transformation properties of the Poisson process can be used to assess distance effects. Diggle (1990) described an intensity transformation which yields such results. In addition, it is also possible to assess the differences between the cumulative distance distribution of cases and controls via such methods as quantile–quantile (Q–Q) plotting. In the second case, resort can be made to Dirichlet tessellation of the events to yield marginal distributional information (Sibson, 1980). For the example of case events with a control disease, it is possible to define the following tessellation characteristics. First, the Dirichlet tessellation of a set of m point locations is defined by a set of *tiles*, one per point for which $\forall\ x \in a_i$. Figure 5.3 displays a tessellation of the Armadale case data. Clearly, areas of high case density are depicted as 'clusters' of small tiles.

The area of each tile surrounding a point is denoted a_i, and it can be shown that $1/a_i$ is a local estimate of the event intensity (Lawson, 1993a). The tile areas are highly correlated. However, their marginal distribution for both case events and control events should be the same under the null hypothesis: that the case events are a random sample from the control distribution. Hence, it would also be possible to compare the empirical distribution functions of the tile areas for both data sets via suitable graphical methods (e.g. Q–Q plots). Note that excesses of small areas will indicate increased clustering relative to the other event process. Hence, in a Q–Q plot of areas, deviations from linear equality supports differences in intensity of case

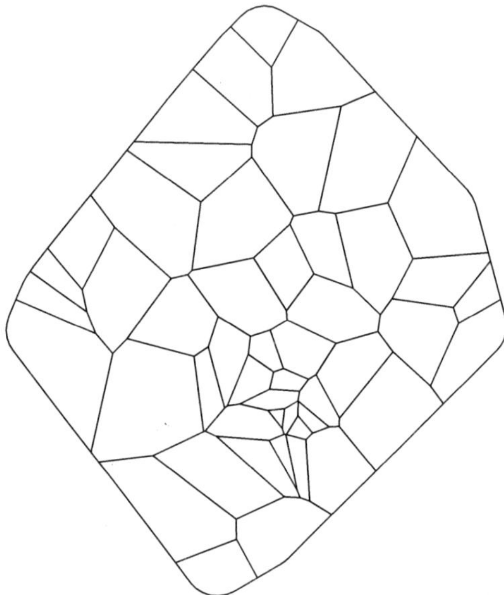

Figure 5.3 Dirichlet tessellation of the Armadale case event realisation (within the convex hull of the data points).

events compared to control events. Edge effects also play a role here, however. At the window boundaries the tile areas will be truncated, as the distribution of events is unknown outside the window. Usually, to construct a tessellation in this case a set of suspension points are defined which are external to the study region. The tessellation is then suspended from these points. The tiles which intersect the boundary are then truncated at the boundary (Berman and Turner, 1992). Hence, any boundary tile area will not be correctly estimated. This edge effect can be compensated for by a variety of methods. The simplest method is to exclude any points which have associated boundary tiles, from the graphical procedures. An alternative method is to include the points but to annotate them to identify their boundary position. Finally, it could be possible to attach weights to each point which describe the extent that tiles intersect the boundary. For instance, a numerical weight defined as the proportion of the tile perimeter which lies on the boundary could be used. This would down weight edge tiles in any computation (Lawson, 1993a). This weighting could be incorporated into the comparison of empirical distribution functions.

The efficient computation of tessellations is the subject of computational geometry (Preparata and Shamos, 1985; Rosenfeld *et al.*, 1998; Mulmuley, 1993). So far the most efficient ($n \log n$ order) is the divide-and-conquer algorithm of Lee and Schacter (1980). This algorithm has been incorporated in the DELDIR program of Berman and Turner (1992). Watson (1981) has also developed an efficient algorithm for such tessellation. Earlier computational methods include the TILE algorithm of Green and Sibson (1978), which does not achieve optimal efficiency. Currently, a range of computational packages include Dirichlet/Voronoi tessellation and Delauney triangulation procedures. Of these packages the commonly used include MATLAB, S-Plus Spatial Stats, and Vertical Mapper, which operates within the Geographical Information System (GIS) MapInfo.

5.1.3 Count Mapping

The exploratory mapping of tract count data has seen a considerable development, not least because this form of data is that which is most readily available. As in the example of case event data, the count of a disease within an arbitrary region should not be viewed without an estimate of the associated 'at-risk' population within the region concerned. A tract count can be regarded as a type of average, obtained by accumulating individual cases over a given area. Hence, this both increases our confidence in the estimation of local rates of disease, due to increased sample size, but also decreases the spatial information available in that individual locations are now unavailable. Figure 1.1 demonstrates this effect clearly.

The estimation of the 'at-risk' population in each tract can be achieved by a variety of means. Conventionally, an 'expected count' is estimated for each tract, either from known national rates for the disease, or from a more local standard population. This standard rate will be broken down into rates for any population strata thought appropriate for the purposes of analysis. Usually, age and sex divisions are used, but other functions of the population could be incorporated, such as deprivation status or other measures of lifestyle choices. A recent review of standardisation of rates is provided by Inskip *et al.* (1983), while the use of deprivation indices is discussed by Carstairs (1981). As such information is now available routinely in many countries from official agencies, it is relatively straightforward to use such expected count information in exploratory mapping of count data.

An alternative source of information concerning the 'at-risk' population within tracts is available. Mirroring the use of a realisation of a control disease in the case event example, it is possible to use the count of a control disease within the tract to estimate this 'at-risk' population. Of course, such a count does not provide stratification of the expected count with regard to the population structure. The immediate advantage of a control disease, that of providing detailed spatial information concerning the 'at-risk' population, is lost here and the absence of other information reduces the attractiveness of this approach.

The representation of the difference between count (n_i) and expected count (e_i) is usually carried out for each tract by either forming a ratio of the form n_i/e_i or, less commonly, by forming a difference such as $n_i - e_i$. The first ratio form is suggested by the idea that any difference in disease incidence from the standardised expected count is multiplicatively linked to that count. This parallels the case event example where the cases contain both population information *and* disease effect information, whereas the control disease or other background data type purely reflects the population information. Hence, the tract count of disease of interest represents both the background population and its resultant rate, whereas the expected count represents the background population effect only. The difference form, on the other hand, assumes that the disease effect is additively linked to the expected count. The ratio form will result in a map of tract ratios ranging from 0 to ∞ with the value 1 where $n_i = e_i$. On the other hand, the additive form will result in a map of tract differences ranging from large negative to large positive values and equalling 0 where $n_i = e_i$. Further modifications are often made to these basic forms. First, the ratio form represents the *relative risk* of the disease for a tract and it is sometimes easier to interpret the form $\log\{n_i/e_i\}$. The ratio form arises naturally as the result of estimation within commonly used models for count data and the log relative risk also has an natural interpretation in that it centres the risk on the 0 value with equal ranges on either side. Note that this also parallels the use of the log density ratio in case event data. In addition to the log transformation, other modifications arise naturally in the context of models for count data. Perhaps the most commonly used modification is to augment the count and the expected count with predefined constants. For example, the form

$$\frac{n_i + a}{e_i + b} \tag{5.3}$$

is often used, and this form arises from a Bayesian model for tract counts using empirical Bayesian (EB) methods. The values of the constants can be estimated naturally within the EB context. Otherwise, the choice of constants is somewhat arbitrary and without some prior rationale for the choice this latitude could lead to considerable distortion in the resulting mapped surface. One arbitrary choice often made is to set both constants to the same small positive constant, to avoid singularities when making transformations (e.g. log transformations).

Finally, it should be noted that a great variety of different forms can be used to represent the relation of disease count to expected count. These are based on different mathematical forms or on different ways of estimating the expected count. It is not the purpose of this work to review in detail these different approaches and the reader is referred to Inskip *et al.* (1983) and Breslow and Day (1987) for more comprehensive reviews. However, it is important to note that the ratio form n_i/e_i is termed a standardised mortality ratio (SMR) when disease mortality is being assessed and standardised morbidity ratio (SMR) when disease morbidity is being assessed. In both cases, these ratios are usually associated with standardisation of rates to provide expected counts. This standardisation could be based on national, regional or study window total rates. These categories correspond with the usual *external* and *internal* standardisation of rates. If a control disease is used to estimate e_i, then this ratio can still be regarded as an SMR. We define the difference form $(n_i - e_i)$ to be the standardised mortality/morbidity difference (SMD).

Assume that each tract now has an estimate of the risk difference, and it is appropriate to map the spatial distribution of SMR or SMD. These measures are continuous variates. Usually, they are represented at some fixed point within each tract, such as the tract centroid (however defined). However, they represent the disease difference over the whole tract and are therefore a type of tract average and *not* a measurement made at a single location. The representation of this variate, then, can be considered

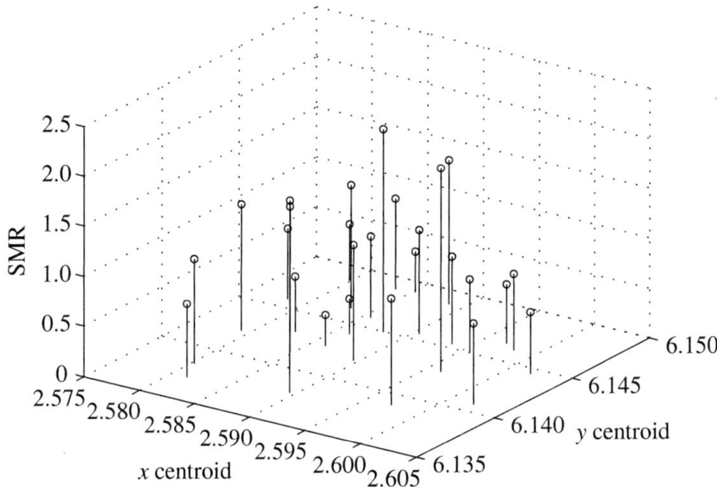

Figure 5.4 Needle plot of the SMRs for respiratory cancer in the Falkirk example. The needles are plotted at the centroids of the tracts.

in a variety of ways. First, it is tempting to simply represent this variate by a needle plot, with needles located at centroids.

Figure 5.4 displays such a plot. The problem of the variation in size and shape of tracts suggests that this information should be included within the representation. In addition, it may be assumed that some form of random noise or error is found within the observations which can be removed by smoothing the tract counts. This smoothing operation would allow interpolation of values to locations other than the centroids and thus attempts to represent the variation in disease differences continuously over a study window. Breslow and Day (1987, pp. 193, 198) describe the use of smoothers applied to SMRs observed over time. It is possible to extend this approach to the spatial domain. A variety of smoothing methods are available for continuously distributed spatial data. Within geostatistics, the method of ordinary kriging has been developed for such data (Cressie, 1993). However, it is strictly *inapplicable* to continuous data on $\mathbb{R}^+$ as negative interpolant values are allowed within kriging. This could be avoided via log transformation of a modified ratio (avoiding singularities). A simpler method to implement that is widely available is kernel smoothing, a special case of non-parametric regression (Härdle, 1991). This method involves a smoothing operation with a two-dimensional kernel function which is controlled via a bandwidth parameter h. The value of h controls the degree of smoothness of the resulting surface. Large values lead to greater smoothness. Define the true SMR or SMD as $\theta(\boldsymbol{x})$. The kernel estimate of $\theta(\boldsymbol{x})$ is given by

$$\hat{\theta}(\boldsymbol{x}) = \frac{1}{m} \sum_{i=1}^{m} w\left(\frac{\|\boldsymbol{x} - \boldsymbol{x}_{n_i}\|}{h} \right) \frac{n_i}{e_i}, \tag{5.4}$$

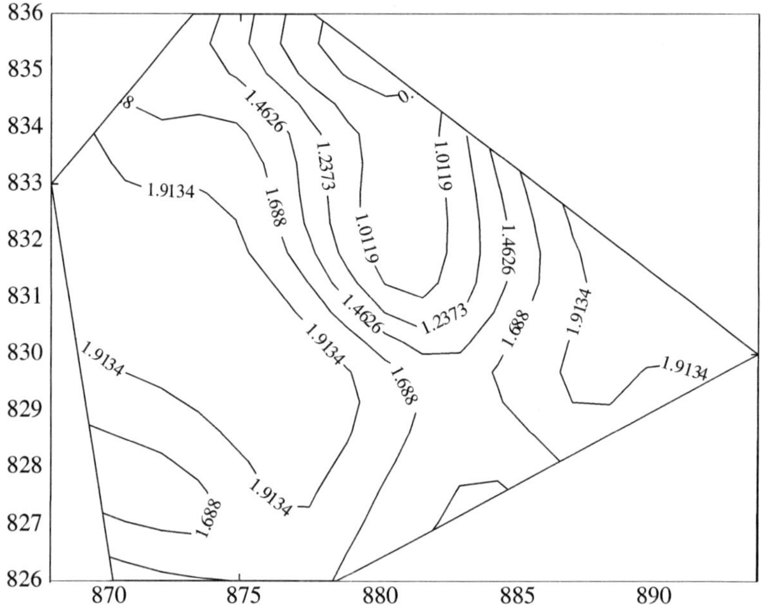

Figure 5.5 The kernel-smoothed SMR surface for the Falkirk example. An idealised boundary has been employed.

where $w(\cdot)$ is a normalised function of a two-dimensional kernel function, $\|\boldsymbol{x} - \boldsymbol{x}_{n_i}\|$ is the Euclidean distance of $\boldsymbol{x}$ from the tract centroid $\boldsymbol{x}_{n_i}$. The conditional standard error surface of this estimate is given by (see Härdle (1991, p. 136))

$$\operatorname{se}(\hat{\theta}(\boldsymbol{x})) = \left[\frac{1}{m}\left\{\sum_{i=1}^{m} w\left(\frac{\|\boldsymbol{x} - \boldsymbol{x}_{n_i}\|}{h}\right)\left(\frac{n_i}{e_i} - \hat{\theta}(\boldsymbol{x})\right)^2\right\}\right]^{1/2}, \tag{5.5}$$

and this surface can also be computed and displayed. Figure 5.5 displays an example of a smoothed SMR surface.

Lawson (1993c) gives examples of the application of this smoothing approach. Note that edge effects occur within this estimator since, at any $\boldsymbol{x}$ close to a boundary of the study window, $\hat{\theta}(\boldsymbol{x})$ will be estimated only from the points internal to the study window. Hence, the bias of this estimator will be less at the interior of the window than at the edges. Methods which attempt to circumvent this problem are (1) use of an internal or external guard area, or (2) edge correction of the estimator. The simplest approach to (1) is to regard a proportion of the tracts as guard area tracts not to be included in the exploratory analysis. For example, all tracts which have a boundary with the study window external boundary, or are within a defined distance of that boundary, could be used. An external boundary could only be used if extra tracts were available outside the study region. Limited work has been carried out concerning edge corrections for two-dimensional kernel smoothers. It may be possible to employ methods akin to those applied to point processes (Kelsall and Diggle, 1995b).

An alternative to the conditional standard error (5.5) is to consider pointwise tolerance intervals for the kernel smoother based on a Monte Carlo procedure. For example, under the null hypothesis, it could be assumed that, conditional on N_t, the total window count, that the observed counts follow a probability distribution where the probability of an event in the ith tract is $e_i / \sum_{k=1}^{m} e_k$. Hence, it is possible to generate s realisations of this count distribution and then it is possible to construct a pointwise ranking for the observed $\hat{\theta}(\boldsymbol{x})$ compared to the $\hat{\theta}(\boldsymbol{x})_j^*$ computed from the $j = 1, s$ realisations. This can yield a 'p-value' surface, computed by counting the proportion of $\hat{\theta}(\boldsymbol{x})_j^* s$ which are less than $\hat{\theta}(\boldsymbol{x})$. As will be noted later in Section 5.4, this also provides a general method for Monte Carlo testing of hypotheses related to tract counts.

As in the example of case events, particular methods can be devised to assess some aspect of the spatial distribution of counts. For example, the empirical cumulative distribution of counts with distance from a known location (or nearest known location) could be compared to the empirical cumulative distribution of expected counts via appropriate graphical methods (e.g. Q–Q plots). In addition, such plots could be used to check the *marginal* distribution of the counts compared to the expected counts. However, as in the Dirichlet tile example above, this does not use the spatial information in the data set.

The graphical display of tract information can be achieved within a variety of packages. Standard statistical or graphics packages do *not* provide facilities to display arbitrarily regionalised data, and resort must usually be made to Geographical Information System (GIS) packages. Amongst these, the packages ArcView and MapInfo are possibly the best known, and both allow interactive computation of tract variates and geometrical manipulation of the region structure. For the purposes of producing interpolated surfaces, with tract boundaries overlaid, resort should then be made to the transfer of graphical objects to such platforms as S-Plus or AXUM. Comments referring to the stages of graphical processing in Section 3.2 also apply here.

5.2 PARAMETER ESTIMATION

In this section, basic methods of estimation for the range of standard models for case event and count data are described. It is not the purpose here to describe all models used in particular areas of application, but rather to outline the methods used for simple and commonly used models. In the following sections methods of estimation commonly used for likelihood models will be discussed. In addition, the use of Bayesian models will be discussed and methods for the exploration of the posterior distribution within these models will be examined.

5.2.1 Case Event Likelihood Models

For the likelihood models described in Chapter 4, it is straightforward to derive maximum-likelihood (ML) estimators for the basic parametrisations of (4.4). There are two components to this intensity specification and each component must be considered for estimation. The exception to this is if the conditional logistic model (4.6) is used. In that case only the parametrisation of $m(F\alpha)$ need be considered, where $F \equiv F(\boldsymbol{x})$ for brevity. Usually, the intensity is defined as

$$\lambda(\boldsymbol{x}) = \rho g(\boldsymbol{x}) m(F\alpha), \tag{5.6}$$

where the ρ parameter is specifically excluded from α. This parameter is a constant representing the constant rate or level of the process over the whole region. Intuitively, this parameter measures the total density of points over the region and is not spatially dependent. The log likelihood for a realisation of m events in T is given by

$$l(\boldsymbol{x} \mid \alpha, \rho, g) = m \log \rho + \sum_{i=1}^{m} \log g(\boldsymbol{x}_i) + \sum_{i=1}^{m} \log m(F_i\alpha) - \rho \int_T g(\boldsymbol{u}) m(F(\boldsymbol{u})\alpha)\, \mathrm{d}\boldsymbol{u}, \tag{5.7}$$

where it is assumed that F contains spatially dependent covariates, and this dependency is denoted by $F(\boldsymbol{u})$. Immediately, it is clear that the ML estimate of ρ is

$$\hat{\rho} = \frac{m}{\int_T g(\boldsymbol{u}) m(F(\boldsymbol{u})\alpha)\, \mathrm{d}\boldsymbol{u}}. \tag{5.8}$$

This is the standard ML estimator for the constant rate parameter of a spatial Poisson process. Further, it is straightforward to show that, if $\hat{\rho}$ is substituted back into the likelihood function, to yield a profile likelihood, then bar a constant depending only on m, this yields the likelihood, conditional on m events in T. This is just

$$l_c(\boldsymbol{x} \mid \alpha, m, g) = -m \log \int_T g(\boldsymbol{u}) m(F(\boldsymbol{u})\alpha)\, \mathrm{d}\boldsymbol{u} + \sum_{i=1}^{m} \log g(\boldsymbol{x}_i) + \sum_{i=1}^{m} \log m(F_i\alpha) \tag{5.9}$$

given by the log of (4.3). Hence, the conditional likelihood is a parsimonious description of the *spatial* structure of the window. The use of (5.9) instead of the unconditional likelihood can lead to computational savings, and excludes a nuisance parameter from the analysis of the spatial structure. This can become important when more complex models are considered. However, the ease with which (5.7) can be maximised for relatively simple models, leads us to consider mainly the unconditional model.

The estimation of $g(\boldsymbol{x})$ has been considered in Section 4.3.2. This function is usually estimated from data related directly to the local 'at-risk' population distribution, such as a control disease distribution or the distribution of an expected rate for the case disease. To proceed with ML estimation in the above likelihoods, a decision has to be made about how to estimate $g(\boldsymbol{x})$ within the estimation procedure. The simplest approach is to estimate $g(\boldsymbol{x})$ separately and to use this estimated $g(\boldsymbol{x})$ surface as a 'plug-in' estimator within the likelihoods. Subsequent estimation of ρ or α is then made conditional on this estimate. This method ignores the variation in estimation of $g(\boldsymbol{x})$, and it has been shown that this method can be very sensitive to the method of smoothing used in the estimation of $g(\boldsymbol{x})$ (Lawson and Williams, 1994). Usually, the estimation of $g(\boldsymbol{x})$ involves the estimation of a smoothing parameter, h say, and its estimation involves an optimisation stage. One alternative approach is to include the estimation of h with the estimation of other parameters. This can be achieved by extending the model specified above and using a prior distribution for h within a Bayesian model framework. However, this approach extends beyond the scope of the current model.

The use of the 'plug-in' method for $g(\boldsymbol{x})$ has an advantage in that it is possible to obtain ML estimates for the ρ, α parameters within conventional GLM software. For example, the two-dimensional integral in (5.7) can be approximated by a weighting system, based on the Dirichlet tile areas of the data points, and these weights can be used in a Poisson likelihood model fit with $\log \hat{g}(\boldsymbol{x})$ as offset within GLIM or S-Plus. This integration method was first proposed by Berman and Turner (1992) and was applied to examples in spatial epidemiology by Lawson (1992). In the following, we assume that $\hat{g}(\boldsymbol{x})$ has been estimated and is available at arbitrary locations.

The likelihood (5.7), with $\hat{g}(\boldsymbol{x})$ replacing $g(\boldsymbol{x})$, can be maximised by considering the solution of the normal equations. At this point it is useful to generalise the parametrisation in (5.6) to demonstrate the connection between these models and the generalised linear model framework. Define the linear predictor $\eta_i = F_i\alpha$, the sum of linear contributions from design variables for the ith observation. Also specify the parameter $\mu_i = m(\eta_i)$, which specifies the link between the linear predictor and the intensity function. In addition, as the design matrix F can be spatially dependent then either μ or η can also be spatially dependent. The likelihood (5.7) can be re-expressed with this notation as

$$l(\boldsymbol{x} \mid \alpha, \rho, g) = m \log \rho + \sum_{i=1}^{m} \log g(\boldsymbol{x}_i) + \sum_{i=1}^{m} \log \mu_i - \rho \int_T g(\boldsymbol{u})\mu(\boldsymbol{u})\, \mathrm{d}\boldsymbol{u}, \tag{5.10}$$

where $\eta_i = m^{-1}(\mu_i)$. In addition, it is useful to note that

$$\frac{\partial \mu_i}{\partial \alpha_k} = \frac{\partial \mu_i}{\partial \eta_i}\frac{\partial \eta_i}{\partial \alpha_k} = \frac{\partial \mu_i}{\partial \eta_i} F_{ik}$$

and hence the normal equations are given by

$$\frac{m}{\rho} - I = 0,$$

$$\sum_{i=1}^{m} F_{ik}\frac{1}{\mu_i}\frac{\partial \mu_i}{\partial \eta_i} - \rho I'_{\alpha_k} = 0 \qquad \forall\, k,$$

where $'$ denotes differentiation with respect to the subscript, and $I = \int_T \hat{g}(\boldsymbol{u})\mu(\boldsymbol{u})\, \mathrm{d}\boldsymbol{u}$.

This yields the usual estimate of ρ, and for particular link functions $m(\cdot)$ some simple results are found for the solution of these normal equations. Table 4.1 describes the functions which are commonly used to link the population background $g(\boldsymbol{x})$ to specific spatial and non-spatial covariates. The most common link functions are the multiplicative-log ($\exp F\alpha$) and the additive-log ($1+\exp F\alpha$). The exponentiation is used to ensure positivity of the resulting intensity. The choice of link affects subsequent inference and it is important to consider how this choice is informed. First, the multiplicative-log link suggests that any difference in observed incidence of the case disease compared to the background is proportional to the local background rate. This implies that the local background population will determine any disease outcomes. One difficulty with this link is that when $\exp F\alpha \to 0$, then $\lambda(\boldsymbol{x}) \to 0$, which would be unattractive if this situation were to arise in applications. This problem does arise in putative hazard source estimation problems (see Section 7). The alternative additive-log link does not suffer from this problem, but describes the *amount* of disease difference as proportional to the local background 'at-risk' population and *adds* this amount to the local background. The choice of link will be determined by any particular application. From a computational viewpoint the multiplicative-log link can be easier to implement, especially as it can be represented by a standard GLM link function in such packages as GLIM.

The choice of the $m \times p$ design matrix F will also depend on the application. Amongst the p variates, there will usually be variates describing the spatial location of cases and also some variates relating to measurements made at spatial locations. In addition, there could also be covariates which do not have spatial dependence. In the simplest case, where there is no prior motivation to include specific spatial variates, then it is usual to include low-order spatial trend components. For example, the x and y coordinates of the events can be included. This inclusion will provide a linear spatial trend component in the analysis. Further higher-order terms, with powers of the coordinates and cross products can be included also. If a constant rate parameter is included in F, then the ith row of F will be

$$\{1, x, y, x^2, y^2, xy, x^2y^2, x^3, y^3\}.$$

As a simple example of ML estimation, we will examine a multiplicative-log link with $\{x, y\}$.

Notice that it is not necessary to include a constant rate parameter here, as this is already included as ρ. It is useful to re-express the functions included within $\lambda(\boldsymbol{x})$ as functions of $\{x, y\}$ rather than $\boldsymbol{x}$. The normal equations now become

$$\rho - \frac{m}{\int_T \hat{g}(x, y)\mathrm{e}^{\alpha_1 x+\alpha_2 y}\,\mathrm{d}x\,\mathrm{d}y} = 0,$$

$$\sum_{i=1}^{m} x_i - \rho \int_T \hat{g}(x, y)x\mathrm{e}^{\alpha_1 x+\alpha_2 y}\,\mathrm{d}x\,\mathrm{d}y = 0,$$

$$\sum_{i=1}^{m} y_i - \rho \int_T \hat{g}(x, y)y\mathrm{e}^{\alpha_1 x+\alpha_2 y}\,\mathrm{d}x\,\mathrm{d}y = 0.$$

Notice that by substitution of $\hat{\rho}$ into the other equations, these reduce to the solution of

$$\overline{x} = E_T(x), \qquad \overline{y} = E_T(y),$$

where $E_T(\cdot)$ is the expectation over the area T. Evaluation of these expectations, in practice, requires the evaluation of two-dimensional integrals. This can be facilitated by use of numerical integration weighing schemes. Two-dimensional weights can be based on simple one-dimensional schemes in each dimension, e.g. Simpson's rule or quadrature. An alternative is the use of Dirichlet tile areas, as these yield single point weights, and excepting edge effects, lead to a much reduced storage requirement for weights.

The observed information matrix can also be derived for the model (5.7). It is given by

$$\begin{array}{cc} \dfrac{m}{\rho^2} & I'_{\alpha_k} \\[2ex] I'_{\alpha_k} & \displaystyle\sum_{i=1}^{m} \frac{F_{ij}F_{ik}}{\mu_i^2}\left(\frac{\partial \mu_i}{\partial \eta_i}\right)^2 + \rho I''_{\alpha_j\alpha_k} \\ \vdots & \vdots \end{array}$$

Using the observed or expected information, it is possible to use asymptotic ML theory (see, for example, Cox and Hinkley (1974, pp. 279–344)) to assess the reliability of the ML estimates via the computation of standard errors or classical confidence intervals. For the example above, with ML estimates replacing parameters, this leads to

$$\begin{array}{ccc} \dfrac{I^2}{m} & \cdot & \cdot \\[2ex] \displaystyle\int_T \hat{g}(x, y)x\mathrm{e}^{\alpha_1 x+\alpha_2 y}\,\mathrm{d}x\,\mathrm{d}y & \displaystyle\sum_{i=1}^{m} x_i^2 + mE(x^2) & \cdot \\[2ex] \displaystyle\int_T \hat{g}(x, y)y\mathrm{e}^{\alpha_1 x+\alpha_2 y}\,\mathrm{d}x\,\mathrm{d}y & \displaystyle\sum_{i=1}^{m} x_i y_i + mE(xy) & \displaystyle\sum_{i=1}^{m} y_i^2 + mE(y^2). \end{array}$$

The use of a control disease to represent the local variation in the 'at-risk' population background can lead to a conditional logistic likelihood model for the m cases and n control events. In that case the log likelihood, expressed in the GLM notation given above, is

$$l(\boldsymbol{x} \mid \rho, \alpha) = m \log \rho + \sum_{i=1}^{m} \log \mu_i - \sum_{i=1}^{m} \log\{1 + \rho\mu_i\} - \sum_{j=m+1}^{m+n} \log\{1 + \rho\mu_j\}. \tag{5.11}$$

The normal equations are now

$$\frac{m}{\rho} - \sum_{i=1}^{m} \frac{\mu_i}{1+\rho\mu_i} - \sum_{j=m+1}^{m+n} \frac{\mu_j}{1+\rho\mu_j} = 0,$$

$$\sum_{i=1}^{m} F_{ik}\left(\frac{\partial\mu_i}{\partial\eta_i}\right)\left[\frac{1}{\mu_i} - \frac{\rho}{1+\rho\mu_i}\right] - \sum_{j=m+1}^{m+n} F_{jk}\left(\frac{\partial\mu_j}{\partial\eta_j}\right)\frac{\rho}{1+\rho\mu_j} = 0,$$

and the observed information matrix elements are

$$-l''_{\rho\rho} = \frac{m}{\rho^2} - \sum_{i=1}^{m}\left\{\frac{\mu_i}{1+\rho\mu_i}\right\}^2 - \sum_{j=m+1}^{m+m}\left\{\frac{\mu_j}{1+\rho\mu_j}\right\}^2,$$

$$\begin{aligned}-l''_{\rho\alpha_k} &= -\sum_{i=1}^{m}\left\{F_{ik}\left(\frac{\partial\mu_i}{\partial\eta_i}\right)\left[\frac{1}{1+\rho\mu_i} - \frac{\rho\mu_i}{(1+\rho\mu_i)^2}\right]\right\} \\ &\quad + \sum_{j=m+1}^{m+n}\left\{F_{jk}\left(\frac{\partial\mu_j}{\partial\eta j}\right)\left[\frac{1}{1+\rho\mu_j} - \frac{\rho\mu_j}{(1+\rho\mu_j)^2}\right]\right\},\end{aligned}$$

$$\begin{aligned}-l''_{\alpha_k\alpha_l} &= \sum_{i=1}^{m} F_{ik}F_{il}\left(\frac{\partial\mu_i}{\partial\eta_i}\right)^2\left[\frac{1}{\mu_i^2} - \frac{\rho^2}{(1+\rho\mu_i)^2}\right] \\ &\quad - \sum_{j=m+1}^{m+n} F_{jk}F_{jl}\left(\frac{\partial\mu_j}{\partial\eta j}\right)^2\left[\frac{\rho^2}{(1+\rho\mu_j)^2}\right].\end{aligned}$$

Similar derivations are possible for the hybrid model of Section 4.3.3, but for brevity these are not described here.

Finally, it is appropriate to note that in some studies, notably those regarding putative sources of health hazard or general clustering of disease, the design matrix may include measurements of distances from arbitrary locations to other spatial locations within the window. In that case it is useful to be able to compute such distances efficiently. Borgefors (1986) discusses such algorithms in image processing applications.

5.2.2 Count Event Likelihood Models

As in the example of case event data, likelihood models for count data can be utilised in parameter estimation. In this case, it is convenient to restrict attention to the Poisson likelihood model alone, as the multinomial model of (4.17) can be obtained by straightforward conditioning, and the parameter estimation issues related to the Poisson model are encountered frequently in applications. It is first assumed that the basic parametrisation of λ_j given in (4.18) is appropriate. However, it is assumed, without loss of generality, that both spatially dependent and non-spatially dependent variates are included in the specification of F. Hence, the expected count in the jth tract is now

$$E\{n_j\} = \lambda_j = \rho \int_{a_j} g(\boldsymbol{u})\mu(\boldsymbol{u})\,\mathrm{d}\boldsymbol{u},$$

and this leads to the log likelihood:

$$\begin{aligned} l(\boldsymbol{n} \mid \rho, \alpha) &= \sum_{j=1}^{m} \left\{ n_j \log\left[\rho \int_{a_j} g(\boldsymbol{u})\mu(\boldsymbol{u})\,\mathrm{d}\boldsymbol{u}\right] - \rho \int_{a_j} g(\boldsymbol{u})\mu(\boldsymbol{u})\,\mathrm{d}\boldsymbol{u} \right\} \\ &= n_T \log \rho + \sum_{j=1}^{m} n_j \log \int_{a_j} g(\boldsymbol{u})\mu(\boldsymbol{u})\,\mathrm{d}\boldsymbol{u} - \rho \int_{W} g(\boldsymbol{u})\mu(\boldsymbol{u})\,\mathrm{d}\boldsymbol{u}. \end{aligned}$$

Based on this log likelihood it is possible to derive ML estimates for the parameters of interest. The normal equations are in this case given by

$$\frac{n_T}{\rho} - \int_W \hat{g}(\boldsymbol{u})\mu(\boldsymbol{u})\,\mathrm{d}\boldsymbol{u} = 0,$$

$$\sum_{j=1}^{m} n_j \frac{\int_{a_j} \hat{g}(\boldsymbol{u}) F_k(\boldsymbol{u})(\partial\mu/\partial\eta)\,\mathrm{d}\boldsymbol{u}}{\int_{a_j} \hat{g}(\boldsymbol{u})\mu(\boldsymbol{u})\,\mathrm{d}\boldsymbol{u}} - \rho \int_W \hat{g}(\boldsymbol{u}) F_k(\boldsymbol{u}) \frac{\partial\mu}{\partial\eta}\,\mathrm{d}\boldsymbol{u} = 0, \qquad \forall\, k.$$

Notice that, as in the case event example, the ML estimate of ρ is the ratio of total count to integrated intensity, i.e. $n_T / \int_W \hat{g}(\boldsymbol{u})\mu(\boldsymbol{u})\,\mathrm{d}\boldsymbol{u}$. It follows straightforwardly that the observed information matrix is given by

$$\begin{aligned} -l''_{\rho\rho} &= \frac{n_T}{\rho^2}, \\ -l''_{\rho\alpha_k} &= \int_W \hat{g}(\boldsymbol{u}) F_k(\boldsymbol{u}) \frac{\partial\mu}{\partial\eta}\,\mathrm{d}\boldsymbol{u}, \\ -l''_{\alpha_k\alpha_l} &= \sum_{j=1}^{m} n_j \left\{ \frac{(\int_{a_j} \hat{g}(\boldsymbol{u}) F_l(\boldsymbol{u})(\partial\mu/\partial\eta)\,\mathrm{d}\boldsymbol{u})(\int_{a_j} \hat{g}(\boldsymbol{u}) F_k(\boldsymbol{u})(\partial\mu/\partial\eta)\,\mathrm{d}\boldsymbol{u})}{(\int_{a_j} \hat{g}(\boldsymbol{u})\mu(\boldsymbol{u})\,\mathrm{d}\boldsymbol{u})^2} \right. \\ &\qquad \left. - \frac{\int_{a_j} \hat{g}(\boldsymbol{u}) F_k(\boldsymbol{u})(\partial/\partial\alpha_l)(\partial\mu/\partial\eta)\,\mathrm{d}\boldsymbol{u}}{\int_{a_j} \hat{g}(\boldsymbol{u})\mu(\boldsymbol{u})\,\mathrm{d}\boldsymbol{u}} \right\} \\ &\quad + \rho \int_W \hat{g}(\boldsymbol{u}) F_k(\boldsymbol{u}) \frac{\partial}{\partial\alpha_l}\left(\frac{\partial\mu}{\partial\eta}\right)\mathrm{d}\boldsymbol{u}. \end{aligned}$$

Notice that for the case of a simple multiplicative link ($\mu_i = \exp(\eta_i)$), then the normal equations and observed information elements have a particularly simple form:

$$\frac{n_T}{\rho} - \int_W \hat{g}(\boldsymbol{u}) \exp\{\eta(\boldsymbol{u})\}\,\mathrm{d}\boldsymbol{u} = 0,$$

$$\frac{\sum_{j=1}^{m} n_j E_{a_j}\{F_k(\boldsymbol{u})\}}{\sum_{j=1}^{m} n_j} - E_W\{F_k(\boldsymbol{u})\} = 0,$$

$$
\begin{aligned}
-l''_{\rho\rho} &= \frac{\int_W \hat{g}(\boldsymbol{u})\mu(\boldsymbol{u})\,\mathrm{d}\boldsymbol{u}}{\sum_{j=1}^{m} n_j},\\
-l''_{\rho\alpha_k} &= \int_W \hat{g}(\boldsymbol{u})\mu(\boldsymbol{u})F_k(\boldsymbol{u})\,\mathrm{d}\boldsymbol{u},\\
-l''_{\alpha_l\alpha_k} &= \sum_{j=1}^{m} n_j\{E_{a_j}\{F_l(\boldsymbol{u})\}E_{a_j}\{F_k(\boldsymbol{u})\} - E_{a_j}\{F_l(\boldsymbol{u})F_k(\boldsymbol{u})\}\}\\
&\quad + \left(\sum_{j=1}^{m} n_j\right)E_W\{F_l(\boldsymbol{u})F_k(\boldsymbol{u})\}.
\end{aligned}
$$

The use of a simple spatial linear predictor of the form used in the case event example, namely $F : \{x, y\}$, also leads to straightforward score and information terms, and these are not pursued here for brevity.

In addition to the count model, which includes the estimated 'at-risk' background function $g(\boldsymbol{x})$, it is also possible to condition on the counts of both the case disease within tracts and on the control disease count when this is available. Using the conditional log likelihood given in (4.19), it is possible to define a joint log likelihood as

$$
l(\boldsymbol{n}, \boldsymbol{n}_{\mathrm{c}} \mid \rho, \boldsymbol{\alpha}) = \sum_{j=1}^{m} n_j \log\left\{\frac{\lambda_j}{\sum_{k=1}^{m}[g_k + \lambda_k]}\right\} + \sum_{j=1}^{m} n_{\mathrm{c}j} \log\left\{\frac{g_j}{\sum_{k=1}^{m}[g_k + \lambda_k]}\right\}, \tag{5.12}
$$

where

$$
g_j = \int_{a_j} g(\boldsymbol{u})\,\mathrm{d}\boldsymbol{u}, \qquad \lambda_j = \int_{a_j} \lambda(\boldsymbol{u})\,\mathrm{d}\boldsymbol{u}, \qquad \lambda(\boldsymbol{u}) = \rho g(u)\mu(u).
$$

5.2.3 Approximations

While the above likelihood models can be applied quite generally in a variety of situations, it has often been expedient to make approximations to the likelihood to allow easier estimation. In addition, in the case of count event likelihoods, it has often been practice to make integral approximations within each tract to simplify the expectation of the counts within tracts.

Likelihood Approximations

It is possible to approximate likelihoods in such a way that they can be represented by a symmetric Gaussian form. This has often been pursued within Bayesian modelling when difficulties have been encountered in exploration of the posterior distribution. The usual approximation employed for this purpose is a Taylor series, up to the quadratic term, usually about an estimated value (Clayton and Kaldor, 1987; Breslow and Clayton, 1993; Lawson *et al.*, 1996a). Press (1989, pp. 70–73) discusses this normal approximation, as well as other types of approximation. Bernardo and Smith (1994, Section 5.3.2) discuss the general results pertaining to the asymptotic normality of a parameter vector $\boldsymbol{\theta}$-based ML estimation ($\hat{\boldsymbol{\theta}}$) and the observed information matrix evaluated at $\hat{\boldsymbol{\theta}}$. This type of approximation will only be valid for $m \longrightarrow \infty$, and the rate of convergence will vary depending on the likelihood model used. For example, a Poisson point process likelihood would only be well approximated if $\lambda(\boldsymbol{x}) \gg 0$, $\forall\, \boldsymbol{x} \in T$, whereas for the Poisson distribution of tract counts this would apply to $\int_T \lambda(\boldsymbol{u})\, \mathrm{d}\boldsymbol{u}$.

Tract Integral Approximations

The approximation of $\lambda_i = \int_{a_i} \lambda(\boldsymbol{u})\, \mathrm{d}\boldsymbol{u} = \text{const.}$, has been used in many examples of analysis in spatial epidemiology. Indeed it is commonly assumed without question in most analyses. However, it can be shown that this approximation could seriously bias parameter estimation where highly heterogeneous tract geometries are found and, with small-scale maps, inevitably this heterogeneity will be more commonly found. This approximation leads to step functions being estimated across tracts instead of a continuous underlying intensity. This discretisation, sometimes termed the *decoupling* approximation, will affect the estimation of spatially dependent covariates. It can be shown that the covariance structure of the covariate field will be incorrectly modelled in this case (Lawson and Waller, 1996; Diggle, 1993; Diggle and Elliott, 1995). Specific applications of approximations will be discussed in later sections dealing with applications (Part II).

5.2.4 Bayesian Models

The application of Bayesian models has an important role to play in modelling the complexity of data structures found in spatial epidemiology. It is a natural approach to the analysis of random effects, for example, to employ distributions to describe the random variation of the effects, which are not themselves observed (see Section 4.3.4). Indeed, it is often the ingredient of spatial autocorrelation, fundamental to many spatial statistical applications, which is naturally modelled by a prior distribution. The application of Bayesian models, however, differs from that of frequentist likelihood modelling. Besides the specification of prior distributions for parameters in a likelihood model, the Bayesian paradigm also differs in its inferential procedures. Hence, the objective in a likelihood modelling exercise is to estimate the model parameters and to provide estimates of their reliability. However, in the Bayesian paradigm the model parameters have a posterior distribution and hence do not provide a single estimated value (except by summarising the posterior information). Often, within a Bayesian analysis, the posterior distribution of the parameters is sampled to provide a realisation of parameter values. In the likelihood case, this would be equivalent to sampling the likelihood surface to yield a realisation, rather than finding the value at which that surface is maximised. The definition of confidence intervals for parameters also differs between the two paradigms. In the Bayesian case, an interval can be obtained from the computation of *highest density regions* of the posterior surface. Whereas in the frequentist paradigm, assumptions about repeatability of the experimental model are used to compute appropriate intervals. The assessment of goodness-of-fit also differs between the two paradigms: the use of tests in the frequentist domain is replaced by the assessment of posterior probabilities and Bayes factors (Gelman *et al.*, 1995). In addition, the comparison of fitted models, which can often be achieved by forming functions of likelihood ratios in the frequentist paradigm, is replaced by comparison of *predictive* distributions. In the frequentist example, a parameter estimate can be substituted in a model and a fitted value of the dependent variable can be computed. Often, goodness-of-fit can then be carried out by comparing data items with fitted values. The fitted values are usually defined as an estimated expectation, i.e. $\hat{y}_i = \hat{\mu}_i = E(y_i \mid \hat{\boldsymbol{\theta}})$. However, under a Bayesian model there are a number of possible values for $\boldsymbol{\theta}$ under the posterior distribution. Define

$$P_0(\boldsymbol{\theta} \mid \boldsymbol{y}) \propto \boldsymbol{L}(\boldsymbol{y} \mid \boldsymbol{\theta})g(\boldsymbol{\theta}) = \prod_{i=1}^{m} f(y_i \mid \boldsymbol{\theta})g(\boldsymbol{\theta}), \tag{5.13}$$

the posterior distribution of $\boldsymbol{\theta}$ given the data $\boldsymbol{y}$, where $g(\boldsymbol{\theta})$ are the prior distributions for $\boldsymbol{\theta}$. The predictive distribution of an observation y^*, say, is defined as

$$p(y^* \mid \boldsymbol{y}) = \int f(y^* \mid \boldsymbol{\theta}) P_0(\boldsymbol{\theta} \mid \boldsymbol{y})\, \mathrm{d}\boldsymbol{\theta}. \tag{5.14}$$

Hence, a sample of y^* values could be obtained from (5.14) and these could be compared to the y data. This approach is advocated by Gelman *et al.* (1995) for model goodness-of-fit assessment. This approach uses the distribution of the data, given the observed sample, integrated over the possible values of the parameters. In a full Bayesian analysis, (5.13) would be used to provide a sample or samples of parameter values. Usually, the joint and marginal posterior distributions of parameters are of interest and these can be estimated from these sample values. Hence, unlike ML estimation in the frequentist paradigm, which leads to single parameter estimates, considerably more information is available to inform decisions concerning model appropriateness. Given such posterior information, it is subsequently possible to examine functionals of the posterior distributions such as the maximum with respect to $\boldsymbol{\theta}$ of $P_0(\boldsymbol{\theta} \mid \boldsymbol{y})$ or $E(\boldsymbol{\theta} \mid \boldsymbol{y})$. The use of modal estimates of the posterior distribution is sometimes known as *maximum a posteriori* (MAP) estimation. This form of estimation is often found in image processing examples (Besag, 1986). It should be noted that ML estimation results when MAP is used when $g(\boldsymbol{\theta}) = 1 \ \forall\ \theta_j$. Computational methods useful in full Bayesian analyses are discussed in Appendix B. A variety of methods have been proposed for MAP estimation and the EM algorithm has been developed specifically to deal with such and related problems (see Gelman *et al.* (1995, Chapter 9)).

A number of methods exist which have been developed to provide intermediate estimation stages, and which avoid the full Bayesian approach. These methods were developed partly due to the difficulty in sampling from posterior distributions, which has only recently been overcome by iterative simulation methods such as Markov chain Monte Carlo (MCMC) (Robert and Casella, 1999; Gilks *et al.*, 1996). These intermediate methods are often termed *empirical Bayes* (EB) methods. They consist of procedures which allow for parameter point estimation as an intermediate stage. In current usage this means approximation of some aspect of the posterior distribution by replacement of a distribution by, say, the parameter value mostly likely under that distribution. Hence, the hyperparameters, as the prior distribution parameters are called, could be replaced by point estimates obtained by maximisation, given the current sample data observed. The example in Chapter 4, of a Poisson likelihood for independent counts within census tracts, with a gamma prior distribution for the relative risk within each tract, is an example of such intermediate estimation.

Detail of specific Bayesian models for application areas will be given in the relevant sections (Part II). Here, it is important to consider the type of prior distributions which are appropriate or characteristic of models within spatial epidemiology. The types to be discussed here are those relating to random effects which are associated with the spatial locations of observations, those related to integral approximations over tracts and frailty effects related to individuals. These effects characterise the type of random effects commonly associated with such data.

Correlated and Uncorrelated Heterogeneity

Heterogeneity can arise in a wide variety of ways in spatial epidemiological data. By heterogeneity we mean extra variation occurs in the observations which is not included within the likelihood model. This variation could lead to greater variation alone in the data (uncorrelated heterogeneity (UH)) or to variation which exhibits spatial correlation (correlated heterogeneity (CH)). In addition, both effects could occur within one example. Many reasons exist for such effects. First, it is *always* possible for unobserved variation (e.g. unmeasured covariates) to induce both or either UH or CH. This is true in any study, but particularly true in studies examining only a small subset of possible explanatory covariables. For example, many studies of small-area health hazard around putative sources of risk confine their modelling to distance-from-source variates and do not include general spatial trend components or clustering terms. The inclusion of census-based additional information, such as deprivation indices, makes some allowance for *some* of the variation, but cannot hope to capture its totality. Second, the disease of interest could have a tendency to cluster in space, even after allowance for the background 'at-risk' population. This clustering could be due to genetic causes, i.e. the result of similar genetic groupings in the population being located closely in space. A family grouping located in a single house could lead to a clustering due to genetic predisposition. Another possible cause of the clustering is a viral aetiology. That is, the disease manifests itself in spatial groupings due to an infectious agent being present or close to susceptible individuals. For some diseases, the exact mechanism for clustering is as yet unknown and hence viral aetiology cannot be discounted. For example, childhood leukaemia may have a viral aetiology, and is known to form weak spatial clusters at an appropriate scale (Cuzick and Hills, 1991). At a large spatial scale, clustering could also be induced by drug prescription side effects (Lawson and Wilson, 1974).

However, regardless of the origin of the heterogeneity, the spatial information alone will not provide enough evidence to distinguish between real clustering and apparent clustering (due to unobserved factors). Unless specific components of the model are structured to capture specific forms of clustering, the origin of the heterogeneity will be uncertain.

The basic form of model for UH ascribes a prior distribution for the rate parameter of the likelihood. For example, in the case of a Poisson process model, dropping the covariate dependence for simplicity of exposition, we could have

$$\lambda(\boldsymbol{x}) = g(\boldsymbol{x})\xi, \qquad \xi \sim G(\upsilon, \beta). \tag{5.15}$$

That is, the local rate of the process is imparted with extra variation by the parameter ξ, which has a prior gamma distribution (for positivity). Note that this prior distribution could force any extra variation to occur in an asymmetric manner, i.e. often the gamma distribution will have a longer upper tail. The choice of prior distribution is largely dependent on the application and its particular requirements. For example, this random effect could also be specified as an *individual* frailty effect, and in that case the effect could be flexibly modelled by a log-normal distribution, which allows the straightforward inclusion of individual covariate information. The hyperparameters could also have hyperprior distributions associated with them.

In the case of a Poisson model for tract counts, then

$$\lambda_j = \xi \int_{a_j} g(\boldsymbol{u})\,\mathrm{d}\boldsymbol{u}, \qquad \xi \sim G(\upsilon, \beta). \tag{5.16}$$

Note that if the integral in (5.16) is approximated by a constant rate, then this can lead to a gamma posterior distribution and negative binomial predictive distribution (Clayton and Kaldor, 1987). Variants of this result have been suggested by Manton *et al.* (1981), Tsutakawa (1988) and Marshall (1991a).

The simple UH random-effect model cannot be easily extended if specified as above. First, a gamma distribution does not easily provide for extensions into covariate adjustment or modelling, and, second, there is no simple and adaptable generalisation of the gamma distribution with spatially correlated parameters. Wolpert and Ickstadt (1998) provided an example of using correlated gamma fields. However, the advantages of incorporating a Gaussian specification are many. First, a random effect which is log-Gaussian behaves in a similar way to a gamma variate, but the Gaussian model can include a correlation structure. Hence, for the case where it is suspected that random effects are correlated, then it is simpler to specify a log Gaussian form for *any* extra variation present. Define

$$\begin{aligned}\lambda(\boldsymbol{x}) &= g(\boldsymbol{x})m_1\{F\alpha + \xi(\boldsymbol{x})\} \qquad (5.17)\\ &= g(\boldsymbol{x})\exp\{\xi(\boldsymbol{x})\}m_2\{F\alpha\},\end{aligned}$$

where m_1 and m_2 are link functions. In this case the spatial dependence of ξ is explicitly included in the model specification. Here $\xi(\boldsymbol{x})$ is regarded as a spatial stochastic process. Hence, conditional on the realisation of this process the case events can still be modelled as a heterogeneous (modulated) Poisson process. For a spatial Gaussian process (see Ripley, 1981, p. 10), any finite realisation has a multivariate normal distribution with mean and covariance inherited from the process itself, i.e. $\boldsymbol{\xi} \sim \text{MVN}(\boldsymbol{\mu}, K)$, where $\boldsymbol{\mu}$ is an m length mean vector and K is an $m \times m$ positive definite covariance matrix. Note that this is not the only possible specification of a prior structure to model CH (see also Møller *et al.* (1998)). Instead, it is possible to specify a standard hierarchical model prior distribution for the random-effect vector $\boldsymbol{\xi}$, which is defined as $\text{MVN}(\boldsymbol{\mu}, K)$. This allows the definition of ξ within the intensity (5.17) as $g(\boldsymbol{x})\exp\{\xi\}m_2\{F\alpha\}$.

In the case of tract counts, the above model can be specified as

$$\begin{aligned}\lambda_j &= \int_{a_j} g(\boldsymbol{u})m_1\{F\alpha + \xi(\boldsymbol{u})\}\,\mathrm{d}u \\ &= m_2\{F\alpha\}\int_{a_j} g(\boldsymbol{u})\exp\{\xi(\boldsymbol{u})\}\,\mathrm{d}u,\end{aligned} \tag{5.18}$$

where for simplicity we assume that the design matrix is not spatially dependent. In principle, this is a straightforward extension of (5.17) above. However, an integral of a function of a random field is now required for each tract. In many previous analyses, the integral has been approximated by a constant term, and hence a simpler random-effect structure can be assumed, i.e. $\lambda_j = g_j \exp\{\xi_j\}$. Using this model, a standard spatial correlation prior distribution can be assumed for $\boldsymbol{\xi}$. Of course, the comments above about the appropriateness of such an approximation must also be considered.

There are many ways of incorporating such heterogeneity in models, and some of these are reviewed here. First, it is often important to include a variety of random effects in a model. For example, both CH and UH might be included. One flexible method for the inclusion of such terms is to include a log-linear term with additive random effects. Besag *et al.* (1991b) first suggested, for tract count effects, a rate parametrisation of the form,

$$\exp\{t_j + u_j + v_j\},$$

where t is a trend component, u and v are correlated and uncorrelated heterogeneity, respectively. These components then have separate prior distributions. An alternative specification involves only one random effect for both CH and UH. This can be achieved by specifying a prior distribution having two parameters governing these effects. For example, the covariance matrix of an MVN prior distribution can be parametrically modelled with such terms (Lawson, 1994b; Lawson *et al.*, 1996a; Diggle *et al.*, 1998). This approach is akin to universal kriging (Wackernagel, 1995; Cressie, 1993), which employs covariance models including variance and covariance range parameters. Usually, these parameters define a multiplicative relation between CH and UH. The full Bayesian analysis for this model requires the use of posterior sampling algorithms. However, when a quadratic likelihood approximation is used, then MAP estimation leads to generalised least-squares (GLS)-type estimators. Define the data likelihood evaluated at $\tilde{\eta}$ as ψ, where $\tilde{\eta}$ is a saturated estimate of η. By adopting a second-order Taylor expansion of the data likelihood about $\tilde{\eta}$, it is possible to integrate out η from the posterior distribution. If a spatial Gaussian prior distribution is assumed with $\pi(\eta) \sim \text{MVN}(F\alpha, K)$, where F is an $n \times p$ design matrix, α is a $p \times 1$ vector of parameters, and K is a covariance matrix, then the predictive density of $\tilde{\eta}$ leads to GLS estimates for α:

$$\hat{\alpha} = (F'K_*^{-1}F)^{-1}F'K_*^{-1}\tilde{\eta}, \tag{5.19}$$

where $K_* = K - (\psi'')^{-1}$ and ψ'' is the second derivative of ψ with respect to η. The parameter covariances, based conditionally on $\tilde{\eta}$, are

$$\text{cov}(\hat{\alpha}) = (F'K_*^{-1}F)^{-1}. \tag{5.20}$$

This is just the regression of $\tilde{\eta}$ on F with covariance matrix K_*. This general result can be applied to a range of data likelihoods, and details can be found in Lawson *et al.* (1996a) and Lawson (1997).

The validity of the approximation will depend on the closeness of the quadratic approximation.

Under the full posterior distribution, the MAP estimate of η, η^m say, is given by

$$\eta^m = R^{-1}T, \tag{5.21}$$

where $R = K^{-1} - \psi''$ and $T = K^{-1}F\alpha - \psi''\tilde{\eta} + \psi'$. Hence, the MAP estimate can be directly evaluated by substitution of $\hat{\alpha}$ and estimated covariance parameters in K. Crude residuals can be computed as

$$\hat{e}_i = \tilde{\eta}_i - \eta_i^m,$$

and their variance can also be estimated. Assessment of residual diagnostics can always be carried out by generating a residual envelope from samples of residuals from the fitted model and comparing the observed residuals with this envelope.

In the parametric approach of Diggle *et al.* (1998) or Lawson (1997), the first-order intensity can be specified as

$$\lambda(\boldsymbol{x}) = g(\boldsymbol{x})\exp\{\beta + S(\boldsymbol{x})\},$$

where β is a non-zero mean level of the process, and $S(\boldsymbol{x})$ is a zero mean Gaussian process with, for example, a correlation function $\rho(u) = \exp\{-(\alpha u)^\delta\}$ and variance σ^2. In this case, the parameter vector $\theta = (\beta, \sigma, \alpha, \delta)$ is updated via a Metropolis–Hastings (M–H) step, followed by pointwise updating of the S surface. Conditional simulation of S surface values at arbitrary spatial locations (non-data locations) can be achieved by inclusion of an additional step once the sampler has converged. Covariates can be included in this formulation in a variety of ways.

Frailty Effects

Frailty is the term used to describe individual variation in susceptibility to disease, and can be considered as an additional effect within models for individual risk. At the individual level, this unobserved variation can be considered to be unobserved heterogeneity, and the random-effect components used for that modelling can also be used. Clayton (1991) has considered a general modelling approach to frailty effects which includes the use of MCMC methods for posterior sampling.

In applications within spatial epidemiology, it would be appropriate to consider frailty when case event models are employed. For example, one can specify a first-order intensity evaluated at a case event location as

$$\lambda(\boldsymbol{x}_i) = g(\boldsymbol{x}_i)\xi_i, \qquad \xi_i \sim G(\upsilon, \beta),$$

so that the individual case can have associated a random frailty response to the disease in question.

Random-Object Effects

So far we have only considered random effects in the intensity of the process or the data space. An alternative approach is to consider random effects in the locations of events, i.e. random-object effects. A natural interpretation of such effects arises in the analysis of clusters of disease. One interpretation of disease clusters is that cluster locations are unobserved random objects which require to be estimated. In this way we can use random objects as random effects and it follows that prior distributions for the locations must be assumed, as in standard random effects modelling. This modelling does require the use of special prior distributions, which arise in the area of stochastic geometry (see Cressie (1993, Chapter 8.5) and Barndorff-Nielsen *et al.* (1999)). In disease cluster modelling, the locations of disease events are assumed to be distributed independently around a set of disease centres, which are themselves unobserved. Define the conditional intensity of events as

$$\lambda(\boldsymbol{x}) = g(\boldsymbol{x})m\left\{\sum_{j=1}^{n_x} h(\boldsymbol{x} - \boldsymbol{y}_j)\right\},$$

where $m\{\cdot\}$ is a link function, and $h(\cdot)$ is a cluster distribution function describing the relation of events to centres. In this definition, the $\{\boldsymbol{y}_j\}$ are unobserved and must be estimated or sampled. The number of centres is also unknown. With suitable prior distributions this problem can be sampled as a mixture problem. Further details of this approach are discussed in the section on clustering (Chapter 6).

Tract Integral Approximation Effects

If the tract integral approximation is employed, it is then possible to make some allowance for this approximation by using random effects at the tract level to provide extra variation at this level. For example, the use of an intensity specification, such as $\lambda_j = g_j \exp\{\xi_j\}$, where ξ_j is a random effect (either CH or UH), may make some allowance for the failure to estimate the tract integral correctly. However, the irregular geometries often encountered in small-area data may not always be adequately represented by such an approximation. An alternative approach would be to employ tract areas to modify the intensity, or, failing that, to use random-object effects, as described above.

5.3 RESIDUAL DIAGNOSTICS

The analysis of residuals and summary functions of residuals forms a fundamental part of the assessment of model goodness-of-fit in any area of statistical application. In the case of spatial epidemiology there is no exception, although full residual analysis is seldom presented in published work in the area. Often, goodness-of-fit measures are aggregate functions of piecewise residuals, while measures relating to individual residuals are also available. A variety of methods are available when full residual analysis is to be undertaken. We define a piecewise residual as the standardised difference between the observed value and the fitted model value. Usually, the standardisation will be based on a measure of the variability of the difference between the two values.

Within a frequentist paradigm, it is common practice to specify a residual as

$$r_{1i} = \{y_i - \hat{y}_i\} \quad \text{or} \quad r_{2i} = \{y_i - \hat{y}_i\}/\sqrt{\text{var}(y_i - \hat{y}_i)}, \tag{5.22}$$

where $\hat{y}_i$ is a fitted value under a given model. When complex spatial models are considered, it is often easier to examine residuals, such as $\{r_{1i}\}$ using Monte Carlo methods. In fact it is straightforward to implement a parametric bootstrap (PB) approach to residual diagnostics for likelihood models. The simplest case is that of tract count data, where for each tract an observed count can be compared to a fitted count. In general, when Poisson likelihood models are assumed with $n_i \sim \text{Poisson}\{\int_{a_i} g(\boldsymbol{u})\mu(\boldsymbol{u})\,\mathrm{d}\boldsymbol{u}\}$, it is then straightforward to employ a PB approach by generating a set of simulated counts $\{n_{ij}^{\text{s}}\}$, $j = 1, \ldots, J$, from a Poisson distribution with mean $\int_{a_i} \hat{g}(\boldsymbol{u})\hat{\mu}(\boldsymbol{u})\,\mathrm{d}\boldsymbol{u}$. In this way, a tract-wise ranking, and hence p-value, can be computed by assessing the rank of the residual within the pooled set

$$\left\{n_i - \int_{a_i} \hat{g}(\boldsymbol{u})\hat{\mu}(\boldsymbol{u})\,\mathrm{d}\boldsymbol{u};\ \left\{n_{ij}^{\text{s}} - \int_{a_i} \hat{g}(\boldsymbol{u})\hat{\mu}(\boldsymbol{u})\,\mathrm{d}\boldsymbol{u}\right\},\ j = 1, \ldots, J\right\}.$$

Denote the observed residual as r_{1i} and the simulated residuals as $\{r_{1ij}^{\text{s}}\}$. Note that it is now possible to compare functions of the residuals as well as making direct comparisons. For example, in a spatial context, it would be appropriate to examine the spatial autocorrelation of the observed residuals. Hence, a Monte Carlo assessment of degree of residual autocorrelation could be made by comparing Moran's I statistic for the observed residuals, say, $M(\{r_{1i}\})$, to that found for the simulated count residuals $M(\{r_{1ij}^{\text{s}}\})$.

In the situation where case events are available, then it is not straightforward to define a residual. As the data are in the form of locations, it is not possible to directly compare observed and fitted values. However, by a suitable transformation, it is possible to compare *measures* which describe the spatial distribution of the cases. A model which fits the data well should provide a good fit to the spatial distribution of the cases. It is therefore possible to examine the difference between a local estimate of the case density, $\hat{\lambda}(x_i)$, and that predicted from a fitted model, $\hat{\lambda}^*(x_i)$, i.e. at the ith location:

$$r_i = \hat{\lambda}_i - \hat{\lambda}_i^*. \tag{5.23}$$

This approach has been proposed in the derivation of a deviance residual for modulated heterogeneous Poisson process models (Lawson, 1993a). Essentially, a saturated estimate of $\hat{\lambda}_i$ based on the Dirichlet tile area of the ith event is employed, while a model-based estimate of $\hat{\lambda}_i^*$ is used in the comparison. This residual can incorporate estimated expected rates. It is possible to simulate J realisations from the fitted model $\{x_{kj}^{\mathrm{s}}\}, k = 1, \ldots, m, j = 1, \ldots, J$, and the local density of these realisations could be compared pointwise with $\hat{\lambda}_i^*$. Of course, these proposals rely on a series of smoothing operations. More complex alternative procedures could be pursued.

In a Bayesian setting it is natural to consider the appropriate version of (5.22). Carlin and Louis (1996) describe a Bayesian residual as

$$r_i = y_i - \frac{1}{G}\sum_{g=1}^{G} E(y_i \mid \theta_i^{(g)}), \tag{5.24}$$

where $E(y_i \mid \theta_i)$ is the expected value from the posterior predictive distribution, and (in the context of MCMC sampling) $\{\theta_i^{(g)}\}$ is a set of parameter values sampled from the posterior distribution.

In the tract count modelling case, this residual can therefore be approximated, when a constant tract rate is assumed, by

$$r_i = n_i - \frac{1}{G}\sum_{g=1}^{G} e_i\theta_i^{(g)}. \tag{5.25}$$

This residual averages over the posterior sample. An alternative possibility is to average the $\{\theta_i^{(g)}\}$ sample, $\hat{\theta}_i$ say, to yield a posterior expected value of n_i, say $\hat{n}_i = e_i\hat{\theta}_i$, and to form $r_i = n_i - \hat{n}_i$. A further possibility is to simply form r_{2i} at each iteration of a posterior sampler and to average these over the converged sample (Spiegelhalter *et al.*, 1996).

Deletion residuals and residuals based on conditional predictive ordinates (CPOs) can also be defined for tract counts (Stern and Cressie, 2000). To further assess the distribution of residuals, it would be advantageous to be able to apply the equivalent of the PB approach in the Bayesian setting. With convergence of an MCMC sampler, it is possible to make subsamples of the converged output. If these samples are separated by a distance (h) which will guarantee approximate independence (Robert and Casella, 1999), then a set of J such samples could be used to generate $\{n_{ij}^{\mathrm{s}}\}$ $j = 1, \ldots, J$, with $n_{ij}^{\mathrm{s}} \leftarrow \text{Poisson}(e_i\hat{\theta}_{ij})$, and the residual computed from the data r_i can be compared to the set of J residuals computed from $n_{ij}^{\mathrm{s}} - E(n_i)$, where $E(n_i)$ is the predictive expected value of n_i. In turn, these residuals can be used to assess functions of the residuals and goodness-of-fit measures.

When the constant tract rate (decoupling) approximation is not appropriate, then an integral Poisson expectation must be evaluated.

In the situation where case events are examined it is also possible to derive a Bayesian residual as we can evaluate $E\{\lambda(x \mid \theta^{(g)})\}$ based on the $\{\theta_i^{(g)}\}$ posterior samples. Hence, it is possible to examine

$$r_i = \hat{\lambda}_i - \frac{1}{G}\sum_{g=1}^{G} \hat{\lambda}_i^{*(g)},$$

where $\hat{\lambda}_i^{*(g)}$ is the fitted model estimate of intensity corresponding to the gth posterior sample. Further it is also possible, with subsampling for approximate independence, to use a PB approach to residual significance testing.

5.4 HYPOTHESIS TESTING

While an approach to the analysis of spatial epidemiology problems based on flexible modelling of disease incidence is usually to be preferred, in situations where a restricted comparison of models is to be made, then it can be useful to consider an approach based on the testing of hypotheses. This type of approach is commonly found in epidemiological applications in which only a small number of effects are to be considered. These effects could be specifically spatial, e.g. a distance effect between locations of cases of disease and the location of cluster centres, or could be related to the inclusion of covariates, e.g. the relation of disease incidence to spatially referenced socio-economic variables (percentage unemployment, age, gender, amongst others). In either case a restricted set of effects are to be examined, and there is no requirement to examine a wide range of possible models for the disease incidence. In this case it is possible to structure hypothesis tests to assess these effects.

It is the intention of this chapter to outline the main approaches to hypothesis testing available in this study area, and to reserve discussion of specific techniques or tests to sections dealing with specific applications.

When non-parametric methods are pursued, then a range of possibilities exist for simple hypothesis testing. Here we interpret non-parametric methods as comprising the exploratory methods outlined in Section 5.1. For both the case event and count examples, we can proceed by examining hypotheses relating to disease excess of unspecified form within a mapped realisation of events. Such tests can be based on individual events or groups of events (such as counts in small areas), and their null distribution can be simulated via event simulation from a non-parametric density estimate (Silverman, 1986) or via multinomial generation from the normalised probabilities of an event arising within given small areas.

In general, the need to pursue such non-parametric testing is due to the difficulties arising in conventional hypothesis testing for spatial data. Often, in the analysis of spatially distributed data, assumptions concerning sampling distributions, which could be made in conventional aspatial studies, are not tenable. For example, large-sample (asymptotic) sampling distributions are often inappropriate due to the inherent correlation found in observations which are spatially contiguous. Further, in many examples particularly where counts of rare diseases are to be studied, the sparseness of the spatial count distribution may invalidate asymptotic properties of test statistics (see Zelterman (1987) for a discussion of sparse multinomial distributions). Diggle (1990) described an example involving case event data where, even in the case where a simple log-link regression model parameter is estimated using likelihood methods, its sampling distribution does not correspond to that expected under conventional likelihood theory.

Thus, for a variety of reasons, it may be appropriate to resort to Monte Carlo testing of hypotheses in such spatial applications. Such testing can be achieved as long as realisations of events or counts can be simulated under the null hypothesis for the test considered. Appendix A describes procedures which can be implemented for such testing.

5.5 EDGE EFFECTS

The importance of the assessment of edge effects in any spatial statistical application cannot be underestimated. Edge effects play a larger role in spatial problems than in, say, time-series. Specifically, we define edge effects as 'any effect upon the analysis of the observed data brought about by the proximity of the window edges'. The effect of the edges of a window are largely the result of the effects of *spatial censoring*. That is, the fact that observations outside the window are not observed and therefore cannot contribute to analysis within the window. This mirrors the effects of temporal censoring in say, survival analysis, where, for example, the outcome for some subjects may not be observed because the observation period has stopped prior to the outcome appearing.

Of course, all censoring depends on the idea that observations are dependent in *some* way. That is, the occurrence of observations outside the window of observation relies on observations within the window. For example, the outcome example above relies on an individual appearing on study within the window and the time dependence of the outcome process. In the spatial case, it is easily possible for individual disease response to relate to 'missing' observations outside the window. For example, it may be that an environmental health hazard is located outside or, in the case of viral aetiology, an infected person or carrier is located outside. For diseases which have uncertain aetiology, it could be possible that factors underlying the incidence of the disease have a spatial distribution that is spatially dependent and hence the disease incidence reflects this structure even when individual responses are independent. If, in addition, some unknown genetic aetiology underpinned the disease incidence, then if this has spatial expression, the incidence of disease could relate to unobserved genetically linked subjects outwith the observation region.

In addition, such spatial censoring can affect estimation procedures, even when no explicit spatial dependence is proposed. For example, spatial smoothing methods, including non-parametric regression and density estimation, use data from different regions of the observed window to estimate a value at a location. In the particular case of kernel density estimation, a sum over all observations is taken to estimate a density value at a point. At or close to an edge, the density value is likely to be similar to values immediately outside the window, but cannot be estimated from such data. Hence, if no correction is pursued for this effect at the edges, then some edge distortion will result. In other cases parametric estimation may require the computation of averages of values in neighbourhoods of a chosen point. Hence, close to edges there could be considerable distortion induced by missing values. This edge problem can not only induce bias in estimation, but also tends to lead to considerable increases in estimator variance at such locations, and hence to low reliability of estimation.

A number of methods have been proposed to deal with such edge effects. These methods have been in part developed within stochastic geometry, where it is often assumed that the process under study is first- and second-order stationary and isotropic (Ripley, 1988). These methods vary from (1) correction methods applied to smoothers or other estimators, for example, using weights relating to the proximity of the external boundary, (2) employing guard areas to provide external information to allow better boundary area estimation within the window, (3) simulation of missing data outside the window and iterative re-estimation or model fitting. (The use of toroidal correction is not usually appropriate in the analysis of disease incidence data, as it is not usually appropriate to make the appropriate stationarity assumptions.) This final method has significant advantages if used within iterative simulation methods such as data augmentation (Gilks *et al.*, 1996; Tanner, 1996; Robert and Casella, 1999) or general MCMC algorithms, as the external data can be treated as parameters in the estimation sequence.

5.5.1 Edge Effects in Case Events

Define a study region W within which we observe m case event locations of a disease of interest. The locations are usually case address locations. We denote the locations as $\{\boldsymbol{x}_i\}$, $i = 1, m$. Also define an arbitrary region T which completely encloses W. Figure 1.4 displays the geographical relations of these regions. For simplicity, we assume that the area of T outwith W lies completely external to the study region. It is possible that for some study regions there may be areas internal to the main study region where no observations are possible. These external and internal areas can be regarded as areas where censoring of observations has occurred and we can apply appropriate methods to either type of area.

A variety of effects can arise due to the proximity of the external boundary of the region W to the observed data. First, if the case locations are spatially interdependent, then any measure which depends on this interdependence will be affected by the fact that observations are unavailable external to the study region. For example, if a measure of autocorrelation is to be applied over the study region, then the censoring of information at boundaries will affect this estimation process. Second, even when observations are independent, the estimation method used can induce edge effects in estimators. For example, a bias will be induced when a smoothing operation is applied to the event distribution. This is due to the unavailability (censoring) of information beyond the edge regions. A larger variance will also be found in edge areas due to the low proportion of small inter-event distances found in that area. While edge effects may be minor when estimation of *global* parameters is considered, they may become severe when *local* estimates in regions close to the study boundary are to be made. Ripley (1981) discusses some aspects of the edge-effect problem for point processes on the plane, and also notes the edge distortion with trend surface fitting to continuous data.

5.5.2 Edge Effects in Counts

In the case of counts within arbitrary tracts, similar considerations apply. Define the count of disease within the ith tract as n_i. We assume there are m tracts within the study region. The inclusion criteria for tracts is an important issue and is discussed more fully in Section 4.4.

We denote tracts which have a common boundary with the external region as n_k^*, whereas if we can also observe or otherwise estimate counts in external tracts, then we denote these counts as n_e^*. Here the external region is defined to be any area *not* included within the study window. Usually, this area lies adjacent to the window, but this is not a fundamental requirement. In addition, the external region may lie *within* the tracts where counts are observed. In that sense the external region may be regarded as having a missing observation. Comments above concerning global and local estimation apply here. The estimate of tract relative risks at or near boundaries can be affected by edge position, by the requirement to use counts from neighbouring tracts in the estimation process, i.e. $\{n_e^*\}$ are censored. Even without the assumption of interdependence between events, any conventional smoothing operation applied to the $\{n_i\}$ will also induce edge effects due to their use of neighbourhoods. Cressie (1993) has discussed this problem for lattice data, and an early reference to the problem appears in Griffith (1983).

5.5.3 Edge Weighting Schemes and MCMC Methods

The two basic methods of dealing with edge effects are (1) the use of weighting/correction systems, which usually apply different weights to observations depending on their proximity to the study boundary, and (2) the use of guard areas, which are areas outwith the region which we analyse as our study region. The original study region could have as its guard area all the $\{n_k^*\}$ and so these areas are not reported, although they are used in the estimation of parameters relating to the internal tracts.

Another edge correction procedure is available for stationary Poisson point processes and that is wrapping of the realisation on a torus (Ripley, 1981). However, this is inappropriate for case event or count data in epidemiology as non-stationarity could be quite common.

Weighting systems Usually, it is appropriate to set up weights which relate the position of the event or tract to the external boundary. These weights, $\{w_i\}$ say, can be included in subsequent estimation and inference. The weight for an observation is usually intended to act as a surrogate for the degree of missing information at that location and so may differ depending on the nature and purpose of the analysis. Some sensitivity to the specification of these weights will inevitably occur and should be assessed in any case study. Some basic weights are

$$\text{for case events:} \qquad w_i = \begin{cases} 1 & \text{if } \boldsymbol{x}_i \notin \{\boldsymbol{x}_k^*\}, \\ m(d_i) & \text{if } \boldsymbol{x}_i \in \{\boldsymbol{x}_k^*\}, \end{cases}$$

$$\text{for tract counts:} \qquad w_i = \begin{cases} 1 & \text{if } n_i \notin \{n_k^*\}, \\ m(d_i) & \text{if } n_i \in \{n_k^*\}, \end{cases}$$

where $m(d_i)$ is a function of the distance (d_i) of the observation to the external boundary, and the $\{\boldsymbol{x}_k^*\}$ is the set of all events closer to the boundary than to any other event in the study region. The distance (d_i) could be the event-boundary distance for case events or the tract-centroid–boundary distance for tract counts. Another possible surrogate for (d_i) in the case of tract counts is to use $m(l_{\mathrm{b}i}/l_i)$, where l_i is the length of the tract perimeter and $l_{\mathrm{b}i}$ is the length of the perimeter of the tract which is in common with the external boundary. A simple choice would be $w_i = 1 - l_{\mathrm{b}i}/l_i \; \forall \, i$, which can be used for all tracts as non-boundary tracts will have $w_i = 1$.

Since the events are generated by a modulated heterogeneous Poisson process, weights could also be specified as functions not only of the distance from the boundary but also of the modulating population density. For example, defining an indicator for closeness to the boundary for each area, when in the tract count case, some external standardised rates are available, it is possible to structure an expectation-dependent weight for a particular tract, e.g. based on the ratio of the sum of all adjacent area expectations to the sum of all such expectations within the study window. Other suitable weighting schemes could be based on the proportion of the number of observed neighbours.

Guard areas An alternative approach is to employ guard areas. These areas are external to the main study window of interest. These areas could be boundary tracts of the study window itself or could be added to the window to provide a guard area, in the case of tract counts. In the case event situation, the guard area could be some fixed distance from the external boundary (Ripley, 1988). The areas are used in the estimation process but they are excluded from the reporting stage, as they will be prone to edge effects themselves. If boundary tracts are used for this, then some loss of information must result. External guard areas have many advantages. First, they can be used *with* or *without* their related data to provide a guard area. Second, they can be used within data augmentation schemes in a Bayesian setting. These methods regard the external areas as a missing data problem (Tanner, 1996).

MCMC and Other Computational Methods

It is usually straightforward to adapt conventional estimation methods to accommodate edge-weighted data. In addition, if guard areas are selected and observations are available within the guard area, then it is possible to proceed with inference by using the whole data but selectively reporting those areas not within the guard area. Note that this is not the same as setting $w_i = 0$ for all guard area observations in a weighting system.

When external guard areas are available but no data are observed, resort must usually be made to missing data methods. An intermediate situation arises when in the tract count case some external standardised rates are available. In that case it is possible to structure an expectation-dependent weight for a particular tract, e.g. based on the ratio of the sum of all adjacent area expectations to the sum of all such expectations within the study window. This can be used as an edge-weight within such a weighting system.

With limited external information it is possible to proceed either via the use of the EM algorithm or full Gibbs–Metropolis sampling. In the EM approach it is possible to iteratively draw missing counts $\{n^{\mathrm{M}}\}$ from the expectation of the conditional distribution of the counts given current relative risk estimates $\{\theta^{\mathrm{C}}\}$, in the expectation (E)-step, and to sample the full conditional distribution of $\{\theta^{\mathrm{C}} \mid n^{\mathrm{C}}\}$. An alternative approach is to regard the missing counts as parameters within a hierarchical model and to sample these iteratively within a full Gibbs–Metropolis sampling algorithm. When the expected rates are unknown in the external regions, then it is simpler to regard the relative risks $\{\theta^{\mathrm{M}}\}$ as the target parameters (without further evaluating the associated missing counts), and to employ the above algorithms as before on this smaller parameter hierarchy.

5.5.4 Discussion

In the situation where case events are studied, then if censoring is present and could be important (i.e. when there is clustering or other correlated heterogeneity), it is advisable to use an internal guard area, or an external guard area with augmentation via MCMC. In cases where only a small proportion of the study window is close to the boundaries and only general (overall) parameter estimation is concerned, then it may suffice to use edge weighting schemes. If residuals are to be weighted, then it may suffice to label the residuals only for exploratory purposes.

In the situation where counts are examined, then it is also advisable to use an internal guard area or external area with augmentation via MCMC. In some cases, an external guard area of *real* data may also be available. This may often be the case when routinely collected data are being examined. In this case, analysis can proceed using the external area *only to correct internal estimates*. Edge weighting can be used also, and the simplest approach would be to use the proportion of the region *not* on the external boundary. Residuals can be labelled for exploratory purposes.

The assumptions underlined in any correction method are that the model be correctly specified and that it could be extended to the areas not observed. In particular, it is questionable if an adjustment can really be obtained when ignoring the information on the outer areas. Edge-effect bias should be less prominent when an unstructured exchangeable model is chosen. Since each area relative risk would be regressed toward a grand mean, the information lacking for the unobserved external areas is very small compared to those from the observed areas. Of course, such a simple model where common expectation is found is highly unlikely to be a good model in this area.

Extending the edge-effect problem to consideration of space-time data, the situation is more complex as spatial edge effects can interact with temporal edge effects. The use of sequential weighting, based on distance from time and space boundaries, may be appropriate (Lawson and Viel, 1995). For tract counts observed in distinct time periods only, the most appropriate method is likely to be based on distance from time and space boundaries, although it may be possible to provide an external spatial and/or temporal guard area either with real data or via augmentation and MCMC methods.

The use of augmentation methods (Tanner, 1996) can also be fruitfully employed in this context. If the external areas are known, but information concerning the disease of interest is not available in these external areas, then it is possible to regard such missing/censored data as parameters which can be estimated within an iterative sampling algorithm, such as an MCMC algorithm. In addition, if partial information were known (for example the standardised rates in the external areas), then we could condition these missing data count estimates on the known information. In the next section, an example of a comparison of edge correction methods is discussed.

5.5.5 The Tuscany Example

Here we examine an example of the analysis of edge effects first considered by Lawson *et al.* (1999b).

A selection of edge compensation/correction methods has been applied to a tract count example from the region of Tuscany, Italy. Municipality tract counts of gastric cancer mortality data in Tuscany (Italy) for males over 35 years have been routinely collected at municipality levels (287 units) from 1980 to 1989. This choice was made as gastric cancer displays high relative risks along the northeastern border of the region, so there may be great interest in the potential distortion due to edge effects when such a raised incidence is displayed. This distortion could appear in the estimation of 'true' relative risks within the study area.

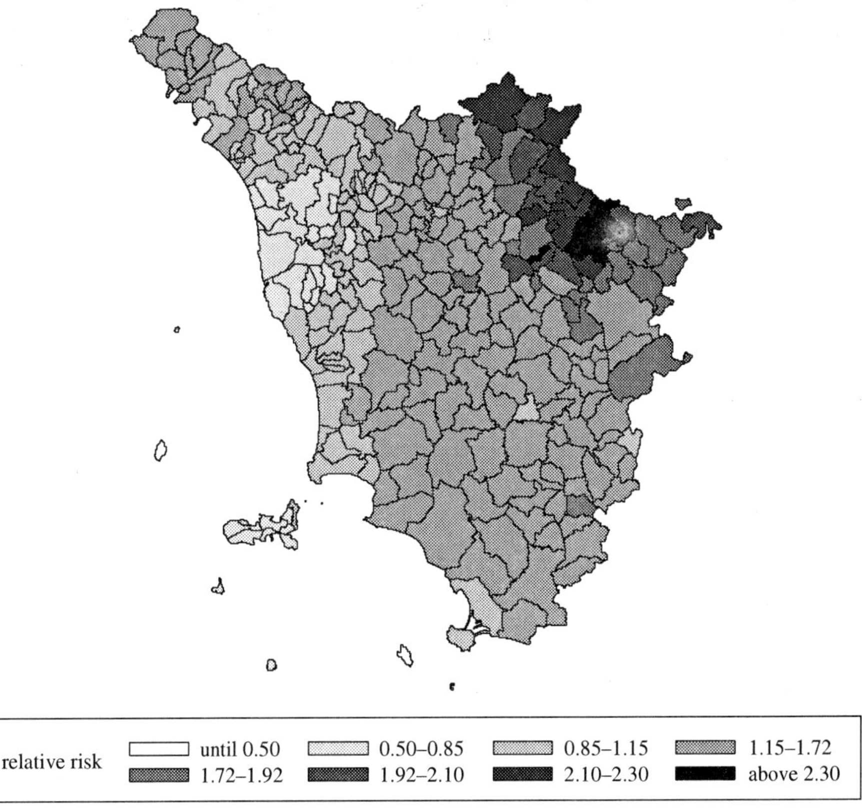

Figure 5.6 Bayesian estimates of relative risks (absolute levels) for Tuscany gastric cancer using the study region only.

In what follows we examined four different scenarios for the data set:

(1) full Bayesian analysis of relative risk with structured and unstructured heterogeneity as specified by Besag *et al.* (1991b) for the augmented region set using $\{n_e^*\}$, $\{e_e^*\}$ and $\{n_i\}$, $\{e_i\}$;

(2) the same analysis applied to $\{n_i\}$, $\{e_i\}$ alone;

(3) edge weighting based on the data-dependent ratio of adjacent expected rates specified above and a diagonal matrix of weights was introduced into the analysis, where the weight is the proportion of observed adjacent area expectations over the sum of the total adjacent area expectations; and

(4) the edge-augmentation method discussed above using an EM algorithm.

In (4) the estimation step consisted of taking the conditional expectation of $\{n_e^*\}$ for each missing area. The maximisation step consisted of sampling the posterior distribution of the relative risks given the augmented data set. The starting values for

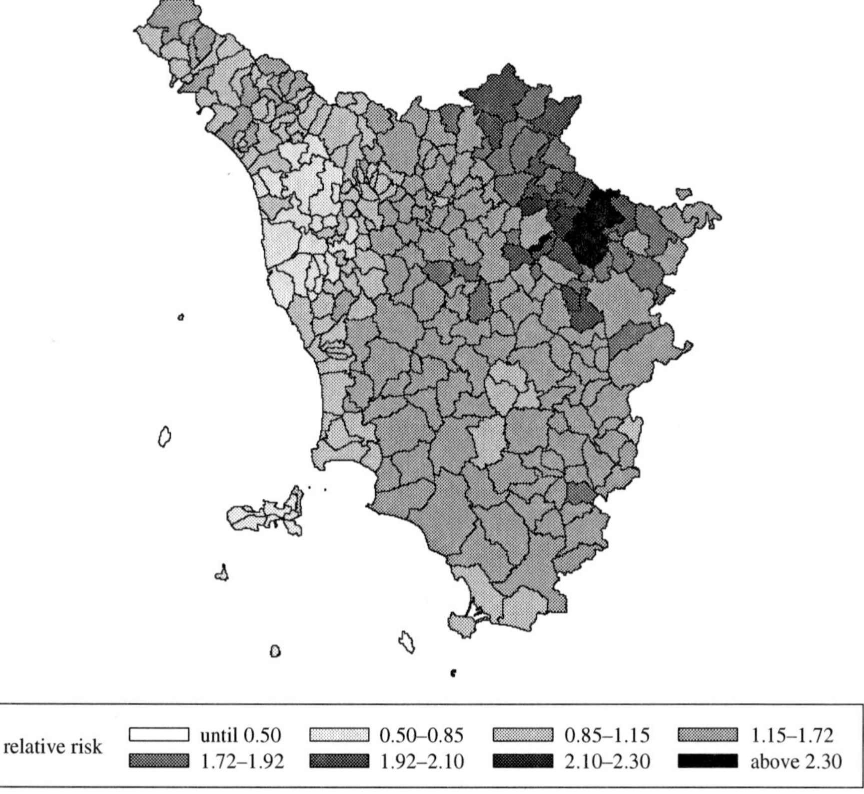

relative risk	until 0.50	0.50–0.85	0.85–1.15	1.15–1.72
	1.72–1.92	1.92–2.10	2.10–2.30	above 2.30

Figure 5.7 Bayesian relative risk estimates (absolute levels) for the Tuscany gastric cancer data set, using counts in external regions and based on observed data of the areas outside the border.

the E-step were $\{e_e^*\}$. All sampling of conditional distributions was carried out by the BEAM program (see Appendix E).

The map representing the SMRs (i.e. n_i/e_i) for the study region is shown in Figure 1.20. The Bayesian estimates for the study region only are shown in Figure 5.6.

The maps are presented using absolute levels. These levels were chosen by inspection of the distribution of the full Bayesian estimates. As an example of the variation of relative risk map which arises when different methods are employed, Figure 5.7 displays the relative risk map for the region including the external count areas. There is clearly a difference between these figures which relates to the degree of censoring present.

In Table 5.1, the different estimators for the areas along the northeastern border of Tuscany are reported (sorted from north to south). Three subregions are of particular interest: the Tuscan Romagna (Rt), the Casentino valley (Ca) and the River Tiber valley (Ti). Gastric cancer mortality is particularly high in the Casentino valley. The Bayesian estimates based on the complete data (C) showed that the areas in the

Table 5.1 Comparison of different estimators for the area along the northeastern border of the Tuscany region (Italy). Gastric cancer, death certificate relative risk, 1980–1989 males.

Area Name	SMR	I-Bayes	W-Bayes	R-Bayes	C-Bayes
Firenzuola (Rt)	2.73	2.26	2.11	2.09	1.97
Palazzuolo (Rt)	1.69	2.00	1.98	1.98	1.72
Marradi (Rt)	2.42	2.12	2.06	2.07	1.92
S. Godenzo (Rt)	2.01	2.11	2.07	2.07	1.83
Stia (Ca)	2.49	2.27	2.19	2.21	2.07
Pratovecchio (Ca)	1.99	2.17	2.15	2.14	2.04
Poppi (Ca)	3.08	2.62	2.55	2.48	2.59
Chiusi Verna (Ca)	1.60	2.01	2.04	2.01	1.97
Pieve S. Stefano (Ti)	1.71	1.79	1.79	1.83	1.75
Badia Tedalda (Ti)	1.70	1.82	1.80	1.83	1.64
Sestino (Ti)	2.14	1.99	1.91	1.85	1.58

Casentino valley ranked higher together with the far-northeast area of the Tuscan Romagna. The estimates based on the incomplete data (I) failed to highlight this pattern. The weighted (W) and the data-augmented (R) Bayesian estimates more closely approximated the full Bayesian analysis.

While this small example gives only an empirical snapshot of the edge-effect problem displayed in a small data example, it does serve to highlight the importance of considering such effects in any mapping exercise.

Part II

Important Problems in Spatial Epidemiology

CHAPTER 6

Small Scale: Disease Clustering

The analysis of clusters of disease has generated considerable interest within the subject area of public health. This interest grew during the 1980s, partly due to growing concerns about adverse environmental effects on the health status of populations. For example, concerns about the influence of nuclear power installations on the health of surrounding populations have given rise to the development of methods which seek to evaluate clusters of disease. These clusters are regarded as representing local adverse health risk conditions, possibly ascribable to environmental causes. However, it is also true that for many diseases the geographical incidence of disease will naturally display clustering at some spatial scale, even after the 'at-risk' population effects are taken into account. The reasons for such clustering of disease are various. First, it is possible that for some *apparently* non-infectious diseases there may be a viral agent, which could induce clustering. This has been hypothesised for childhood leukaemia (Kinlen, 1995). Second, other common but unobserved factors/variables could lead to observed clustering in maps. For example, localised pollution sources could produce elevated incidence of disease (e.g. road junctions could yield high carbon monoxide levels and hence elevated respiratory disease incidence); alternatively, the common treatment of diseases can lead to clustering of disease side effects. The prescription of a drug by a medical practice could lead to elevated incidence of disease within that practice area (Lawson and Wilson, 1974).

Hence, there are many situations where diseases may be found to cluster, even when the aetiology does not suggest this should be observed. Because of this, it is important to be aware of the role of clustering methods, as even when clustering per se is not the main focus of interest, it may be important to consider clustering as a background effect and to employ appropriate methods to detect such effects.

In this chapter, we consider a number of aspects of the analysis of clustering. First, we examine basic definitions of clustering, and their use in different studies. Second, we consider appropriate models based on these definitions. Third, we examine the estimation of clustering as a background effect in studies where the prime focus is *not* clustering. Finally, we examine the use of testing for clusters and its use in different studies.

6.1 DEFINITION OF CLUSTERS AND CLUSTERING

A wide variety of definitions can be put forward for the definition of clusters. However, it is convenient here to consider two extreme forms of clustering within which most definitions can be subsumed. First, as many epidemiologists may not wish to specify *a priori* the exact form/extent of clusters to be studied, then a non-parametric definition is often the basis adopted. An example of such a definition is given by Knox (1989): 'a geographically bounded group of occurrences of sufficient size and concentration to be unlikely to have occurred by chance'. Without any assumptions about shape or form of the cluster, then the most basic definition would be as follows:

> any area within the study region of *significant* elevated risk.

This definition is often referred to as *hot-spot* clustering. This is a simpler form of Knox's definition but summarises the essential ingredients. In essence, any area of elevated risk, regardless of shape or extent, could qualify as a cluster, provided the area meets some statistical criteria. Note that it is not usual to regard areas of significantly low risk as of interest, although these may have some importance in further studies of the aetiology of a particular disease.

Second, at the other extreme, we can define a parametric cluster form:

> the study region has a prespecified cluster structure.

This definition describes a parametrised cluster form which would be thought to apply across the study region. Usually, this implies some stronger restriction on the cluster form and also some region-wide parameters which control cluster form. Both the above extremes can be modified by modelling approaches which borrow from either extreme form. For example, it is possible to model cluster form parametrically, but also to include a non-parametric component in the cluster estimation part which allows a variety of cluster shapes across the study region. As implied above, these two extremes represent the spectrum of modelling from non-parametric to parametric forms and associated with these forms are appropriate statistical models and estimation procedures.

Besag and Newell (1991) first defined a classification of types of clustering study and associated cluster definition. We will extend their definitions here to include some extra classes. First of all, those authors defined *general* clustering as the analysis of the overall clustering tendency of the disease incidence in a study region. As such, the assessment of general clustering is closely akin to the assessment of autocorrelation. Hence, any model or test relating to general clustering will assess some overall/global aspect of the clustering tendency of the disease of interest. This could be summarised by a model parameter (e.g. an autocorrelation parameter in an appropriate model) or by a test which assesses the aggregation of cases of disease. For example, the correlated prior distributions used by Besag *et al.* (1991b), Clayton and Bernardinelli (1992) or Lawson *et al.* (1996a) incorporate a single parameter which describes the correlation of neighbouring locations on a map. The methods of Cuzick and Edwards (1990), Diggle and Chetwynd (1991) and Anderson and Titterington (1997) for case events, and Whittemore *et al.* (1987), Raubertas (1988) and Oden (1995) for counts, however, consider testing for a clustered pattern within the study region.

It should be noted at this point that the above general clustering methods can be regarded as *non-specific* in that they do not seek to estimate the spatial locations of clusters, but simply to assess whether clustering is apparent in the study region. Any method which seeks to assess the locational structure of clusters is defined to be *specific.*

An alternative *non-specific* effect has also been proposed in models for count or case event data. This effect is conventionally known as uncorrelated heterogeneity (or overdispersion/extra-Poisson variation in the Poisson likelihood case). This effect gives rise to extra variation in incidence and in the Poisson likelihood case displays variability of observed counts that exceeds the mean of the observed counts. This marginal heterogeneity has traditionally been linked to 'clustering', as is evidenced by the use of negative binomial distributions as 'cluster' distributions (Douglas, 1979). Often, such effects can be considered to be modelled as for correlated heterogeneity except that no neighbourhood effects are included. Hence, log-normal or gamma distributions are often used to model this component of the expected incidence. The result of using such a *non-specific* effect is to mimic cluster intensity variation as a realisation of these distributions over the study region. This will lead to a greater peakedness in intensity variation than that induced by correlated heterogeneity, and the comments above concerning the appropriateness of this approach for cluster structure also apply here.

Besag and Newell's second class of clustering methods are termed *focused* and *non-focused.* These are *specific* methods. These methods are designed to examine one or more clusters and the locational structure of the clusters are to be assessed. Focused clustering is defined to be the study of clusters where the location and the number of the clusters are predefined. In that case, only the extent of clustering around the predefined locations is to be modelled. Examples of this approach mainly come from studies of putative sources of health hazard, e.g. the analysis of disease incidence around prespecified *foci* which are thought to be possible sources of health hazard, such as nuclear power installations, waste dumps, incinerators, harbours, road intersections or steel foundries. In this section we consider only the *non-focused* form of clustering, as focused clustering is discussed in the section concerning putative sources of hazard.

It is very important to consider, within any analysis of geographically distributed health data, the structure of hypotheses which could include cluster components. For example, many examples of published analyses within the areas of disease mapping and focused clustering consider the null hypothesis that the observed disease incidence arises as a realisation of events from the underlying *at-risk* population distribution. The assumption is made that, once this *at-risk* population is accurately estimated, it is possible to assess any differences between the observed disease incidence and that expected to have arisen from the *at-risk* background population. However, if the disease of interest naturally clusters (beyond that explained by the estimated *at-risk* background), then this form of clustering should also be included within the

Table 6.1 The structure of hypotheses relating to cluster studies.

	background only (H_0)	foreground (H_1): non-focused	foreground (H_1): focused
non-parametric	non-parametric regression	extraction mapping	extraction mapping
semi-parametric	?	correlated prior + cluster mixture	distance decline and covariates
parametric (non-specific)	correlated prior	general clustering/ autocorrelation	—
parametric (specific)	mixture models	mixture models	modelling distance and other effects

null hypothesis. As this form of clustering often represents unobserved covariates or confounding variables, then it is appropriate to include this as heterogeneity. This can be achieved in many cases via the inclusion of random effects in the analysis. Note that such random effects are often *non-specific* in that they do not attempt to model the exact form of clusters but seek to mimic the effect of clustering in the expected incidence of the disease. The correlated and uncorrelated heterogeneity first described by Clayton and Kaldor (1987) and Besag *et al.* (1991b) come under this category. Note also that if clustering of disease incidence is to be studied under the alternative H_1, then not only would heterogeneity be needed under H_0 but some form of cluster structure must be estimable under H_1 as well. Besag *et al.* (1991b) provide an example, in a disease mapping context, where a residual can be computed after fitting a model with different types of heterogeneity. This residual could contain uncorrelated error, trend or cluster structure depending on the application. Hence, such a residual could provide a simple non-parametric approach for the exploration of cluster form in some cases.

One disadvantage of the use of the *non-specific* random effects so far advocated in the literature is that they do not exactly match the usual form of cluster variation in geographical studies. At least in rare diseases, clusters usually occur as isolated areas of elevated intensity separated by relatively large areas of low intensity. In that case, the use of a log transformed Gaussian random-effect model fitted to the whole region will not closely mimic the disease clustering tendency. Table 6.1 describes methodology appropriate under different clustering hypotheses.

6.2 MODELLING ISSUES

The development of models for clusters and clustering has seen greater development in some areas than in others. For example, it is straightforward to formulate a non-specific Bayesian model for case events or tract counts which includes heterogeneity (Besag *et al.*, 1991b; Clayton and Bernardinelli, 1992; Lawson, 1994b, 1997). However, specific models are less often reported. It is possible to formulate specific clustering models for the case event and tract count situation. If it is assumed that the intensity of case events, at location $\boldsymbol{x}$, is $\lambda(\boldsymbol{x})$, then by specifying a dependence in this intensity on the locations of cluster centres, it is possible to proceed. For example,

$$\lambda(\boldsymbol{x}) = \rho g(\boldsymbol{x}) m\left\{\sum_{j=1}^{k} h(\boldsymbol{x} - \boldsymbol{y}_j)\right\} \tag{6.1}$$

describes the intensity of events around k centres located at $\{\boldsymbol{y}_j\}$. The distribution of events around a centre is defined by a cluster distribution function $h(\cdot)$. Conditional on the cluster centres, the events can be assumed to be governed by a heterogeneous Poisson process, and hence a likelihood can be specified. As the number (k) and the locations of centres are unknown, then with a suitable prior distribution specified for these components, it is possible to formulate this problem as a Bayesian posterior sampling problem, with a mixture of components of unknown number. This type of problem is well suited to reversible-jump MCMC sampling (Green, 1995). The approach can be extended to count data straightforwardly, as

$$E(n_i) = \rho \int_{a_i} g(\boldsymbol{u}) m\left\{\sum_{j=1}^{k} h(\boldsymbol{u} - \boldsymbol{y}_j)\right\} \mathrm{d}\boldsymbol{u}, \tag{6.2}$$

under the equivalent Poisson distributional model, where a_i is the area of, and n_i is the count in, the mth tract. Making a piecewise constant assumption over the tract area (the decoupling approximation) and $m\{u\} = u$, (6.2) becomes

$$E(n_i) = \rho g_i |a_i| \sum_{j=1}^{k} h(\boldsymbol{x}_{ni} - \boldsymbol{y}_j). \tag{6.3}$$

Note that this specification is similar to a conventional mixture model with equal component weights. Examples of the use of these models in case event data are provided in Lawson (1995, 1996a) and Lawson and Clark (1999c). The application of such cluster models to count data (the Falkirk example) is found in Lawson (1997) and Lawson and Clark (1999a). Variants of this specification can be derived for specific purposes or under simplifying assumptions. For example, it is possible to associate weights with each centre, which can define the degree of excess at that locale (Lawson and Clark, 1998). In addition, it is possible to allow the cluster variance to vary spatially across the study region, thereby allowing a parsimonious description of variation in cluster size (Lawson, 1995). The wide applicability of this formulation can be appreciated by the fact that $h(\cdot)$ could be non-parametrically estimated, in which case a data-dependent cluster form will prevail. This provides a modelling framework which can allow both vague prior beliefs about cluster form and also highly parametric forms. Further extensions of these methods have been suggested where both point cluster centres (P-centres) and line cluster centres (L-centres) are allowed, to enable the definition of linear forms of clusters (Lawson *et al.*, 2000b) with intensity specification,

$$\lambda(\boldsymbol{x} \mid \boldsymbol{y}, \boldsymbol{l}) = \rho g(\boldsymbol{x}) \left[1 + \sum_{j=1}^{n} h_p(\boldsymbol{x} - \boldsymbol{y}_j) + \sum_{j=1}^{k} h_l(\boldsymbol{x} - \boldsymbol{l}_j) \right],$$

where $\boldsymbol{l}_j$ denotes the jth line segment. Recent developments in perfect sampling may allow greater use of such cluster models (Loizeaux and McKeague, 2000).

Other approaches to parametric cluster modelling have been proposed, which employ more arbitrary methods to define cluster forms. For example, Banfield and Raftery (1993) have proposed Gaussian cluster models (in general applications) while Guidici *et al.* (2000) and Knorr-Held and Rasser (2000) have proposed partitioning methods for isolating areas of common risk. These methods often have edge-effect problems associated with their use, and these problems have not been addressed so far. In addition, the assumption that the incidence of a disease is characterised by a small number of non-overlapping uniform intensity groups may be questionable on epidemiological grounds.

While parametric models are useful, it is often the case that the form of cluster to be estimated is not well defined and that the analysis is only concerned with areas of raised incidence. In this connection it is possible to employ non-parametric relative-risk estimation methods as described in Section 7.3.1. Define the log relative risk as

$$\hat{r}(x) = \log(\hat{R}(\boldsymbol{x})) = \log\left\{ \frac{\hat{\lambda}(\boldsymbol{x})}{\hat{g}(\boldsymbol{x})} \right\},$$

where $\hat{\lambda}(\boldsymbol{x})$ and $\hat{g}(\boldsymbol{x})$ are non-parametric estimates of the intensity of cases and of the background respectively. It is possible to obtain a probability surface (p-value surface) by simulation of a set of s log relative risks $\{\hat{r}_i(x) : i = 1, \ldots, s\}$ under H_0, and comparing these values with the computed value $\hat{r}_0(x)$. Kelsall and Diggle (1995b) suggested using re-allocations of cases and events from a control disease to provide these sets under the null hypothesis of random labelling. Areas of the resulting p-value surface which exceed a critical value could be treated as clusters. Alternative methods of computing the realisations under the null could be proposed, which do not require a control realisation. For example, it is possible to obtain an estimate of $g(\boldsymbol{x})$ from expected rates within tracts and to subsequently simulate case event realisations from this surface. These realisations should represent the spatial distribution of the at-risk population under H_0.

Figure 1 of Kelsall and Diggle (1995b) provides an illustration of the p-value surface for the Chorley–Ribble data.

For count data, a similar procedure could be adopted, whereby the log relative risk in a census tract is defined as

$$\hat{r}_i(x) = \log(\hat{R}_i(\boldsymbol{x})) = \log\left\{ \frac{S(n_i)}{S(e_i)} \right\}, \tag{6.4}$$

where $S(\cdot)$ denotes a non-parametric smoothing operation (e.g. non-parametric regression). This operation can be applied to the numerator and denominator separately and so a tract count version of the Kelsall–Diggle (KD) estimator can be derived (Lawson *et al.*, 2000a). Similar p-value surfaces can be derived by simulation of a set of count realisations from the distribution of the $\{e_i\}$. This can also be used to isolate hot-spot clusters within count data.

One concern related to the use of this method for cluster assessment is that it has been found that the count KD estimator (using the Nadaraya–Watson kernel regression smoother with common bandwidth cross-validation) yields a very poor recovery of true relative risk (based on fitting to a range of simulated true relative risk models (Lawson *et al.*, 2000a)), and so it is currently not clear whether this method will be useful beyond an exploratory analysis.

6.3 HYPOTHESIS TESTING FOR CLUSTERS

The literature of spatial epidemiology has developed considerably in the area of hypothesis testing and, more specifically, in the sphere of hypothesis testing for clusters. Very early developments in this area arose from the application of statistical tests to spatio-temporal clustering, a particularly strong indicator of the importance of a *spatial* clustering phenomenon. The early seminal work of Mantel (1967) and Knox (1964) in the field of space-time cluster testing, predates most of the development of *spatial* cluster testing. As noted above, distinction should be made between tests for general (non-specific) clustering, which assess the overall clustering pattern of the disease, and the specific clustering tests where cluster locations are estimated.

For case events, a few tests have been developed for non-specific clustering. Cuzick and Edwards (1990) developed a test based on a realisation of cases and a *sample* of a control realisation. Functions of the distance between case locations and k 'nearest' cases were proposed as test statistics (as opposed to controls). The null hypothesis of random labelling is tested against clustered alternatives, although not specifically of the form (6.1). The test takes the form,

$$T_k = \sum_{i=1}^{n_t} \delta_i d_i^k, \tag{6.5}$$

where δ_i is a 1/0 label for a case (1) or control (0), d_i is a 1/0 variable denoting whether the nearest neighbour is a case (1) or control (0), and k is the order of the neighbourhood (e.g. $k = 1$ denotes first neighbours). The statistic can be computed for different values of k and an example of applying such a test for different neighbourhoods was given by the authors. Variants of the test were also described. Diggle and Chetwynd (1991) extended stationary point process model descriptive measures ($K(t)$ functions) to the case where a modulated population background is present. Their method uses a complete control disease realisation and provides a measure of scale of clustering also. Their test statistic is of the form,

$$D = \sum_{k=1}^{m} \hat{D}(s_k)/\sqrt{\text{var}\{\hat{D}(s_k)\}}, \tag{6.6}$$

where $\hat{D}(s_k) = \hat{K}_{11}(s_k) - \hat{K}_{22}(s_k)$ and

$$\left.\begin{aligned} \hat{K}_{11}(s_k) &= |A|\{n_1(n_1-1)\}^{-1} \sum_{i=1}^{n_1}\sum_{j=1}^{n_1} w_{ij}\delta_{ij}(s_k), \\ \hat{K}_{22}(s_k) &= |A|\{n_2(n_2-1)\}^{-1} \sum_{i=n_1+1}^{n}\sum_{j=n_1+1}^{n} w_{ij}\delta_{ij}(s_k), \end{aligned}\right\} \tag{6.7}$$

and $w(\boldsymbol{x}_i, d_{ij}) = w_{ij}$ (for $j \neq i$ and $w_{ii} = 0$) is the reciprocal of the proportion of the circumference of a circle with centre at $\boldsymbol{x}_i$ and radius d_{ij} which lies within A. Here, $d_{ij} = \|\boldsymbol{x}_i - \boldsymbol{x}_j\|$, and $\delta_{ij}(s_k)$ is the indicator of the event $d_{ij} \prec s_k$, where s_k, $k = 1, \ldots, m$, are a discrete set of equally spaced values. The separate K_{ij} functions refer to n_1 cases (K_{11}) and n_2 controls (K_{22}), respectively. A variety of test variants were also proposed. Under random labelling the approximate sampling distribution of D is normal, but the authors perform Monte Carlo tests for random labelling without resort to the approximate distribution. It is possible to compute approximate tolerance intervals for $\hat{D}(s_k)$ using $\pm 2\sqrt{\text{var}\{\hat{D}(s_k)\}}$. In addition, a plot of $\hat{D}(s_k)$ against values of s_k can be made and this plot can include tolerance intervals. Thereby, some information concerning the scale of clustering can also be obtained by this method. There may also be some clustering situations which cannot be detected by this test procedure, as there are a number of such patterns where $\hat{D}(s) = 0, \forall\ s$ (Tango, 1999).

Neither of these methods allows for first-order non-stationarity which may be present in many examples. Anderson and Titterington (1997) have proposed the use of a simple integrated squared distance (ISD) statistic for cluster assessment. This is closely related to the analysis of density ratios in exploratory analysis (e.g. the KD method), and could be regarded as a type of non-parametric assessment of clustering. This approach is based on the form,

$$T = \int \{\hat{\lambda}(\boldsymbol{u}) - \hat{g}(\boldsymbol{u})\}^2\, \mathrm{d}\boldsymbol{u}, \tag{6.8}$$

where the integration is over the study area, and $\hat{\lambda}(x)$ is a non-parametric density estimate based on the case event distribution, and $\hat{g}(x)$ is a non-parametric density estimate of the control distribution. These estimates are based on separate smoothing operations and have different bandwidths in general. Alternative forms of (6.8) can be suggested, based for example on generalised Kullback–Leibler distance or simple ratio forms. The advantage of this approach is that the assessment is not tied to a specific cluster model but detects overall departures from background. The major disadvantage, shared with all such statistics, is its low power against specific forms of clustering. However, the ISD statistic can be used more widely than the Cuzick and Edwards or Diggle and Chetwynd forms, as it does not require that the two processes studied are in the form of point events.

Other simple forms of global test can be proposed where density estimates of cases are compared to density estimates of case events simulated from the control background. These could provide pointwise confidence intervals as well as global tests. There appears to have been little development of tests which detect uncorrelated heterogeneity in the intensity of the case process as a form of spatial clustering. It is unclear what aetiological difference would be inferred when uncorrelated rather than correlated forms of heterogeneity were found.

The general tests for overall clustering so far proposed, suffer from the problem that often underlying unobserved heterogeneities are common in such data and the above tests do not provide mechanisms for the incorporation of such effects. For example, if first-order non-stationarity were present in the case events, then this effect could be confounded with cluster effects. One solution to this is to adopt a full clustering model such as (6.1), which can be expanded easily to include such effects as non-stationarity and heterogeneity, and to test for inclusion of effects within MCMC algorithms.

General clustering tests for tract counts, so far developed, can be classified into tests for correlated heterogeneity and tests for uncorrelated heterogeneity. The latter tests are not *spatial* in origin but are included here for completeness. We also consider the possibility of general cluster tests based on cluster sums. In the case of correlated heterogeneity, Whittemore *et al.* (1987) developed a quadratic form test statistic which compared observed counts and expected counts for all tracts weighted by a covariance matrix. The test statistic can be derived from a multinomial distribution. Define n_{T} as the total incidence of cases of disease over all tracts, and $r = \{n_i/n_{\mathrm{T}}, \ldots, n_m/n_{\mathrm{T}}\}^{\mathrm{T}}$ the vector of tract relative frequencies, and D as the $m \times m$ matrix of distances between the tract centroids. Also, define the probability vector

$$\pi = \{e_1, \ldots, e_m\} \Big/ \sum_{j=1}^{m} e_j \tag{6.9}$$

and $U = \{\mathrm{diag}(\pi) - \pi\pi^{\mathrm{T}}\}/n^{\mathrm{T}}$ the multinomial covariance matrix of r. The resulting statistic,

$$\tfrac{1}{2}\sqrt{n}\{r^{\mathrm{T}}Dr - \pi^{\mathrm{T}}D\pi\}/\sqrt{\{\pi^{\mathrm{T}}DUD\pi\}},$$

has a standard normal distribution asymptotically. This test was found to have reduced power in some situations (Turnbull *et al.*, 1990), and it has been noted that its asymptotic distribution could be far from normal under certain conditions on the asymptotic infill of the incidences in the tracts. Clearly, a Monte Carlo test procedure could be employed to evaluate this test statistic, instead of the asymptotic result. Subsequently, Tango (1995) developed a modified general class of tests for general and focused clustering, which are similar to the above test, but which use SMR vectors or different distance matrix elements. Alternative procedures based on Moran's I statistic, modified to allow tract-specific expected rates, have also been proposed (Oden, 1995; Assuncao and Reis, 1999). All these tests make approximating assumptions (e.g. that counts are independently Poisson distributed with constant expectation within each tract, choice of distance weighting in the covariance matrix), and are unlikely to perform well against specific clustering forms. Also they assume that clusters yield a total increase in divergence between count and expectation, while other forms of process could yield equivalent degrees of divergence, and hence this could lead to misinterpretation.

As mentioned above, some use has been made of tests for uncorrelated heterogeneity to assess clustering of tract counts. For example, the Euroclus project (Alexander *et al.*, 1996) has tested for such heterogeneity across European states using the Potthoff–Whittinghill test (Potthoff and Whittinghill, 1966) and score tests for Poisson versus negative binomial distributions for the marginal count distribution (Collings and Margolin, 1985). As noted above these tests are approximate, in that they assume constant within region expected rate, and they may suffer from considerable interpretational problems when *a priori* there is likely to be some non-specific heterogeneity in small-area data. In addition, the evidence of Euroclus suggests that for certain important forms of non-Poisson alternatives within the negative binomial family these tests perform poorly (Alexander *et al.*, 1996). In addition, as noted above, at least for rare diseases, it is easily possible that the marginal count distribution would not follow a negative binomial distribution and could even display multimodality.

Specific cluster tests address the issue of the location of putative clusters. These tests produce results in the form of locational probabilities or significances associated with specific groups of tract counts or cases. Openshaw *et al.* (1987) first developed a general method which allowed the assessment of the location of clusters of cases within large disease maps. The method was based on repeated testing of counts of disease within circular regions of different sizes. Whenever a circle contains a significant excess of cases, it is drawn on the map. After a large number of iterations, the resulting map can contain areas where a concentration of overlapping circles suggests localised excesses of a disease. The statistical foundation of this method has been criticised and an improvement to the method proposed by Besag and Newell (1991). Their method involves accumulating events (either cases or counts) around individual event locations. These could be cases or tracts. Accumulation proceeds up to a fixed number of events or tracts (k). The number k is fixed in advance. The method can be carried out for a range of k values. The distance to the kth case around each case is measured and the corresponding number of individuals at risk within that distance is noted. If the number at risk falls below a threshold value, then there is evidence for excess risk around that case location. The test can also be applied to tract counts, and in that case each tract has associated a number m of tracts which contain the k nearest cases and a comparison made between the counts and expected counts within these areas, based on the cumulative probability of k or more events from a Poisson distribution with mean given by the total expected rate. There are some problems which can arise with this test procedure, such as discretisation of the centroid locations (Tango, 1999). While the local alternative for this test is increased intensity, there appears to be no specific clustering process under the alternative, and in that sense the test procedure is non-parametric, except that a monotone cluster distance distribution is implicit. One advantage of the test is that it can also be applied to focused clusters, while a disadvantage is that an arbitrary choice of k must be made and the results of the test must depend on this choice.

An alternative statistic has been proposed by Kulldorff and Nagarwalla (1995), who employ a likelihood ratio test for the comparison of an overall binomial likelihood for the study region for number of cases out of a total population (the null hypothesis), to a likelihood which has different binomial components depending on being inside or outside a circular zone of defined size. The test can be applied to both case events and tract counts. The advantage of the test is that it examines a potentially infinite range of zone sizes and does rely on a formal model of null and alternative hypotheses. However, some limitations of the method relate to the use of circular regions, which tends to emphasise *circular* clusters (as does the Openshaw or Besag and Newell procedures), and the choice of crude population as the expression of the background 'at-risk' structure.

It is also possible to apply two extreme forms of test for *either* a non-parametric (hot-spot) cluster specific test or a fully parametric form. First, if we assume n_i is the tract count of disease, and e_i is the expected rate in the ith tract, then we can compare $n_i - e_i$ with $n^*_{ij} - e_i$ for each tract, where n^*_{ij}, $j = 1, \ldots, 99$, are simulated counts for each tract based on the given expectation for that tract. If any tract count exceeds the critical level within the rankings of the simulated residuals, then we accept the tract as 'significant'. The resulting map of 'significant' tracts displays clusters of different forms. This does not use contiguity information. In the case event situation, pointwise comparison of $\hat{\lambda}_i - \hat{\lambda}^*_i$, where $\hat{\lambda}_i$ is a density estimate based on the case events only and $\hat{\lambda}^*_i$ is a density estimate based on the controls only (assuming a control realisation is available), can be made. This could be compared to a set of events simulated from the density estimate of the controls and their density estimates. Clearly, it is possible to employ a form of parametric bootstrap in these cases, where residuals from realisations of the fitted model are compared to the residuals found for the data example.

At the other extreme, it is possible to test for specific cluster locations via the assumption of a cluster sum term of the form (6.1) in either the intensity of case events or, in the case of tract counts, the specification of the expected rate in each tract, as in (6.2). As the cluster locations and number of locations are random quantities, it would be necessary to employ either approximations which involve fixed cluster numbers, or to include testing within MCMC algorithms (Besag and Clifford, 1989) which sample the joint posterior distribution of number and locations of centres.

6.4 SPACE-TIME CLUSTERING

While spatial clustering is of great importance in geographical epidemiology, it is also clear that such clustering is but one component of the dynamic behaviour of disease within a framework of spatial and temporal variation. Usually, spatial clustering is assessed on the spatial distribution of incidence within a fixed time period. By ignoring

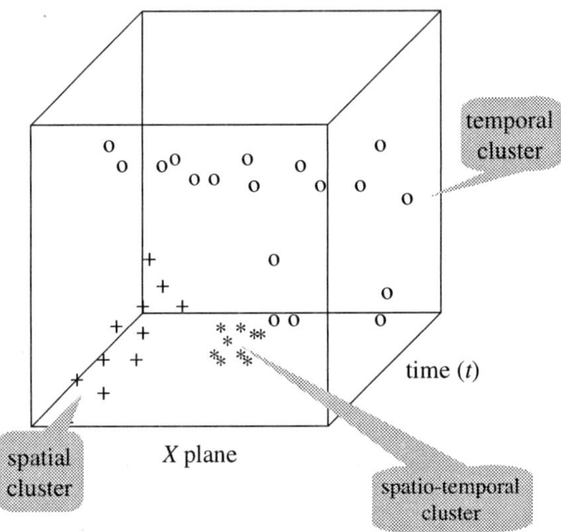

Figure 6.1 The three components of clustering in space-time: spatial, temporal and spatio-temporal.

the potential for temporal variation within such a period, or over other time frames, some evidence for the variation in spatial distribution will be lost. Clearly, within the context of surveillance of disease this temporal component is often central to any analysis (see Section 9).

6.4.1 Modelling Issues

It is possible to construct parametric models for spatio-temporal clustering in disease (Lawson and Clark, 1998). One approach is to extend the parametric models defined for spatial clusters, to include temporal and spatio-temporal cluster terms. Figure 6.1 displays a pictorial representation of these terms within a space-time cube.

These terms can be included by defining an extended intensity function. Define the intensity at space-time location x, as

$$\lambda(\boldsymbol{x} \mid \boldsymbol{\theta}) = \rho g(\boldsymbol{x}) m\{f_1(\boldsymbol{x}^{\mathrm{s}}; \theta^{\mathrm{s}}) f_2(\boldsymbol{x}^{\mathrm{t}}; \theta^{\mathrm{t}}) f_3(\boldsymbol{x}^{\mathrm{s}}, \boldsymbol{x}^{\mathrm{t}}; \theta^{\mathrm{st}})\},$$

where ρ is a constant background rate (in space $\times$ time units), $g(\boldsymbol{x})$ is a modulation function describing the spatio-temporal 'at-risk' population background in the study region, $\boldsymbol{\theta} = (\theta^{\mathrm{s}}, \theta^{\mathrm{t}}, \theta^{\mathrm{st}})$, $m\{\cdot\}$, is a link function, f_k are appropriately defined functions of space, time and space-time, and $\theta^{\mathrm{s}}, \theta^{\mathrm{t}}, \theta^{\mathrm{st}}$ are parameters relating to the spatial, temporal and spatio-temporal components of the model.

Here each component of the f_k can represent a *full* model for the component, i.e. f_1 can include spatial trend, covariate and covariance terms, and f_2 can contain similar terms for the temporal effects, while f_3 can contain *interaction* terms between the components in space and time. Note that this final term can include *separate* spatial structures relating to interactions which are not included in f_1 or f_2. The exact specification of each of these components will depend on the application, but the separation of these three components is helpful in the formulation of components.

The above intensity specification can be used as a basis for the development of likelihood and Bayesian models for case events; if it can be assumed that the events form a modulated Poisson process in space-time, then a likelihood can be specified as in the spatial case.

Note that the above case event intensity specification can be applied in the space-time case where small-area counts within regions $\{S_i\}$ are observed within fixed time periods $\{t_j\}$, $j = 1, \ldots, l$, by noting that

$$E\{n_{it_j}\} = \int_{t_j} \int_{S_i} \lambda(\boldsymbol{x} \mid \boldsymbol{\theta})\, \mathrm{d}\boldsymbol{x}^{\mathrm{s}}\, \mathrm{d}x^{\mathrm{t}}, \tag{6.10}$$

under the usual assumption of Poisson process regionalisation. In addition, the counts are independent conditional on the intensity given, and this expectation can be used within a likelihood modelling framework or within Bayesian model extensions. In previous published work in this area, cited above, the expected count is assumed to have constant risk within a given small-area/time unit, which is an approximation to the continuous intensity defined for the underlying case events. The appropriateness of such an approximation should be considered in any given application.

In the example of specific cluster modelling, it is important to parametrise the f_* functions with specific terms relating to cluster structures. To do this we assume that each cluster type has a cluster distribution function relating data to a notional cluster centre. For the purposes of exposition, we here assume that the $g(\boldsymbol{x}) \equiv 1$, although the incorporation of this function in a real example would be important.

We assume that we have a uniform background population, and so our intensity is

$$\begin{aligned}\lambda(\boldsymbol{x} \mid \boldsymbol{y}_1, \boldsymbol{y}_2, \boldsymbol{y}_3, \boldsymbol{\theta}) = 1 + \alpha_1 \sum_{i=1}^{nsc} K_1(\boldsymbol{x}^{\mathrm{s}} - y_{1i}) \\ + \alpha_2 \sum_{i=1}^{ntc} K_2(\boldsymbol{x}^{\mathrm{t}} - y_{2i}) + \alpha_3 \sum_{i=1}^{nstc} K_3(\boldsymbol{x} - y_{3i}),\end{aligned}$$

where $\boldsymbol{x}^{\mathrm{s}}$ is the spatial coordinate of $\boldsymbol{x}$, $\boldsymbol{x}^{\mathrm{t}}$ is the temporal coordinate of $\boldsymbol{x}$, $y_1 = \{y_{1i}\}_{i=1}^{nsc}$ are the spatial cluster centres, $y_2 = \{y_{2i}\}_{i=1}^{ntc}$ are the temporal cluster centres and $y_3 = \{y_{3i}\}_{i=1}^{nstc}$ and θ is a vector of parameters that specify the cluster distribution functions (K_1, K_2 and K_3). The number of centres are nsc, ntc and $nstc$ in space, time and space-time respectively. A series of weights $\{\alpha_1, \alpha_2, \alpha_3\}$ are also included within the formulation. Here the number of centres and centre locations are unknown, and so we must regard this problem as one of unknown parameter dimensionality. Inference and estimation can proceed via methods akin to those proposed for spatial cluster models.

6.4.2 Hypothesis Testing

A variety of test procedures have been developed to assess the extent of spatio-temporal clustering within geographical disease data. Early examples of these tests, which address the issue of space-time *interaction* (rather than clustering), are those of Knox (1964) and Mantel (1967). A review and comparison of these tests is made in Chen *et al.* (1984). These tests are based on the idea that the combination of geographical and temporal closeness of cases of disease represents space-time clustering of disease. This certainly represents space-time interaction, but space-time clustering can occur even when this interaction does not occur (see Kulldorff and Hjalmars (1999) for a good example of this effect). The structure of these test statistics are of the form,

$$T = \sum_i \sum_j d_{ij} \Delta t_{ij}, \qquad \forall\, i < j,$$

where d_{ij} is the spatial distance between the ijth case pair, and Δt_{ij} is the time difference between these pairs. Knox proposed a method where threshold values were used in determining the level of interaction. This method was extended by Diggle *et al.* (1995) to provide a general K-function approach to spatio-temporal analysis, which provides for edge correction as well as the inclusion of a range of threshold values in the Knox procedure. The procedure relies on the theory of stationary point processes and is based on inter-event distances, and if the non-stationarity assumption were violated, then this method may have difficulty in distinguishing certain forms of trend from interaction. Scales of space-time interaction can be examined in the K-function approach, but the method is descriptive and cannot provide specific information about the location of such interaction. In addition, as noted above some forms of clustering may not be well detected by these interaction tests.

Alternative tests for space-time clustering which do detect a range of clustering types are the space-time scan statistic (Kulldorff *et al.*, 1998; Kulldorff and Hjalmars, 1999), a space-time test devised for imprecise locational information (Jacquez, 1996), and a test employing directional-linear correlation (Lawson and Viel, 1995). The space-time scan statistic is a straightforward development of the spatial scan statistic, where instead of testing within a series of circles a series of cylinders are used, the height of the cylinder representing the time window. Some disadvantages of these testing procedures lie in the use of circular areas and the need to test specific effects with different statistics. The Lawson–Viel test uses only time-ordered observations and exploits the idea that certain forms of directional-linear correlation must be found when space-time clustering is evident.

Clearly, borrowing strength from cluster parametric modelling, conditioning on the given spatio-temporal cluster centres, then we can consider a statistic of the form,

$$T = \sum_i \sum_j \hat{g}(\boldsymbol{x}_i, t_i) h_x(\boldsymbol{x}_i - c_{x_j}) h_t(t_i - c_{tj}),$$

where $h_x(\cdot)$ and $h_t(\cdot)$ are distance functions in space and time, respectively, and $\{x_i, t_i\}$ are the spatial and temporal location of the ith case, and the $\{c_{xj}, c_{tj}\}$ are the spatial and temporal coordinates of the jth space-time cluster centre. For any configuration of the centres, this statistic will yield evidence of support for these centres, by large values of T. As the centres must be given to compute this statistic, it would be most suited to Monte Carlo testing within an MCMC algorithm which sampled cluster centres (Besag *et al.*, 1991b). Tests of this type could also be constructed for spatial and/or temporal clustering separately.

6.5 A CLUSTER MODELLING EXAMPLE

As an illustration of a model-based approach to clustering, I will consider the analysis of a case event data set which has been previously assessed by Cuzick and Edwards (1990) and Diggle and Chetwynd (1991). The data set consists of the residential locations of 62 cases of childhood leukaemia and lymphoma in the north Humberside region of England for the period 1974–1986 (see Figures 1.14 and 1.15). Cuzick and Edwards first analysed and published this data, and applied their test statistic (6.5) to this realisation of cases employing a random sample of 141 birth addresses from the birth register for the study region for the same period. The authors computed their T_k statistics for $k = 1, \ldots, 10$. They noted that the greatest significance is attained for 'a value of k near 3, corresponding to a cluster of about size 4'. However, the choice of k is arbitrary and is usually fixed in advance. Hence, the wrong choice of k could easily miss important clustering scales. The method does not provide any insight into *where* the cluster or clusters can be found. Diggle and Chetwynd subsequently applied their statistic $\hat{D}(s)$ to this data set. They applied the statistic with $s_k = 0.001k$, with $k = 1, \ldots, 10$, and produced 95% tolerance limits from $\pm 2\surd[\text{var}\{\hat{D}(s)\}]$. The tolerance limits are exceeded by $\hat{D}(s)$ in the vicinity of $s \approx 0.005$, and the authors suggest that there is mild evidence of spatial clustering, i.e. 'some degree of spatial clustering within a range of about 500 m'. This approach yields an overall test for clustering as in the Cuzick and Edwards approach, but also provides evidence for the scale of clustering. However, the location of any putative clusters cannot be provided by this method. Neither of these methods can provide for non-stationarity if, for example, spatial trends were also underlying the cluster pattern.

In contrast to the testing approaches described above, a cluster modelling approach has also been applied to this data set, assuming a full parametric-modelling approach. A more detailed account of the modelling described here is given elsewhere (Lawson, 2000).

Here, our aim is to model the clustering tendency of the case events given the local population structure. To do this a cluster model of the form (6.1) is assumed:

$$\lambda(x \mid \underline{y}) = \rho g(x) m \left\{ \sum_{j=1}^{k} h(x - y_j) \right\}.$$

Hence, we assume k and $\{\boldsymbol{y}_j\}$, $j = 1, \ldots, k$, are unknown and we are interested in the joint posterior marginal distribution and conditional distribution of $\boldsymbol{y}$ given k. This distribution is useful when conditioning on the modal posterior value of k. It is also assumed that $m(\cdot) = \varsigma(\boldsymbol{x})\{1 + \sum_{j=1}^{k} h(\boldsymbol{x} - \boldsymbol{y}_j)\}$, where the additive form is used to allow for the cases where there are no clusters. The $\varsigma(\boldsymbol{x})$ term is a spatially structured random effect, which is included to allow for extra background variation. Identifiability of this term and the cluster term can be a concern in general, although in this example the clustering absorbs most of the structured variation and is of a different spatial scale from the non-specific random variation. At a case event location the intensity is defined as

$$\lambda(\boldsymbol{x}_i \mid \underline{y}) = g(\boldsymbol{x}_i)s(\boldsymbol{x}_i)\left\{1 + \sum_{j=1}^{k} h(\boldsymbol{x}_i - \boldsymbol{y}_j)\right\}.$$

It is assumed that the case locations have occurred within a heterogeneous population, and that given the local population structure clusters will then follow a cluster process. In this case the realisation of the intensity process consists of a background process, $g(\boldsymbol{x})$, which represents the 'at-risk' population, and a cluster distribution, $h(\cdot)$, is defined to be the Gaussian form,

$$h(\boldsymbol{x} - \boldsymbol{y}) = \frac{1}{2\pi\kappa} \mathrm{e}^{-[\|\boldsymbol{x}-\boldsymbol{y}\|]^2/2\kappa},$$

with the spread of the clusters defined by the cluster variance κ.

The likelihood conditional on $\{k, (\boldsymbol{y}_j)\}$ and m is given by

$$L(\boldsymbol{x} \mid \boldsymbol{y}, \boldsymbol{\theta}) = \left\{\prod_{i=1}^{m} \lambda(x_i \mid \underline{y})\right\}\left\{\int_T \lambda(\boldsymbol{u} \mid \underline{y})\, \mathrm{d}\boldsymbol{u}\right\}^{-m}.$$

Within the intensity a number of parameters are specified, other than those relating to the cluster centre locations and number. The cluster model must also include prior distributions for the centre locations and number, the cluster variance, and also parameters in prior distributions, if appropriate. Here, we assume that the centre locations and number have a Strauss inhibition prior distribution where the probability of any configuration of k centres is given by

$$p(\underline{y}) \propto \rho\gamma^{n_R},$$

where n_R is the number of R-close pairs of centres in the configuration, γ is an inhibition parameter, R is an inhibition distance parameter, and ρ is the rate of the process. The process is CSR if $\gamma = 1$, and a γ value below 1 yields inhibited configurations. Both γ and R are highly correlated and it is simplest to fix one or both parameters in any example. The prior distribution for other parameters $\boldsymbol{\theta}$ (such as the cluster variance) is defined as $g(\boldsymbol{\theta})$. In the example here we have assumed an inverse exponential distribution for the cluster variance. For the structured random variation, we have assumed an intrinsic Gaussian prior distribution (Kunsch, 1987) with $\varsigma_i = \exp\{u_i + v_i\}$. The components represent structured/correlated (u) and uncorrelated (v) heterogeneity, respectively, with intrinsic Gaussian prior distribution,

$$p_i(u_i \mid \cdots) \propto \exp\left\{-\sum_{k\in\partial_i} w_{ij}(u_i - u_j)^2\right\},$$

where the weights are specified as $w_{ij} = \exp(-d_{ij})/\{2r\}$, where r is a range parameter and ∂_i is a fixed distance neighbourhood. In our example the distance neighbourhood is taken as half the maximum distance within the study region. The prior for $\{v\}$ is a zero mean normal with variance σ^2. Both r and σ have inverse exponential hyperprior distributions:

$$\text{prior}(r, \sigma) \propto \mathrm{e}^{-\epsilon/2r}\mathrm{e}^{-\epsilon/2\sigma}, \qquad \sigma, r \succ 0,$$

where ϵ is taken as 0.001.

Usually, inference concerning cluster parameters is made conditionally on $\hat{g}(\boldsymbol{x})$, separately estimated from the birth register sample. An alternative method that can be used is the approach of Diggle and Rowlingson (1994), where a conditional logistic likelihood is specified and $g(\boldsymbol{x})$ factors out of the likelihood. This approach applied to cluster modelling has been explored by Lawson and Clark (1999a). It is also possible to sample the values of the smoothing constant h_s, within an MCMC context, if a suitable prior distribution can be used. This has the advantage of not requiring the use of a profile likelihood, and can be applied quite generally, even when control realisations are not available. Here, the latter approach is adopted and an inverse exponential distribution has been used as a prior distribution for h_s.

The full posterior distribution can be specified by

$$P(\underline{y}, k, \boldsymbol{\theta} \mid \boldsymbol{x}) \propto L(\boldsymbol{x} \mid \underline{y}, \boldsymbol{\theta})p(\underline{y})g(\boldsymbol{\theta}),$$

where $\boldsymbol{\theta} : \{\kappa, \rho, \sigma, r, h_s\}$. The posterior sampling for the various parameters was carried out using a Metropolis–Hastings sampler, which, in the special case of the cluster centres, includes reversible-jump transitions. This reversible-jump step, and associated proposal distributions, is described in Appendix C. Besides the centre parameters, the proposal distributions for the other parameters were based on normal distributions with mean equal to the previous parameter value and large fixed variance, to allow better exploration of the surface.

In all the example runs, it was assumed that $W = T$, to allow for the problem of seaward boundaries, and we have used $p = 1$, $q = 0.5$, a death rate of $1/k$ and a uniform birth rate in a disc of radius 0.01. The Strauss prior parameters are $\gamma = 0.8$ and the interaction distance, $R = 0.25$. These parameter values have been found to yield enough inhibition of centres to prevent multiple response in the sampler. The Metropolis algorithm was run to convergence. This usually took place by 50 000 iterations. Convergence checks were performed using comparisons of summary values from chains. Chains were run from different start configurations. Other diagnostics were also examined including Geweke's posterior monitoring and empirical Q–Q plotting (Cowles and Carlin, 1996; Robert and Casella, 1999).

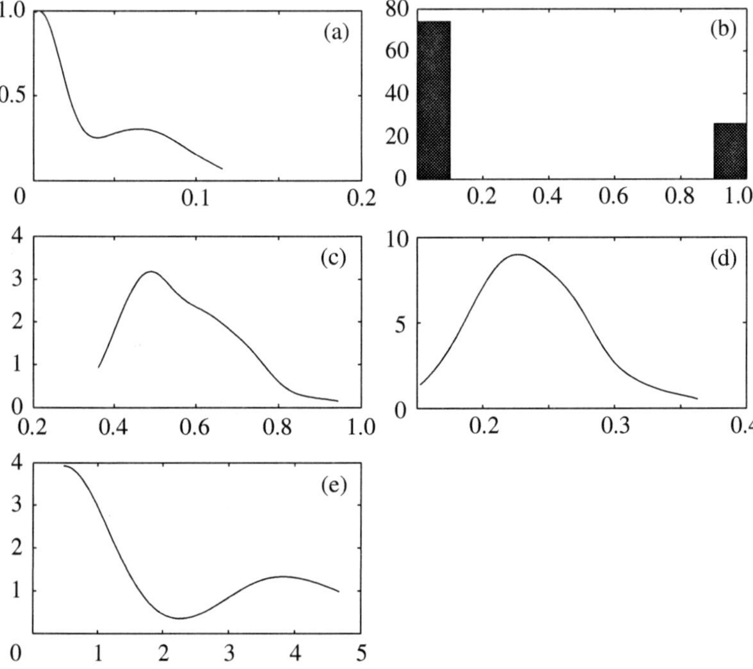

Figure 6.2 Posterior marginal displays of a selection of parameters for the Humberside data example: (a) h_S, (b) k, (c) r, (d) σ, (e) ρ.

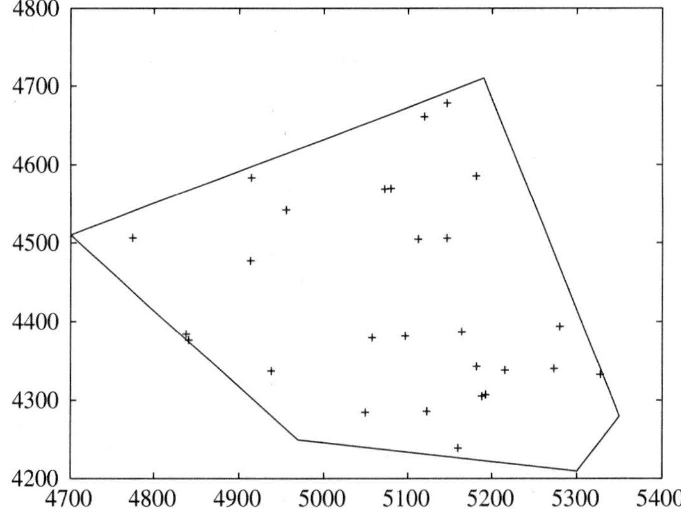

Figure 6.3 The posterior marginal distribution of the cluster centre locations in the converged sample: Humberside data example.

A selection of results from this analysis are presented in Figures 6.2 and 6.3.

The results of this approach appear to confirm that there is little evidence of clustering in this data example. Indeed, the modal value of the number of centres is zero, with a subsidiary mode at one. The spatial distribution of the converged sample centres appears to display little spatial differentiation, although a small concentration of points in the southeast of the area appears as a density peak. A similar analysis of this data which compared the basic cluster model (without random effects) and the Diggle and Rowlingson (DR) likelihood (Lawson and Clark, 1999a) yielded similar results with the DR model yielding a modal value of one for the number of centres. The difference between these results is marginal, and it should be borne in mind that apparent modal peaks in the density estimates of posterior parameter distributions can be affected by edge effects. Hence, the difference between zero and one cluster modes may be artefactual.

Overall this cluster analysis seems to confirm that there is little evidence for clustering in the Humberside data example. However, unlike testing for a restricted hypothesis, the cluster modelling approach provides considerably greater amounts of information concerning scales of clustering and location of clusters.

CHAPTER 7

Small Scale: Putative Sources of Hazard

7.1 INTRODUCTION

The assessment of the impact of sources of pollution on the health status of communities is of considerable academic and public concern. The incidence of many respiratory, skin and genetic diseases is thought to be related to environmental pollution (Hills and Alexander, 1989), and hence any localised source of such pollution could give rise to changes in the incidence of such diseases in the adjoining community.

In recent years, there has been growing interest in the development of statistical methods useful in the detection of patterns of health events associated with pollution sources. In this review we consider the statistical methodology for the assessment of putative health effects of sources of air pollution or ionising radiation. We consider study design issues, inference and modelling problems. We concentrate primarily on the data analysis of observed point patterns of events rather than specific features of a particular disease or outcome. Our purpose is to review statistical methods, so some published case studies of sources of pollution hazard may not appear.

A number of studies use data based on the spatial distribution of such diseases to assess the strength of association with exposure to a pollution source. Raised incidence near the source, or directional preference related to a dominant wind direction, may provide evidence of such a link. Hence, the aim of the analysis of such data is usually to assess specific spatial variables rather than general spatial modelling. That is, the analyst is interested in detecting patterns of events near (or exposed to) the focus and less concerned about aggregation of events in other locations. The former type of analysis has been named ‘focused clustering’ by Besag and Newell (1991). To date, most pollution source studies concentrate on incidence of a single disease (e.g. childhood leukaemia around nuclear power stations or respiratory cancers around waste-product incinerators).

The types of data observed can vary from disease event locations (usually residence addresses of cases) to counts of disease (mortality or morbidity) within census tracts or other arbitrary spatial regions. The two different data types lead to different modelling approaches. Spatial point process models are appropriate for event location data. In the case of count data, one may use properties of regionalised point processes. That is, an independent Poisson model for regional counts is often assumed and one typically uses log-linear models and related tests.

The effects of pollution sources are often measured over geographic areas containing heterogeneous population densities (usually both urban and rural areas). As a result, the underlying intensity of the point process model is heterogeneous. For an introduction to heterogeneous spatial point processes, and spatial point processes in general, see Diggle (1983). A review of spatial point process theory appears in Chapter 8 of Cressie (1993). Section 4.3.2 also provides an introduction to these models.

In later sections, statistical issues involved in the design of a study of health events around putative sources of hazard are reviewed. Some problems in statistical inference associated with such studies are reviewed in Sections 7.3 and 7.4. Exploratory and diagnostic techniques are presented in Section 7.3.1. Sections 7.7 and 7.5 deal with estimation and hypothesis testing in models for point event and count data. A recent review of this area of application can be found in Lawson *et al.* (1999a).

7.2 STUDY DESIGN

In what follows, we consider a delimited geographical study area or window within which data concerning disease occurrence and exposure to the pollution source are collected. Issues concerning the strategic aims of the study must be considered prior to detailed consideration of the appropriate study region and data collection requirements.

7.2.1 Retrospective and Prospective Studies

During the 1980s, a number of studies of disease occurrence in geographical regions around putative sources of risk were carried out (Lenihan, 1985; Bhopal *et al.*, 1992). Most of these were 'reactive', in that suspicion of a health risk, due to the past operation of a pollution source, instigated a review of the historical evidence for a link between disease incidence and exposure to the source. In essence, a *retrospective* study of disease occurrence was carried out. In some cases, continued monitoring of the source was also recommended or initiated. However, solely *prospective* studies of sources are seldom encountered. These two approaches and their respective strengths and weaknesses are well-known in the epidemiological literature.

Such studies of effects of pollution have a number of limitations, however. First, typically the emission characteristics of a source are not recorded for a suitable time period. Retrospective data on emissions may not be available and prospective monitoring data are expensive to collect over a long time period for a wide range of substances of interest. Often, no direct information is available on correlation between emission and disease occurrence. Furthermore, exposure and disease data are often collected by separate groups at different levels of resolution (even in prospective studies). Also, the nature of available data may be limited for particular diseases or health status indicators, or for particular time periods. Often, nationally collected data rather than data from a specially designed study must be utilised. In some cases, the level of resolution in available data constrains the analysis considerably. For example, some diseases are reported only as counts from postal zones or census enumeration districts and not as exact addresses due to confidentiality. In that case, methods based on analysis of counts rather than point events are appropriate. Inevitably, such regionalisation leads to some loss of information. For example, very small clusters cannot be detected if they occur within a large census tract as the aggregate disease rate for the tract as a whole may not differ from the background disease rate. Only if the spatial pattern of events occurs at a larger scale than the measurement unit will it be detectable in regionalised data. Finally, for chronic outcomes like cancers, the temporal lag between exposure and an event of interest may be on the order of years or decades. Mobility of individuals over such a time period can confound exposure–outcome relationships and cause prohibitive costs in prospective studies over large areas.

7.2.2 Study Region Design

The design of a study region or window is of great practical importance. Usually, a study will concern the distribution of events (e.g. incident disease cases) within a fixed map area of given size and shape. The choice of size and shape can have considerable impact on study results and, while it is often not possible to choose the most appropriate region, some consideration should be given to these issues.

Region Size

A study region should be defined which is of sufficient size that any effects of a putative source can be measured adequately. As it is often not possible to assess, *a priori*, the spatial scale of pollution effects, it is important that a large region including the pollution source should be used. In many published studies a region is defined and the total incidence in the region is analysed (compared to external 'control' regions). Lenihan (1985) provides an example of this approach. If a region is specified which is larger than the true pollution range, then a localised effect within some part of the region may be diluted. On the other hand, a small region may truncate the evidence and not represent the complete effects in the population. In addition, the use of multiple region sizes may still induce problems in data analysis if a pollution effect occurs at a spatial scale different than those considered (Glick, 1979; Elliott *et al.*, 1992a; Waller *et al.*, 1993).

In previous studies, sizes of region, in radial units from a source, vary from less than 1 km to 10 km. Most study windows have areas between 10 and 100 km^2 (Elliott *et al.*, 1992a). Often, the size of region is defined by a natural break in the underlying population. For example, the boundary of a town (Lawson and Williams, 1994) or physical barriers, such as rivers, mountains or coastlines, may affect the region size (and shape). Practical data-acquisition problems may limit the region size. Furthermore, exposure and outcome data may be available for different regions.

Region Shape

When one assesses exposure to a single pollution source, and one assumes that distance is a surrogate for exposure, then a circular region centred on the source yields the least sampling bias for detecting directional trends, in that sampling is equal in all directions. Square, rectangular or other polygonal regions do not provide such unbiasedness. Of course, if the putative source is not central to the region, then a circular window has no advantage (Lenihan, 1985; Diggle, 1990). If population structure dictates the region shape and size, then a polygonal region may have to be adopted, although some advanced statistical techniques can be used to allow for population-sparse regions in regular windows (Lawson, 1995).

When one examines multiple pollution sources, a rectangular or polygonal region should suffice. However, one should make some effort to provide 'similar' sampling detail in all directions from the sources in case directional anisotropy is present.

7.2.3 Replication and Controls

Few studies examine replicated realisations of disease events near pollution sources. A notable exception is the examination of 10 incinerators of waste solvent in the UK as a pooled sample by Elliott *et al.* (1992b).

The main use of replication in such studies should be to provide estimates of variability not available from single realisations. An alternative use of replication is to study other areas where potential pollution sources exist but where no evidence has been demonstrated for adverse health links to the source or sources. Cook-Mozaffari *et al.* (1989) provide an example and compare nuclear sites in the UK with sites considered for nuclear plants as controls. Here one uses a set of control areas to directly compare with the study area.

If substantial hypotheses concerning an individual source are to be examined, then control areas may be of some use. However, the use of replication to provide increased sample size by pooling, without examination of variability, only provides evidence for hypotheses concerning the sources in general, and not for individual sites. Local effects, which may be 'unusually' marked at an individual site, may be swamped in such a pooled sample.

In any study of disease incidence within a population, one must take some account of population structure. A standard epidemiological case-control design can be used where individuals are selected as controls and matched to cases with respect to confounding factors (e.g. age and occupation) (Breslow and Day, 1984). Another standard approach in the conventional analysis of small-area count data involves the use of strata-specific standardised rates to represent the 'background' population effect. The ratio of observed count to expected count, based on such a standardisation, can be used as a crude estimate of region-specific relative risk.

An alternative approach is to utilise a disease or group of diseases which is thought to represent the 'at-risk' population in the area but is usually unaffected by the type of pollution being considered (Diggle, 1990; Lawson and Williams, 1994). This approach is designed for point event data where a 'background' point event map of a 'control' disease is available. This method could also be used with count data, where counts of 'case' and 'control' diseases are available.

The goal is to find a 'control' disease which affects the same population with respect to possible confounding variables (e.g. age, occupation, smoking, etc.) yet is unrelated to the exposure of interest. While the existence of such a 'control disease' is subject to epidemiological debate, if such data are available, the statistical foundation of the methods is sound.

In many non-geographical studies in epidemiology, it is common to assign *individual* controls to cases, i.e. each case has an individual control who is matched to the case on a selection of variables such as age, gender or exposure history. Such matched case-control studies can be implemented within a geographical setting (see Section 4.3.2). Details of the statistical issues relating to these studies and putative source examples are discussed by Diggle *et al.* (2000).

7.3 PROBLEMS OF INFERENCE

The primary inferential problems arising in putative source studies are (a) post hoc analyses, and (b) multiple comparisons.

The well-known problem of post hoc analysis arises when prior knowledge of reported disease incidence near a putative source leads an investigator to carry out statistical tests or fit models to data to 'confirm' the evidence (Neutra, 1990; Rothman, 1990). Essentially, this problem concerns bias in data collection and prior knowledge of an apparent effect. Hills and Alexander (1989) and Gardner (1989) note that both hypothesis tests and study region definition can be biased by this problem. However, Lawson (1993c) notes that if a study *region* is noted *a priori* to be of interest because it includes a pollution source, one does not suffer from post hoc analysis problems if the internal spatial structure of disease incidence did not influence the choice of region.

Although much recent work examines the statistical methodology appropriate for analysis for single disease types, there is little consideration of how to accommodate multiple 'health markers' in the investigation of putative sources. For example, in the Bonnybridge–Denny Morbidity Review (Lenihan, 1985), the authors examined a group of diseases within a circular window within a fixed time period.

The multiple comparison problem has been addressed in several ways. Bonferonni's inequality may be used to adjust critical regions for multiple comparisons but the conservative nature of such an adjustment is well known. Thomas (1985) discussed multiple comparison problems proposes the use of cumulative p-value plotting to assess the number of diseases yielding evidence of association with a particular source (Schweder and Spjotwoll, 1982; see also Haybrittle *et al.* (1995)).

7.3.1 Exploratory Techniques

The use of exploratory techniques is widespread in conventional statistical analysis and general methods for such analysis are discussed in Section 5.1. However, in

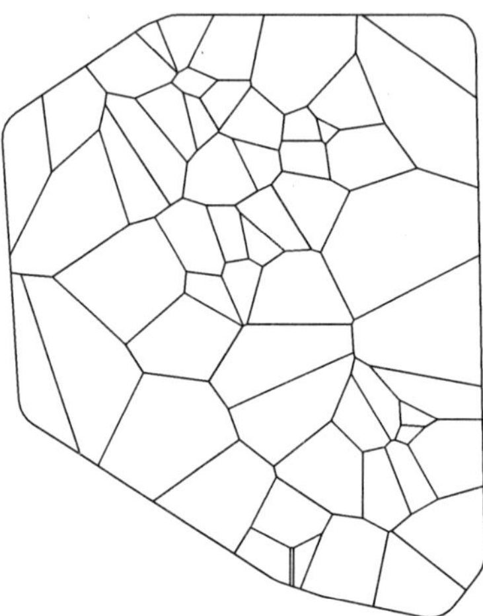

Figure 7.1 Dirichlet tessellation of the larynx cancer data (within the convex hull of the data points).

putative source analysis one must exercise care about how subsequent model design is influenced by exploratory or diagnostic findings. For example, if exploratory analysis isolates a cluster of events located near a pollution source, then this knowledge could lead to a post hoc analysis problem: i.e. inference based on a model specifically including such a cluster is suspect. As long as an analyst predefines the sources of interest and does not include a source simply because of its proximity to a cluster detected during the exploratory phase, many post hoc inference problems may be avoided.

In the case of point event data, one can employ standard point process methods to explore data structure. One often begins by comparing the observed pattern to that from some model of spatial variation. For example, the intensity (i.e. points per unit area) of events can be mapped and viewed as a contoured surface, usually using non-parametric density estimation (Diggle, 1985a). A natural model of spatial variation is a heterogeneous Poisson process (HEPP) with this surface representing the first-order intensity of the process. Additionally, the Dirichlet tessellation or Delauney triangulation of the points can demonstrate overall structure (Sibson, 1980; Ripley, 1981). Figure 7.1 displays an example of a Dirichlet tessellation of the larynx cancer case event data (Chapter 2). This displays the local density of points, and can show areas of high density associated with small tile areas. Tile is the term used to describe the area around a data point which includes all locations nearest to the point. This type of display is limited, however, because it does not include the underlying population background variation.

If the intensity of controls is also mapped, then it is useful to assess whether the cases demonstrate an excess of events beyond that demonstrated by the controls (e.g. in areas of increased risk). Controls could consist of randomly selected individuals from the population at risk (perhaps matched on confounding factors), or a ‘control disease’

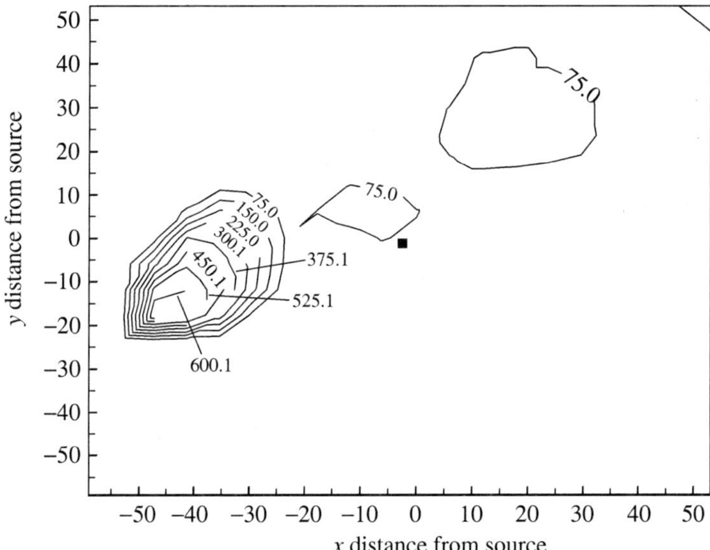

Figure 7.2 Armadale example: extraction mapping of the ratio of respiratory cancer case events and CHD control locations. Reproduced with permission from Lawson and Williams (1994).

as mentioned above. A higher intensity of 'cases' than 'controls' near a pollution source may support a hypothesis of association. The relative-risk estimation methods of Section 5.1.2 were originally developed in connection with the examination of clusters of disease excess.

Bithell (1990) suggested that the ratio of density estimates of cases and controls be used as a map displaying areas of increased risk. Lawson and Williams (1993) proposed a different method based on kernel smoothing and also provided crude standard error surfaces for the resulting map. This type of 'extraction' of a control intensity is akin to the mapping of standardised mortality ratios for count data. Kelsall and Diggle (1995b) further refined the original ratio estimator and describe improved conditions for estimation of smoothing. This form of excess risk analysis can be regarded in more formal terms as the estimation of

$$R(\boldsymbol{x}) = \lambda(\boldsymbol{x})/g(\boldsymbol{x}),$$

where the model for the case intensity consists of a product of the 'at-risk' background effect $g(\boldsymbol{x})$, and the excess risk, i.e. $\lambda(\boldsymbol{x}) = g(\boldsymbol{x})R(\boldsymbol{x})$. Figure 7.2 displays the extraction map for respiratory cancer with CHD (coronary heart disease) as a control disease for Armadale central Scotland (Section 1.4.1). Each event intensity surface has been kernel smoothed using density estimation. The smoothing of each surface is based on the likelihood cross-validated smoothing constant (respiratory cancer: 5.187; CHD: 2.712). Note that in this case a large residual peak is evident in the southwest of the map area. However, this peak lies in an area where there are few control locations

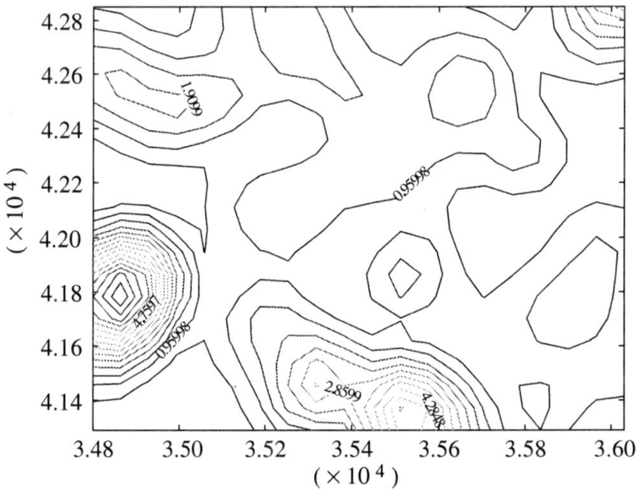

Figure 7.3 Extraction map of larynx cancer to respiratory cancer for Lancashire, UK.

and so must be treated with caution. Figure 7.3 displays the extraction map contour surface for the Lancashire larynx cancer data, with respiratory cancer as the control disease (see Section 1.4.1). As in the Armadale cases each intensity surface has been separately estimated. The residual peaks apparent in the surface must also be treated with caution due to the low intensity of control cases in these areas. However, the peak at the southern edge of the area lies in the vicinity of a waste-product incinerator. This fact may warrant the further analysis of the nature of the excess risk found and in particular the assessment of probability surfaces for relative risk as suggested by Kelsall and Diggle.

While extraction isolates the global structure, some techniques might be developed to isolate particular structural elements, e.g. clusters of given numbers of cases, clusters within a given number of people at risk, or 'within-distance' groups. Such an approach may be similar to the methods for assessing so-called 'general clustering'. A test of 'general clustering' explores the tendency of cases to cluster without regard to where clustering might be expected to occur. Proposals for cluster detection (Besag and Newell, 1991; Turnbull *et al.*, 1990; Openshaw *et al.*, 1987; Schulman *et al.*, 1988) could be regarded as exploratory tools. Second-order models of general clustering have also been explored (Diggle and Chetwynd, 1991), and could be used in an exploratory setting.

In the case of count data, a variety of exploratory methods exist. One can use representation of counts as surfaces and incorporate expected count standardisation (e.g. through a standardised mortality/morbidity ratio (SMR)). The SMR is the saturated maximum likelihood estimate of the relative risk in each tract under a simple Poisson count model.

Figure 7.4 displays a thematic map of the SMRs for respiratory cancer for the Falkirk example. Areas of relatively high SMR are depicted with darker grey intensity.

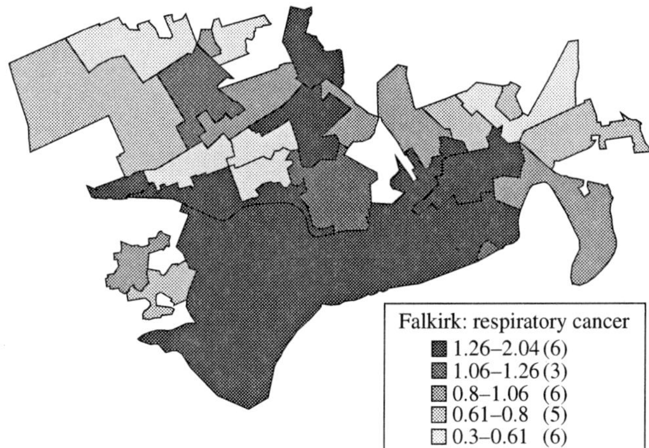

Figure 7.4 Thematic map of the SMRs for respiratory cancer for the Falkirk example.

The map must be interpreted with caution as the greyscale grouping is arbitrary and such a choice can affect interpretation. This is discussed more fully in Chapter 3.

While mapping regional SMRs can help isolate excess incidence, estimates of SMRs from counts in small areas are notoriously variable, especially for areas with few persons at risk. Various methods have been proposed to stabilise these small-area estimates. Two different approaches are non-parametric smoothing and EB 'shrinkage' estimation.

Smoothing approaches have been proposed for the analysis of SMRs over time (Breslow and Day, 1987). A kernel-smoothing approach using a single parameter to describe the surface smoothness has also been proposed (Lawson, 1993c). Figure 7.5 displays a kernel smoothing, using a bivariate Gaussian kernel, of the Falkirk respiratory cancer SMRs, performed at the centroids of the enumeration districts. The contouring itself inherently produces a smoothed view of the variation over the study region, after the kernel-smoothing process is complete.

Carrat and Valleron (1992) and Webster *et al.* (1994) proposed various implementations of geostatistical prediction (kriging) to obtain a risk surface, although some key assumptions implicit in the methodology may not hold for disease data. These approaches yield a smooth, possibly non-stationary relative risk surface which one can subsequently examine for clustering or trend effects. However, two disadvantages of standard kriging estimators is that they can produce *negative* interpolant values, which are invalid for relative risk surfaces, and that they assume a constant variance in the spatial field. Many alternative forms of smoothing could be used (Kafadar, 1996; Mungiole *et al.*, 1999). The relative merits of different smoothing approaches in application to putative hazard source data has not so far been systematically evaluated.

Many researchers have proposed empirical Bayesian estimates of regional rates (Section 4.3.5). The methods are similar to those used for small-area analysis (see Ghosh and Rao (1994) for a review). The EB methods stabilise estimates of SMRs

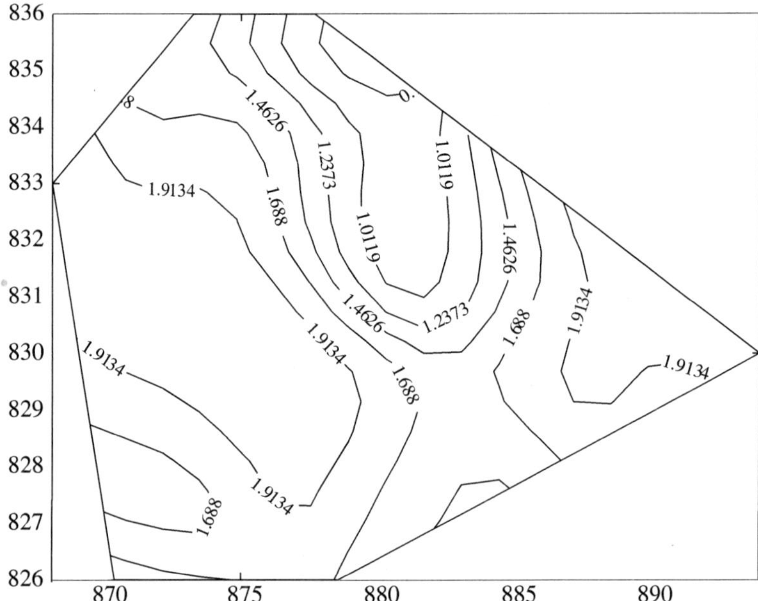

Figure 7.5 A two-dimensional kernel smoothing of the SMRs of Falkirk respiratory cancer, using an approximate polygonal window with $h_x = h_y = 1.45$. No edge correction.

in small areas by adding parameters with spatially correlated prior distributions, or adding uncorrelated random effects to models of disease counts. Application of EB methods including approximations to likelihoods have been made in the context of putative source analyses (Lawson, 1994b; Hoffmann and Schlattmann, 1999).

Recent advances in MCMC algorithms such as the Gibbs sampler allow a fully Bayesian approach (Besag *et al.*, 1991b; Clayton and Bernardinelli, 1992; Lawson *et al.*, 1996a). While Bayesian implementations can involve complicated parametric models of disease rates, one could use simple models incorporating only regional heterogeneity and spatial autocorrelation for exploratory purposes.

Results of the various exploratory techniques provide a starting point for model fitting and assessment. As event data around pollution sources are typically available as either point locations or as regional counts, we address modelling issues for the two types of data. Models for count data are often based on underlying point process models, so it is appropriate to begin with point models in Section 7.5 and outline applications to count data in Section 7.7.

7.4 MODELLING THE HAZARD EXPOSURE RISK

Before considering the detailed modelling of different types of data, it is appropriate to consider the types of evidence, and hence model ingredients, important in the

Table 7.1 Components of the putative source modelling process.

pollution measures		pollution measurement
pollution surrogates		distance and direction from source direction around sources
background estimation	ecological variables	expected cases or control diseases deprivation indices/census variables

specification of models of risk around putative sources of health hazard. These model components can be included under any data type.

Usually, what is fundamental in the conceptualisation of these issues is the assumption that risk at a location or within a tract is related to risk variables measured at the location or interpolated to the location or to represent the tract. This assumption has continued to be made in studies of particular putative sources, and this leads to the formulation of putative source problems as ecological regression studies. That is, the hazard measurements are regarded as explanatory variables, and the analysis proceeds by the assessment of the relation between these variables and the disease incidence. The particular feature of this ecological approach is that only a restricted set of explanatory variables is usually examined, i.e. those variables having a well-defined association with health risk. For example, in a prospective study of respiratory disease morbidity around a waste-product incinerator, it may be useful to monitor air pollution at a network of sites around the incinerator. The relation between disease incidence and air pollution could then be examined, for example, by interpolation of air pollution to case locations or averaging of pollution over tracts. Alternatively, if a retrospective study is to be carried out, then some surrogate pollution measures may be required (as direct measurement may not have been made). Surrogate measures commonly used in this connection are distance from source, direction around source, and functions of these measures. It is also appropriate to employ ecological variables to help to estimate the background 'at-risk' population. However, these variables are not usually regarded as surrogate for pollution measurements. Table 7.1 describes the types of variable appropriate in different types of study.

Exposure modelling here concerns the specification of variables and functions of variables which provide evidence for a link with pollution source or sources. Different potential sources of pollution or health risk can give rise to different forms of exposure evidence. For example, waste dump sites or nuclear power stations may by the nature of the potential pollution risk display only a distance-related effect to cases of disease. That is, only distance of cases from the source (or some function of distance) would be appropriate. This may also be true for electromagnetic fields which may be thought to act without any directional preference. In the case of sources which emit effluent into air or water bodies, then dispersion effects related to the movement of the host body take effect. In the case of air pollution, this means that wind direction and speed must play a role in the modelling of exposure.

In prospective studies, direct measurements of pollution can be made, and so there is less need to consider surrogates and their modelling. However, even in prospective

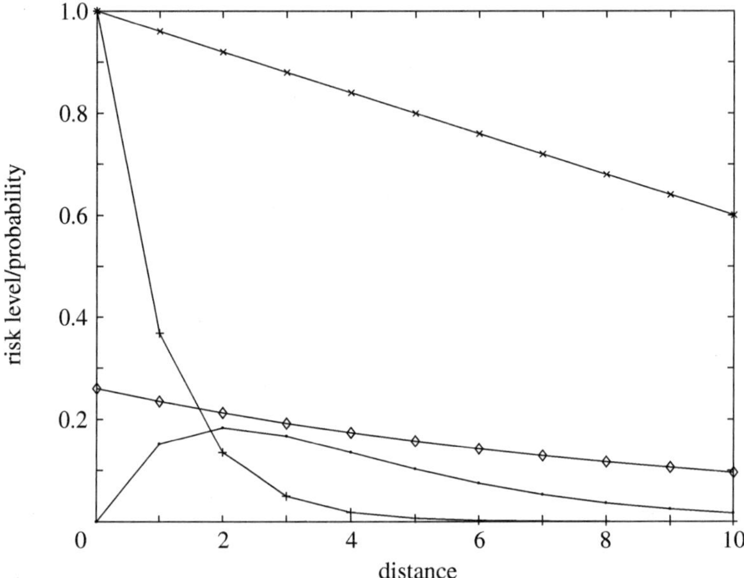

Figure 7.6 Variance of possible distance–risk relations around a putative source of health hazard: -×-, linear decline; -◇-, 'flat' gamma-like decline; -+-, exponential decline; ---, peaked-then-decline.

studies the lack of complete observation of the pollution process and the uncertainty of the aetiology of the disease in the particular example under study could lead to the consideration of exposure modelling to augment the information already available. In retrospective studies, surrogate measures are often the only available evidence and it is then essential to specify the exposure evidence which is to be considered with a model.

Here, we consider three basic forms of exposure evidence: distance based, direction based, and distance–direction interaction. While distance-only effects may be appropriate for waste dump sites, electromagnetic fields or nuclear installations, the inclusion of directional effects and also distance–direction interaction is important for any sites which could have an air pollution risk associated with them.

The distance relations described in Figure 7.6 can be regarded as the models for the possible distance–risk relation when a spatially homogeneous background is present. The patterns are all possible types to be expected around, for example, an air pollution source. Monotonic distance relations are by no means the only patterns possible, and indeed, the results of empirical studies and theoretical studies of dispersal around sources (Panopsky and Dutton, 1984; Esman and Marsh, 1996) support the possibility of peak-then-decline behaviour with increasing distance. The assumption often made, that monotonic decline should be assessed (alone) is therefore potentially quite misleading.

Directional effects are also likely when a wind regime applies, e.g. with air pollution related to incinerator outfall. Time-averaged wind effects could lead to peaks of

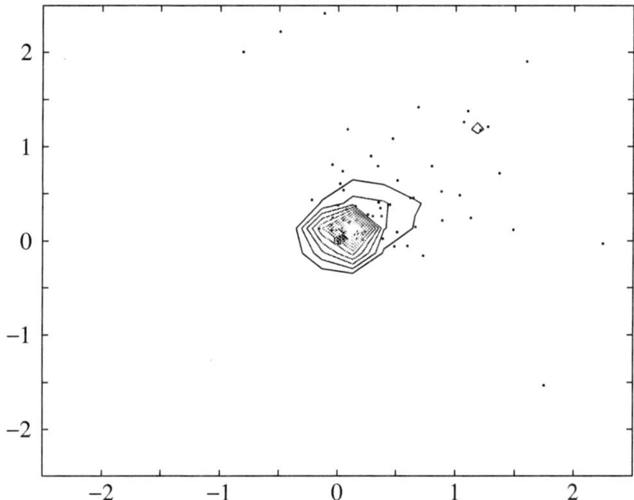

Figure 7.7 A simulation of case events around a source (0,0): 100 events with monotonic distance decline but angular concentration ($\kappa = 3.0$ from a von Mises distribution) around a mean angle (50°).

concentration in certain directions (possibly downwind of the dominant direction). Peaks downwind of the sub-dominant direction may also be possible (Lawson and Williams, 1994). Figures 7.7 and 7.8 display simulations of distance–angular relations found with and without a distance peak.

Figures 7.9 and 7.10 demonstrate a possible time-averaged outfall/risk pattern which can be described by a linear–angular model with correlation between distance and angle. These types of patterns are typically predicted from dispersal models from outfall sources.

One major issue relating to the choice of a small set of explanatory pollution surrogates is that after fitting such variables, much unexplained residual structure may remain in the data. This residual structure is likely to be related to the fact that only a small number of effects are being fitted and no attempt to fully describe the spatial pattern is being made. Hence, if no further attempt is made to provide a description based on known explanatory variables (for example, trend surface components), then there is likely to exist considerable residual effects. These effects could be modelled as unobserved heterogeneity via random-effect modelling, and some consideration should be given to this approach in such studies. However, not all residual *nuisance* structure will be removed by such modelling if long-range effects (trends) are present in the observations. Hence, it may be necessary to model a variety of spatial range effects (both long and short range) as well as pollution surrogates, if the underlying nuisance structure is to be properly isolated. Of course, if considerable nuisance structure remains, then the two main results of this would be to (a) *lower the power of hypothesis tests* employed to assess the role of pollution surrogates, and (b) *increase the variance of parameter estimates* associated with these surrogates. In addition, any

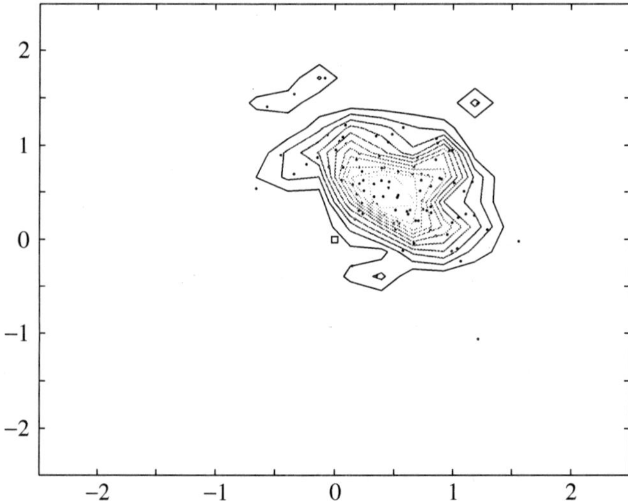

Figure 7.8 A simulation of case events around a source (0,0): 100 events with peaked distance decline but angular concentration ($\kappa = 3.0$ from a von Mises distribution) around a mean angle (50°).

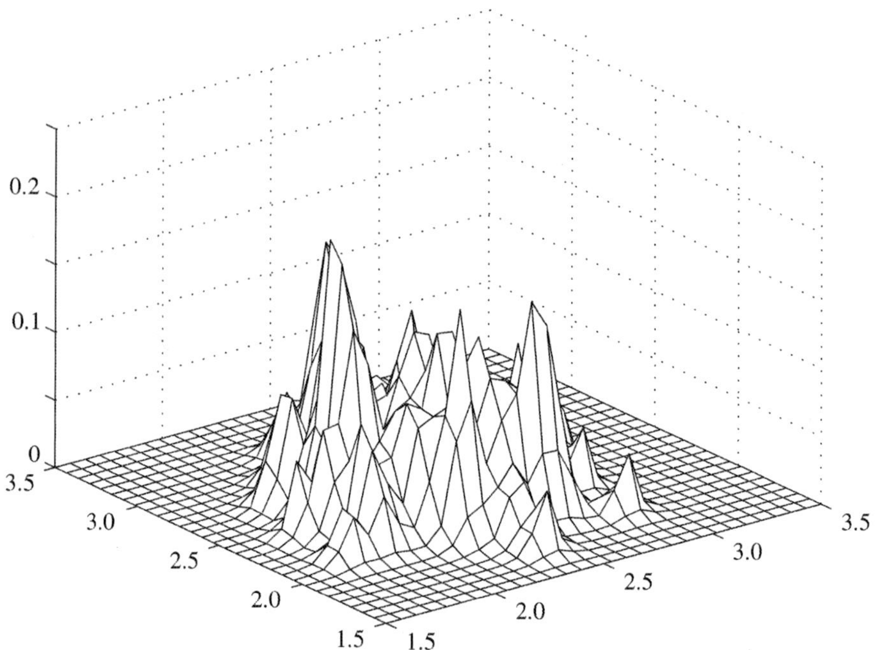

Figure 7.9 Perspective view of Figure 7.8.

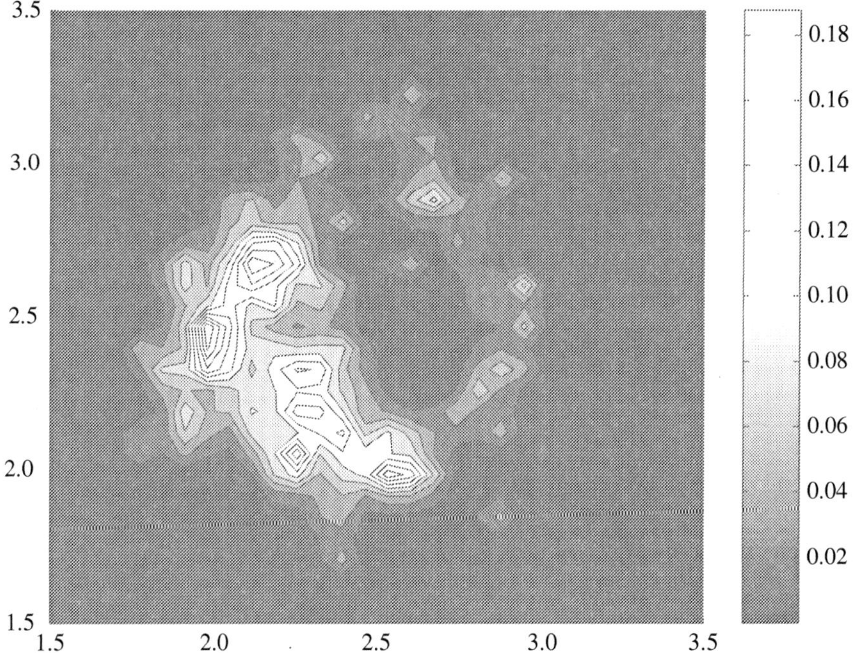

Figure 7.10 Density estimate of a sample of events from a five-parameter Weibull–von Mises distribution where the shape parameter of the Weibull is dependent on angle (source: 2.5,2.5).

pointwise residual analysis carried out will be marred by the presence of nuisance effects confounded with any pure error present.

The Specification of $f(x; \theta)$ in the Case Intensity

The intensity specification employed to describe case event distribution is usually of the form,

$$\lambda(\boldsymbol{x}) = g(\boldsymbol{x}) f(\boldsymbol{x}; \theta),$$

where $f(\boldsymbol{x}; \theta)$ is suitably parametrised to represent the excess risk found due to association with the source and possibly other covariates. It is important to consider the appropriate form for the function $f(\boldsymbol{x}; \theta)$, which usually describes the exposure model used in the analysis of the association of events to a source. Define the location of the source as $\boldsymbol{x}_0$. Usually, the spatial relation between the source and disease events is based on the polar coordinates of events from the source: $\{r, \phi\}$, where $r = \|\boldsymbol{x} - \boldsymbol{x}_0\|$, and ϕ is the angle measured to the source. It is important to consider how these polar coordinates can be used in models describing pollution effects on surrounding populations. In many studies, only the distance measure (r) has been used as evidence for association between a source and surrounding populations (Diggle, 1989; Elliott *et al.*, 1992b; Elliott, 1995; Diggle *et al.*, 1997). However, it is dangerous to pursue distance-only analyses when considerable directional effects are present. The reason for this is based on elementary exposure modelling ideas, which are confirmed by more formal theoretical and empirical exposure studies (Panopsky and Dutton, 1984; Esman and Marsh, 1996). It is clear that differential exposure may occur with change in distance *and* direction, particularly around air pollution sources (such as incinerator stacks or foundry chimneys). Indeed the wind regime which is prevalent in the vicinity of a source can easily produce considerable differences in exposure in different directions. Such directional preference or anisotropy can lead to marked differences in exposure in different directions and hence to different distance–exposure profiles. Figure 7.8 displays such differences clearly. Hence, the collapsing of exposure over the directional marginal of the distribution could lead to considerable misinterpretation, and in the extreme to *Simpson's* paradox. In the extreme case, a strong distance relationship with a source may be masked by the collapsing over directions, and this can lead to erroneous conclusions. Many published studies by the SAHSU (Small Area Health Statistics Unit) in the UK (Elliott *et al.*, 1992b, 1996; Elliott, 1995; Sans *et al.*, 1995; Diggle *et al.*, 1997) have, apparently, ignored directional components in the distribution, and therefore the conclusions of these studies should be viewed with caution. Further, if the analysis of a large number of putative source sites is carried out by pooling between sites ignoring local directional effects at each site, then these studies should also be regarded with caution.

The importance of the examination of a *range* of possible indicators of association between sources and health risk in their vicinity is clear. The first criterion for association is usually assumed to be evidence of a decline in disease incidence with increased distance from the source. Without this distance–decline effect, there is likely to be only weak support for an association. However, this does not imply that this effect should be examined in isolation. As noted above, other effects can provide evidence for association, or could be nuisance effects which should be taken into consideration so that correct inferences be made. In the former category are directional and directional–distance correlation effects, which can be marked with particular wind regimes. In the latter category are peaked incidence effects, which relate to *increases* of incidence with distance from the source. While a peak at some distance from a source can occur, it is also possible for this to be combined with an overall underlying decline in incidence, and hence is of importance in any modelling approach. This peaked effect is a nuisance effect, in terms of association, but it is clearly important to include such effects. If they were not included, then inference may be erroneously made that no distance–decline is present, when in fact a combination of distance–decline and peaked incidence is found. Diggle *et al.* (1997) display data on stomach cancer incidence around a putative source, where peaking of incidence occurs at some distance from the source. Peaks of incidence compounded with distance–decline are clearly found in the Lancashire larynx cancer data also (Elliott *et al.*, 1992b). Further nuisance effects which may be of concern are, for example, random effects related to individual *frailty*, where individual variation of susceptibility is directly modelled or where general heterogeneity is admitted. A recent review of these critical issues appears in Lawson *et al.* (1999a).

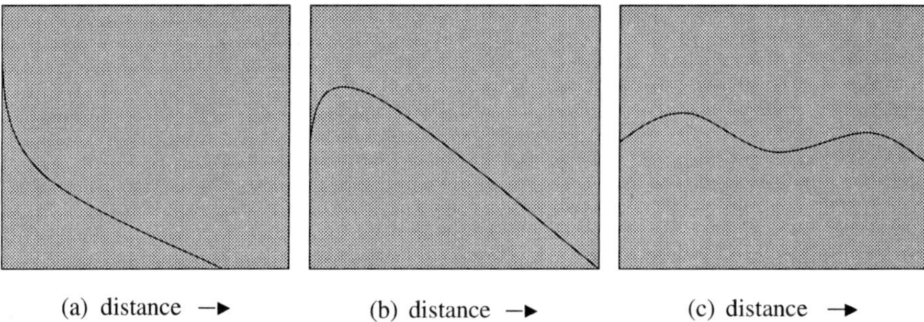

Figure 7.11 Possible exposure patterns over distance from a source: (a) monotone, (b) peaked, (c) clustered.

A general approach to modelling exposure risk is to include an appropriate selection of the above measures in the specification of $f(x; \cdot)$. First it is appropriate to consider how exposure variables can be linked to the background intensity $g(\boldsymbol{x})$. We define $f(\boldsymbol{x}; \theta) = m\{f^*(\boldsymbol{x})'\alpha\}$, where $m\{\cdot\}$ is an appropriate link function, and $f^*(\boldsymbol{x})$ represents the design matrix of exposure variables which is evaluated at $\boldsymbol{x}$. The link function is usually defined as $m\{\cdot\} = 1 + \exp\{\cdot\}$, although a direct multiplicative link can also be used. Usually, each row of $f^*(\boldsymbol{x})$ will consist of a selection of the variables

$$\{r, \log(r), \cos(\phi), \sin(\phi), r\cos(\phi), r\sin(\phi), \log(r)\cos(\phi), \log(r)\sin(\phi)\}.$$

The first four variables represent distance–decline, peakedness and directional effects, while the latter variables are directional–distance correlation effects (Lawson, 1993c). The directional components can be fitted separately and transformations of parameters can be made to yield corresponding directional concentration and mean angle (Lawson, 1992). Figure 7.11 displays different distance-related exposure models which could be used to specify $f(\boldsymbol{x}; \boldsymbol{\theta})$. Note that in Figure 7.11, nuisance effects of peakedness and heterogeneity appear in (b) and (c).

Further examination of dispersal models for air pollution suggest that the spatial distribution of outfall around a source is likely to follow a convolution of Gaussian distributions where in any particular direction there could be a separate mean level and lateral variance of concentration (dependent on r) (Esman and Marsh, 1996). As a parsimonious representation of these effects it is possible to use a subset of the exposure variables listed above to describe this behaviour.

Some simple models which can be proposed lead to the specification of $f(r, \phi)$ as follows:

(1) $f(r, \phi) = 1 + \exp\{-\alpha_1 r\}$, distance decline;

(2) $f(r, \phi) = 1 + \exp\{\alpha_1 \log r - \alpha_2 r\}$, *peaked* distance decline ($\alpha_1, \alpha_2 \succ 0$);

(3) $f(r, \phi) = 1 + \exp\{\alpha_1 \log r - \alpha_2 r + \alpha_3 \cos(\phi) + \alpha_4 \sin(\phi)\}$, *peaked* distance decline with angular concentration;

(4) $f(r,\phi) = 1 + \exp\{\alpha_1 \log r - \alpha_2 r + \alpha_3 \cos(\phi) + \alpha_4 \sin(\phi) + \alpha_5 r \cos(\phi) + \alpha_6 r \sin(\phi)\}$, same as (3) except linear angular correlation is added;

(5) $f(r,\phi) = 1 + \exp\{\delta \log r - \alpha_2 r\}$, where $\delta = \alpha_1 + \delta_1 * \cos(\phi - \mu)$, and μ is the mean angle peaked decline which varies with angle.

The specifications above appear to be flexible enough to model a variety of possible outfall patterns. Model (1) has often been used within models (Diggle, 1990), while variants with an inner area of constant risk have also been proposed by Diggle *et al.* (1997). The use of these simple decline models alone does not appear to be supported by any realistic exposure model for air pollution. In particular, an inner concentric zone of constant risk appears to have little epidemiological foundation *a priori*.

While the models listed above are not the only possible specifications which can describe potential radial and angular variation in risk, they do provide parsimonious descriptions of the qualitative features of exposure zones around pollution sources.

Figure 7.12 displays the result of a simulation for a model which involves both peaked and distance–decline components and directional preference. Time-averaged exposure can be thought to lead to patterns similar to that depicted. Here a northwest direction of concentration is apparent and the simulated exposure intensity surface was obtained from a five-parameter model for the distance and directional components. Note that averaging over the directional marginal of this distribution will lead to considerable attenuation of increased risk at distance from the source due to the anisotropic distance relations found.

7.5 MODELS FOR CASE EVENT DATA

In this section, we consider a variety of modelling approaches available when data are recorded as a point map of disease events. Let $\boldsymbol{x}_i, i = 1, \ldots, m$, denote the locations of events in a realisation of a point process in $\mathbb{R}^2$. In order to distinguish between random points and locations from a given realisation of the process, we follow convention and refer to $\{\boldsymbol{x}_i\}$ as the set of 'events' of the process. Define W to be any planar region and $|W|$ to be the area of W.

In analysing events around a pollution source, one usually defines a fixed window or geographical region and all events which occur within this region within a particular time period are recorded (mapped). Thus the complete realisation of the point process is to be modelled. In the analysis of point events around pollution sources the long-range or trend components of variation are often of primary concern. This leads one to consider heterogeneous (non-stationary) Poisson process (HEPP) models to describe this variation.

Event locations often represent residential addresses of cases and take place in a heterogeneous population which both varies in spatial density and in susceptibility to disease. Diggle (1989) and Lawson (1989), independently, gave a method to accommodate such a population effect within a HEPP model.

Define the first-order intensity function of the process as $\lambda(\boldsymbol{x})$, which represents the mean number of events per unit area in the neighbourhood of location $\boldsymbol{x}$. This

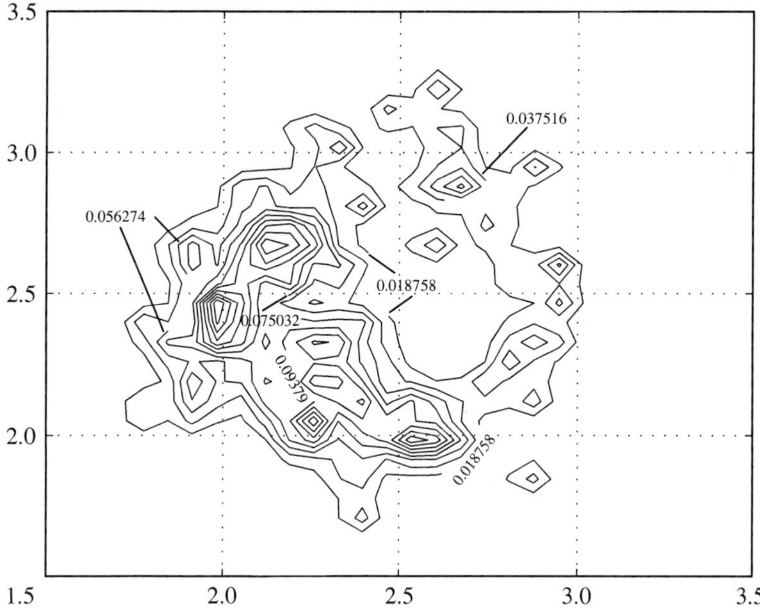

Figure 7.12 Simulation of a five-parameter dispersal model for a putative source, using a Weibull density for the distance marginal with scale and shape parameters and a von Mises with directional linear correlation for the directional component. Source location: {2.5,2.5}.

intensity may be parametrised as

$$\lambda(\boldsymbol{x}) = g(\boldsymbol{x}) f(\boldsymbol{x}; \boldsymbol{\theta}),$$

where $g(\boldsymbol{x})$ is the 'background' intensity of the population at risk at $\boldsymbol{x}$, and $f(\boldsymbol{x}; \boldsymbol{\theta})$ is a parametrised function of risk relative to the location of the pollution source. The focus of interest for assessing associations between events and the source is inference regarding parameters in $f(\boldsymbol{x}; \boldsymbol{\theta})$ treating $g(\boldsymbol{x})$ as a nuisance function. The likelihood of m events in W, conditional on m, is (bar a constant)

$$l_1 = \sum_{i=1}^{m} \log f(\boldsymbol{x}_i; \boldsymbol{\theta}) - m \log \int_W g(\boldsymbol{x}) f(\boldsymbol{x}; \boldsymbol{\theta}) \, \mathrm{d}\boldsymbol{x}. \tag{7.1}$$

In (7.1), parameters in $f(\boldsymbol{x}; \boldsymbol{\theta})$ must be estimated as well as $g(\boldsymbol{x})$. Diggle (1989) and Lawson (1989) propose estimating $g(\boldsymbol{x})$ non-parametrically from the 'at-risk' population. The locations of a 'control' disease (as described above) were proposed to provide a kernel estimate, $\hat{g}(\boldsymbol{x})$, of the background at arbitrary $\boldsymbol{x}$ and Lawson and Williams (1994) illustrate an application where one estimates $g(\boldsymbol{x})$ from the expected death surface using the entire population as controls instead of a control disease.

Inferential problems arise when $g(\boldsymbol{x})$ is estimated as a function and then apparently regarded as constant in subsequent inference concerning $\lambda(\boldsymbol{x})$. As an alternative, Diggle and Rowlingson (1994) proposed avoiding estimation of $g(\boldsymbol{x})$ by regarding the control locations and case locations as a set of labels whose binary value is determined by a position-dependent probability:

$$\Pr(\boldsymbol{x}) = \rho f(\boldsymbol{x}; \boldsymbol{\theta})/(1 + \rho f(\boldsymbol{x}; \boldsymbol{\theta})). \tag{7.2}$$

The binary regression model (7.2) avoids the use of $g(\boldsymbol{x})$ and hence avoids the inferential problems noted above. However, this model can only be applied when a point map of a control disease is available and when multiplicative relative risk is assumed.

An alternative model similar to the binary regression in (7.2) may be proposed. One conditions on the set of locations (cases and controls) and randomly assigns a binary label to each location indicating whether a particular location is a case or a control. Baddeley and Lieshout (1993) consider such a marked point process model. For example, if the points are a realisation of a Markov point process, then conditional on the points, the marks form a binary Markov random field (MRF) (Baddeley and Møller, 1989). Note that a HEPP can be considered as a special case of a Markov point process. The comments above concerning interpolation of local background, however, also apply to this case.

Variants to the above models have been proposed where the observational units are changed. For instance, Lawson and Williams's (1994) estimate of $g(\boldsymbol{x})$ from the expected death surface brings the HEPP model closer to the usual relative risk models for count data, where expected numbers of deaths are compared to observed numbers. In addition, Lawson and Williams (1994) proposed a hybrid model which is directly based on the expected death estimator of $g(\boldsymbol{x})$, and which requires no interpolation.

It is possible that population or environmental heterogeneity may be unobserved in the data set. This could be either because the population background hazard is not directly available or because the disease displays a tendency to cluster (perhaps due to unmeasured covariates). The heterogeneity could be spatially correlated or lack correlation, in which case it could be regarded as a type of 'overdispersion'.

One can include such unobserved heterogeneity within the framework of conventional models as a random effect. For example, a general definition of the first-order intensity could be

$$\lambda(\boldsymbol{x}) = g(\boldsymbol{x}) m(\exp(F\alpha + \zeta(\boldsymbol{x}))),$$

where F is a design matrix dependent on spatial location, α is a parameter vector, $\zeta(\boldsymbol{x})$ is a random effect at location $\boldsymbol{x}$.

In this specification $\zeta(\boldsymbol{x})$ represents a spatial process. If $\zeta(\boldsymbol{x})$ is a spatial Gaussian process, then conditional on the realisation of the process, any finite values of $\{\zeta(\boldsymbol{x}_i)\}$ will have a multivariate normal distribution. This distribution can include variance and covariance parameters representing uncorrelated and correlated heterogeneity respectively. An alternative specification is to assume that the log intensity ($g^*(\boldsymbol{x})$, say) has a multivariate normal prior distribution, MVN($F\alpha$, Σ), where Σ is the covariance matrix. Here, $\lambda(\boldsymbol{x}) \equiv m(\exp(g^*(\boldsymbol{x})))$, possibly with a modulating function $g(\boldsymbol{x})$ included. This is closer in spirit to the specification of a Cox process where the intensity itself is realised from a random process. This approach also leads to GLS estimators for α given Σ, similar to those found for universal kriging in geostatistics (see Section 5.2.4). The approach could be extended to individual region random effects and other types.

7.5.1 Estimation

The parameters of the HEPP and modulated HEPP models discussed above can be estimated by maximum likelihood, conditional on $\hat{g}(\boldsymbol{x})$. In fact, it is possible to use GLIM for such model fitting. Berman and Turner (1992) employ a novel integral approximation method which involves using the Dirichlet tile areas or associated Delauney triangle areas of data points as weights in the approximation.

For the hybrid model of Lawson and Williams (1994) and the binary regression model (7.2) of Diggle and Rowlingson (1994), direct maximum-likelihood methods must be used. For the MRF model of Baddeley and Lieshout (1993), one may use pseudolikelihood directly. In the case of spatially correlated heterogeneity, one may estimate covariance components via restricted maximum likelihood (REML, cf. Searle *et al.* (1992)) and use an iterative algorithm for trend parameter estimation (e.g. the expectation-maximisation, or EM algorithm).

In the above examples, many estimation problems can be overcome by use of MCMC methods. MCMC methods can aid in estimation problems by providing a simulation-based estimate of the likelihood surface (or posterior distribution in Bayesian inference). The main disadvantage to MCMC methods is that different model parametrisations must be run separately in, for example, Gibbs sampler runs. Hence, one may pay a high computational price to find the best subset model. Reversible-jump methods could avoid this problem. However, convergence of MCMC algorithms can be difficult to assess and there is still dispute on the best way to implement MCMC methods (Robert and Casella, 1999).

7.5.2 Hypothesis Tests

While most recent work on point case events has emphasised modelling, the possibility of employing simple hypothesis tests for assessment of spatial effects can be considered. Although statistical modelling is usually preferred as a paradigm, many epidemiologists employ tests or confidence intervals based on summary measures, partly because such results can be simpler to communicate to a non-specialist audience.

For standard HEPP models, Laplace's test can assess simple trend effects (Cox and Lewis, 1966). This is the score test for exponential trend and is uniformly most powerful (UMP) for monotone alternatives (provided a UMP test exists). Cox (1972) discussed tests in modulated HEPP models in one dimension. Lawson (1993b) presents tests for spatial effects in modulated HEPP models. These include a variety of score tests for radial, directional and directional–radial correlation. The score test for radial monotonic trend based on a realisation of $\{r_i, \theta_i\}$ within W is given by

$$W_r = \frac{\bar{r} - E(r)}{\sqrt{\{E(r^2) - E(r)^2\}/n}},$$

where $\bar{r}$ is the average of the distances and

$$E(\cdot) = \int \cdot \hat{g}(r)\, \mathrm{d}\underline{r} \Big/ \int \hat{g}(r)\, \mathrm{d}\underline{r} \quad \text{and} \quad \mathrm{d}\underline{r} = \mathrm{d}r\, \mathrm{d}\theta.$$

The statistics W_r has a standard normal distribution if the model is correct and m is large. However, often some of these conditions may be violated in practice and as a result resort may need to be made to Monte Carlo testing.

Note that both likelihood ratio (LR) and score tests are available in statistical software packages (such as GLIM) if one uses the Berman–Turner approach mentioned above (Lawson, 1992; Berman and Turner, 1992; Lawson and Williams, 1994).

Tests of monotonic radial decline assume that distance acts as a surrogate for exposure. Many proposed tests are based on radial decline models in point data (Lloyd, 1982; Diggle, 1990) and count data (Section 7.7). However, a wide variety of spatial effects could arise due to pollution from a fixed source, and overemphasis on radial decline can yield erroneous conclusions. For example, outfall from stack plumes tends to peak at some distance from a source. Hence, one would expect a peak-and-decline intensity to be present (Panopsky and Dutton, 1984). Simple radial decline tests can have low power when non-monotone effects, such as these, are present (Lawson, 1993c).

The collection of data and spatial modelling of exposure levels should lead to increased power to detect pollution effects. Unobserved heterogeneity in tests may be included as random effects following the generalised linear mixed models described by Breslow and Clayton (1993). Alternatively, the heterogeneity may be formulated as nuisance parameters. One typically structures this approach around a normal approximation, although one could use generalised Monte Carlo tests (based on MCMC algorithms). Lawson and Harrington (1996) examined Monte Carlo tests when spatial correlation is present.

7.5.3 Diagnostic Techniques

The analysis of residual diagnostics for the assessment of goodness-of-fit of a model is common practice in statistical modelling. Usually, such diagnostics are used to assess overall model goodness-of-fit as well as specific features in the data. If a spatial point process model fits well and all relevant covariates are included, we expect spatially independent residuals. Residual analysis for spatial point processes is a developing area and worthy of future research. In Section 5.3, a general discussion of diagnostic methods appears. Here we examine diagnostic methods which have been applied within putative source applications.

Diagnostic techniques display 'outliers' or unusual features not accounted for by a model. If the underlying model assumes no clustering of events, unusually strong clustering can be highlighted by clusters of positive residuals. Clustering may be reflected in positive spatial autocorrelation among residuals, or isolated areas of positive residual clusters.

For point event data it is possible to use a 'transformation' residual (Diggle, 1990) to detect the above effects. This residual relies on the transformation of distance from source and is often used in time domain analysis (Ogata, 1988). A general deviance residual for HEPP models has been proposed (Lawson, 1993a) and applied to pollution source data (Lawson and Williams, 1994). This more general residual takes the form of $r_i = \text{sgn}\{a_i - \tau\hat{\lambda}_i\}\sqrt{d_i}$, where $\tau = n/\sum_i \hat{\lambda}_i a_i$, and $\hat{\lambda}_i$ is the fitted model intensity, and d_i is the deviance contribution at the ith point. Here, a_i is the ith Dirichlet tile area. The deviance contribution is

$$d_i = -\ln\tau - \ln\hat{\lambda}_i a_i - 1 + \tau\hat{\lambda}_i a_i.$$

This crude deviance residual can also be standardised.

The extension of point process residuals to count data may be problematic as the aggregation of residuals will depend on the arbitrary definition of the shape and size of subregions. Standardised Anscombe residuals are available for count data, but many of the usual distributional assumptions relating to these may be violated (McCullagh and Nelder, 1989).

For analysis of Bayesian models where samples from the posterior distribution are available, the Bayesian residuals or other variants described in Section 5.3 could also be employed. The deviance residual specified above could be used in a Bayesian setting where model-based posterior simulations of λ_i are available.

7.6 A CASE EVENT EXAMPLE

As an example of the analysis of a putative source of hazard, we examine the Armadale data example. In this example 49 deaths from respiratory cancer were recorded in a six-year period in a small industrial town for the period 1968–1974. This data set has been analysed with a CHD realisation as control. Detailed discussion of the appropriateness of this as a control is given in Lawson and Williams (1994), where the original analysis was presented. A hypothesised cause of the increased incidence of respiratory cancer was the presence of a steel foundry in the town. The operating practices of the foundry were modified shortly before the study period, and it is thought that forms of tumour promoter in the foundry air emissions could have reduced the latency period for the disease of interest. To analyse the foundry as a putative health hazard, the distance (r) and angle (θ) of cases around the central foundry was recorded. There is no record of occupational confounding in this data nor any deaths related to smoking history. A variety of models have been fitted to this data based on specifications of $f(\boldsymbol{x}; \boldsymbol{\theta})$.

The results of fitting a variety of distance and distance–directional models for the Armadale example are displayed in the above table. The best subset model is displayed for two different background estimates: CHD control disease realisation, and expected deaths computed for 18 enumeration districts. The expected deaths are

Table 7.2 Armadale: ML estimates for the best subset models for CHD and expected death background estimation.

parameter	CHD control	expected deaths
grand mean	2.78 (0.207)	3.064 (0.405)
r	—	0.034 (0.018)
$\cos\theta$	−0.935 (0.275)	—
$\sin\theta$	−0.331 (0.217)	—
$r\cos\theta$	—	−0.001 (0.014)
$r\sin\theta$	—	−0.02 (0.008)
null deviance	92 (78)	77 (78)
deviance (df)	73 (76)	66.5 (75)
AIC	583.6	582.2

only available at a high-resolution level and this affects the final model fitting. As can be seen, different control estimates are associated with different best subset models. For the CHD control, only direction components are included, while under expected deaths, directional-linear components are admitted and there is some evidence for a distance effect also. This lack of invariance between choices of background estimators is due in part to the profile likelihood model which conditions on the estimated control/background. One way round this problem is to incorporate the estimation of the background within the estimation of the likelihood. This has been examined recently within an MCMC approach (Lawson and Clark, 1999b).

Some further criticisms can be made concerning this likelihood-based analysis of the Armadale data. First, it is assumed that there is no unexplained variation in the data. However, it might be assumed that individuals may vary randomly in their propensity to contract the disease of interest and further that unobserved covariates may induce further random variation in the expected intensity of cases. These two situations represent uncorrelated and correlated heterogeneity, respectively. In addition, uncorrelated random susceptibility can be regarded as a form of frailty (see Clayton (1991) and also Lawson (1996b)). In the Armadale example, an analysis of such models has been previously made and the results are presented in Lawson *et al.* (1996a). A comparison of a fully Bayesian analysis and maximum *a posteriori* estimation based on a Taylor approximation was made (see Section 5.2.4). The Taylor expansion was around a saturated estimate of local intensity ($\tilde{\lambda}_i = 1/\{\hat{g}(\boldsymbol{x}_i)a_i\}$) for the Poisson process likelihood specified with $\lambda(\boldsymbol{x}_i) = g(\boldsymbol{x}_i)\exp\{\eta(\boldsymbol{x}_i)\}$. Then, the prior distribution for $\boldsymbol{\eta}$ given by MVN$(F\alpha, K)$ yields the GLS estimator of α:

$$\hat{\alpha} = (F'K_*^{-1}F)^{-1}F'K_*^{-1}\tilde{\boldsymbol{\eta}}, \tag{7.3}$$

$$\tilde{\eta}_i = -\ln\{\hat{g}(\boldsymbol{x}_i)a_i\},$$

$$K_* = K + I_n. \tag{7.4}$$

Table 7.3 Armadale: best BIC model comparing MAP and Metropolis–Hastings posterior expectation.

parameter	MAP estimate (s.e.)	M–H expectation (s.e.*)
1	1.919 (0.8528)	1.6121 (0.8124)
r	−0.269 (0.3248)	−0.3245 (0.3012)
$\log(r)$	−2.629 (0.2368)	−1.9126 (0.6249)
$\cos(\theta)$	−6.468 (0.1962)	−5.9172 (1.5972)
$\sin(\theta)$	0.276 (0.6897)	0.2611 (0.9273)
$r\cos(\theta)$	4.496 (0.7384)	4.0011 (0.9211)
$r\sin(\theta)$	0.426 (0.1498)	0.5213 (0.1917)
σ^2	0.050 (0.0120)	0.6251 (0.3139)
$\boldsymbol{R}$	1.051 (0.4791)	0.00685 (0.01812)

*Empirical estimates: final 100 iterations.

with $\text{cov}(\hat{\alpha}) = (F'K_*^{-1}F)^{-1}$. Estimation with this approach can proceed iteratively by least-squares estimation of α followed by estimation of parameters in K (variance σ^2 and range R), and then re-estimation of α based on (7.3). This is a form of REML estimation. The fully Bayesian approach samples the full posterior distribution with Poisson process likelihood and MVN prior distribution. A Metropolis–Hastings sampler can be employed for this purpose and is described in Lawson *et al.* (1996a) and Diggle *et al.* (1998).

The results above suggest that a model including a distance effect is relevant and some directional components are also present, once the unobserved heterogeneity is accounted for. There is a strong indication that uncorrelated heterogeneity is present although there appears to be little evidence of autocorrelation here. The differences between the estimated covariance structures between the approximate MAP estimates and the full Bayesian estimate warrant further investigation. Residual analysis based on model and saturated estimates of λ_i, for the MAP estimation, demonstrate low autocorrelation (based on Moran's I under conditional randomisation).

7.7 MODELS FOR COUNT DATA

As mentioned above, outcome data may be available only as counts for small census regions rather than event locations for a variety of reasons. As a result, a considerable literature has developed concerning the analysis of such data (Tango, 1995; Clayton and Kaldor, 1987; Whittemore *et al.*, 1987; Cressie and Chan, 1989; Hills and Alexander, 1989; Bithell, 1990; Marshall, 1991a; Lawson, 1993c; Devine and Louis, 1994; Best *et al.*, 1998; Stern and Cressie, 1999).

Let $n_i, i = 1, \ldots, m$, denote the count of disease (or other outcome) events within m arbitrary regions or tracts. We assume the study window includes all m region centres. Other sampling rules may lead to size biases in selection of regions (Miles, 1974). For example, the inclusion rule, 'all regions intersecting the window' (plus sampling), leads to a bias towards larger regions.

The usual model adopted for the region counts assumes $\{n_i\}$ to be independent Poisson random variables with parameters $\{\lambda_i\}$. Any non-overlapping regionalisation of a HEPP leads to independently Poisson distributed regional event counts with means

$$\lambda_i = \int_{a_i} \lambda(\boldsymbol{x})\,\mathrm{d}\boldsymbol{x}, \qquad i = 1, \ldots, m,$$

where $\lambda(\boldsymbol{x})$ is the first-order intensity of the HEPP and a_i is the extent of the ith subregion.

The analysis and interpretation of models based on these assumptions is not without problems. First, many studies of count data assume that λ_i is constant within region a_i so spatial variation between regions follows a step function (Diggle, 1993). When λ_i is parametrised as a log-linear function, one often treats explanatory variables (in particular exposure or radial distance from a pollution source) as constants for the subregions or as occurring at region centres only. While such log-linear models can be useful in describing the global characteristics of a pattern, the differences between a_is and any continuous variation in $\lambda(\boldsymbol{x})$ between and within regions is largely ignored. Second, the underlying process of events may not be a HEPP, in which case the independence assumption may not hold or the Poisson distributional assumption may be violated. Assessments of model assumptions do not usually appear in studies of pollution sources (Bhopal *et al.*, 1992; Elliott *et al.*, 1992b; Waller *et al.*, 1993). Analysis based on regional counts is ecological in nature and inference can suffer from the well-known 'ecological fallacy' of attributing effects observed in aggregate to individuals (see Richardson (1992) for a review and Chapter 10). Finally, extreme sparseness in the data (i.e. large numbers of zero counts) can lead to a bimodal marginal distribution of counts or invalidate asymptotic sampling distributions (Zelterman, 1987).

While the above factors should be taken into consideration, the independent Poisson model is a useful starting point from which to examine effects of pollution sources (Bithell and Stone, 1989). One often uses a log-linear model with a modulating function e_i, say, which acts as the link of the population of subregion i to the expected deaths in subregion i, $i = 1, \ldots, m$. Usually, the expected count is modelled as

$$E(n_i) = \lambda_i = e_i m(\exp(F\alpha)).$$

Here, the e_i, $i = 1, \ldots, m$, act as a background rate for the m subregions. The function $m(\cdot)$ represents a link to spatial and other covariates in the $m \times q$ design matrix F. The parameter vector α has dimension $q \times 1$. Define the polar coordinates of the subregion centre as (r_i, θ_i), relative to the pollution source. Often, the only variable to be included in F is r, the radial distance from the source. When this is used alone, an additive link such as $m(\cdot) = 1 + \exp(F\alpha)$ is appropriate since (for radial distance decline) the background rate (e_i) is unaltered at great distances. However, directional variables (e.g. $\cos\theta$, $\sin\theta$, $r\cos\theta$, $\log(r)\cos\theta$, etc.) representing preferred direction and angular-linear correlation can also be useful in detecting directional preference resulting from preferred directions of pollution outfall.

One may extend this model to include unobserved heterogeneity between regions by introducing a prior distribution for the log relative risks ($\log \lambda_i$, $i = 1, \ldots, m$). This could be defined to include spatially uncorrelated or correlated heterogeneity. The empirical and fully Bayesian methods described in Section 4.3.4 often take this approach.

7.7.1 Estimation

One may estimate the parameters of the log-linear model via maximum likelihood through standard GLM packages, such as GLIM. Using GLIM, one treats the known log of the background hazard for each subregions, e_i, $i = 1, \ldots, m$, as an 'offset'. A multiplicative (log) link can be directly modelled in this way, while an additive link can be programmed via user-defined macros (Breslow and Day, 1984).

Log-linear models are appropriate if due care is taken to examine whether model assumptions are met. For example, Lawson (1993c) suggests avoiding the violation of asymptotic sampling distributions by the use of Monte Carlo tests for change of deviance. If a model fits well, then the standardised model residuals should be approximately independently and identically distributed (i.i.d.). One may use auto-correlation tests, again via Monte Carlo, and make any required model adjustments. If such residuals are not available directly, then it is always possible to compare crude model residuals to a simulation envelope of m sets of residuals generated from the fitted model.

7.7.2 Hypothesis Tests

Most of the existing literature on regional counts of health effects of pollution sources is based on hypothesis testing. Stone (1988) first outlined tests specifically designed for count data of events around a pollution source. These tests are based on the ratio of observed to expected counts cumulated over distance from a pollution source:

$$T = \max \sum_i^j n_i \Big/ \sum_i^j e_i, \qquad 1 \leqslant j \leqslant m.$$

The tests are based on the assumption of independent Poisson counts with monotonic distance ordering. A number of case studies have been based on these tests (Elliott *et al.*, 1992b, 1996; Bithell, 1990, 1995; Waller *et al.*, 1993; Bithell and Stone, 1989).

While Stone's test is based on traditional epidemiological estimates (i.e. SMRs), the test is not UMP for a monotonic trend. If a UMP test exists, it is a score test for particular clustering alternative hypotheses. Such a test can be defined as

$$W_r = \frac{\sum_i r_i(n_i - e_i)}{\sqrt{\{\sum_i r_i^2 e_i - (\sum_i r_i e_i)^2 / \sum_i n_i\}}}. \tag{7.5}$$

Table 7.4 Falkirk example: results of log-linear model fits.

model	deviance (d.f.)
null	14.834 (25)
r	13.789 (24)
Dep	14.704 (24)
Dep $+r$	13.437 (23)
Dep $+ \cos\theta + \sin\theta$	13.460 (22)
$\cos\theta + \sin\theta$	13.835 (23)
$r + \cos\theta + \sin\theta$	12.808 (22)

This test statistic also has a standard normal distribution when the model is correct and m is large. Monte Carlo testing can be used when such conditions are not met. Waller and Lawson (1995) compare the analytic power functions of Stone's test, a score test and focused versions of the method of Besag and Newell (1991) versus monotonic cluster alternatives. The power of Stone's test is typically less than that of the score test, and slower to improve than that of the Besag and Newell method as clusters become more extreme (i.e. higher relative risk of disease within the cluster).

Both Stone's test and a score test for monotonic trend will have low power against non-monotone alternatives. A score test versus a non-monotone, peaked alternative has also been developed (Lawson, 1993c). In summary, if a particular type of clustering (i.e. a particular alternative hypothesis) is of interest, one maximises statistical power by developing score tests (Bithell, 1995).

7.8 A COUNT DATA EXAMPLE

As an example of the type of analysis possible with tract count data, the Falkirk respiratory cancer example (Section 1.4.2) has been analysed with regards to a putative hazard air pollution hazard. The counts of respiratory cancer for 26 enumeration districts have been examined in conjunction with some explanatory variables. The variables examined are the Carstairs deprivation index which is designed to act as a surrogate for lifestyle and socio-economic status variables, and functions of distance and direction from the source (measured to tract centroids). We have used the log of the expected number of cases as an offset within a generalised linear model for the tract counts. This model consists of a Poisson error and log link, which ensures positivity of the expectations. Explanatory variables can be added to the model linearly. This type of analysis was first proposed by Lawson (1993c).

In Table 7.4, the null model deviance (for the log offset model) is 14.834 on 25 degrees of freedom. Addition of a variety of single variable and multiple variable models consisting of deprivation, distance, cosine and sine of angle, and functions of these variables did not produce any 'significant' reduction in deviance from the null model. Deprivation produced the least reduction (0.1301 on 1 df). Distance alone reduced the deviance by 1.045, while in combination with deprivation a further reduction of 0.3 was found. Directional variables also reduced the deviance by similar amount to distance. However, none of these factors were significant. It would appear therefore that a tentative conclusion of this analysis is that the null model (that of counts generated from the local expectations) could be accepted as the best model for this example. It must also be concluded that there is some evidence of distance and directional effects, but these are not strong enough to reach significance, and so there is little evidence of a link between the putative source and respiratory cancer incidence in this example.

A number of concerns arise when considering the analysis just presented. These concerns can be regarded mainly as criticisms of the tenability of the assumptions of the analysis. First, the assumption of piecewise-constant risk within each tract may not be appropriate, and so any substantial analysis should examine models where $\lambda_i = \int_{a_i} e(u)m(F(u)\alpha)\,du$ to ensure correct adjustment for aggregation from case events. Second, the linearity assumption of the log-linear model may be inappropriate. Some or all covariates included in the model may be better modelled via nonlinear functions and this could be examined via generalised Poisson additive models (Hastie and Tibshirani, 1990). One advantage of this approach is that some part of unexplained random variation on the counts may be absorbed by the smoothing operation performed on covariates. In the Falkirk example, spline smoothing of deprivation and inclusion of smoothing of the expected rates for the tracts does produce lower deviances for the same models cited above, but they do not alter the relative goodness-of-fit of the models nor yield any substantially improved absolute fits. Finally, it is always possible that unexplained variation in the tract counts exists (due to unobserved covariates) and this extra effect could be modelled via the inclusion of tract-specific random effects. These effects could be regarded as frailties (to mirror the use of such effects for individuals). Random-effect modelling will usually capture a component of extra variation in the data if such a component exists, and may give insight into the form of lack of fit of the model to the data. In addition, the use of such effects will improve the precision of estimation while providing greater latitude in the specification of model components. An example of such modelling based on approximate maximum *a posteriori* estimation applied to a putative source example is available (Lawson, 1994b). In that example the random effects were assumed to have a log-Gaussian prior distribution with uncorrelated and correlated components.

7.9 OTHER DIRECTIONS

7.9.1 Multiple Disease Analysis

In the analysis of the health status of populations within specific geographical regions, it is often appropriate to examine several diseases simultaneously. For example, in the investigation of health consequences of living near putative sources of air pollution, often a selection of diseases will be thought to have a link with the pollution. A major difficulty is identifying the most appropriate diseases to include in the investigation.

Incinerators, for example, emit an enormous variety of substances: aluminium, antimony, arsenic, beryllium, bismuth, cadmium, cobalt, copper, iron, lead, magnesium, mercury, molybdenum, nickel, selenium, silver, thallium, tin, titanium, tungsten, uranium, vanadium, zinc and zirconium. This lists just the inorganic fraction; the list is equally long for the organic compounds such as polychlorinated biphenyls. The identification of the most appropriate disease to study is further complicated because different chemicals target different organs of the body. Toxicity can vary between the sexes. Also the old, young and immuno-compromised are generally more susceptible to the effects of toxins.

Despite the multiplicity of possible health outcomes, it is usually possible to suggest a ranking of the importance of each disease. The ideal statistical model is one which could accommodate both the competition between diseases as they affect a population (competing risks) and also a method for weighting each disease or health indicator. An added benefit of such a model would be the removal of the need to perform multiple testing on the same data set.

Previous work on multiple disease assessment is limited. The use of cumulative p-value plotting has been suggested for multiple testing of *single* outcomes. Although this method has not been applied to multiple spatial pattern analysis, it could be extended to include prior weighting.

The purpose of this section is to outline a general model for competing risks which could, if required, include prior weighting. The application of the model will be demonstrated by a study of health status in a small town.

The Case Event Situation

In what follows, the methods described are largely those described in Lawson and Williams (2000).

A study window of area A is defined and the locations of disease events of m types are recorded within this window. The window may be delineated according to topographical features or other factors of public health importance. The location of events are $\{\boldsymbol{x}_i\}, i = 1, \ldots, n$. The first-order intensity of disease event j at location i is $\lambda_j(\boldsymbol{x}_i)$. This intensity is defined in the usual way. We assume that the intensity $\lambda_j(\cdot)$ is the realisation of a spatial stochastic process on $\mathbb{R}^+$, and conditional on the realisation of the m-set of intensities, then the ith disease is independently distributed as a modulated heterogeneous Poisson process with intensity $\lambda_i(\boldsymbol{x})$. This does not preclude the possibility of prior, possibly spatially dependent, cross-correlation between the intensities. The detailed modelling of $\lambda_j(\cdot)$ is discussed later.

Denoting the binary labelling variable $c(\boldsymbol{x}_i)$ with $c(\boldsymbol{x}_i) = 1$ representing a case labelling of $\boldsymbol{x}_i$. Also denote the disease type label as t, with $k = 1, \ldots, m$ types.

Given this conditioning, then

$$\Pr(c(\boldsymbol{x}) = 1, t = j) = \Pr(t = j \mid c(\boldsymbol{x}) = 1) \Pr(c(\boldsymbol{x}) = 1).$$

The left-hand term is given straightforwardly by

$$\lambda_j(\boldsymbol{x}) \Big/ \sum_{k=1}^{m} \lambda_k(\boldsymbol{x}), \tag{7.6}$$

while the right-hand term is the total intensity at $\boldsymbol{x}$, times $\partial\boldsymbol{x}$, a small spatial increment,

$$\lambda(\boldsymbol{x})\partial\boldsymbol{x},$$

where

$$\lambda(\boldsymbol{x}) = \sum_{k=1}^{m} \lambda_k(\boldsymbol{x}). \tag{7.7}$$

Hence, the probability of a death at $\boldsymbol{x}$ of cause j simplifies to

$$\lambda_j(\boldsymbol{x})\partial\boldsymbol{x}. \tag{7.8}$$

The likelihood of n events is then

$$L_1 = \prod_{i=1}^{n} \lambda_j(\boldsymbol{x}_i) \exp\left\{-\int_A \sum_{k=1}^{m} \lambda_k(\boldsymbol{u})\,\mathrm{d}\boldsymbol{u}\right\}, \tag{7.9}$$

where the j subscript denotes the death type of the event at $\boldsymbol{x}_i$.

Note that L_1 can be written as

$$L_2 = \prod_{k=1}^{m}\left[\prod_{\phi_k} \lambda_k(\boldsymbol{x}_{ik})\mathrm{e}^{-\int_A \lambda_k(\boldsymbol{u})\,\mathrm{d}\boldsymbol{u}}\right], \tag{7.10}$$

where ϕ_k denotes the death set for the kth disease. Hence, unless prior dependence between disease intensities or other conditioning is included, then each disease can be modelled separately as

$$\ell_2 = \sum_{k=1}^{m}\left[\sum_{\phi_k} \ln \lambda_k(\boldsymbol{x}_{ik}) - \int_A \lambda_k(\boldsymbol{u})\,\mathrm{d}\boldsymbol{u}\right]. \tag{7.11}$$

Intensity Parametrisation

The modelling of $\lambda_k(\boldsymbol{x})$ can be considered separately for each disease type, given the independence inherent in ℓ_2 above. For example, for an intensity defined as a function of distance from a putative source of hazard at $\boldsymbol{x}_0$ we could have

$$\lambda_k(\boldsymbol{x}) = h_k(\boldsymbol{x})\{1 + f(|\boldsymbol{x} - \boldsymbol{x}_0|)\},$$

where $h_k(\boldsymbol{x})$ is a background rate for disease k at $\boldsymbol{x}$, and $f(\cdot)$ is some function of distance from the source. Hence, each disease could have a background or some or all of the diseases could share a background. This latter condition may be assumed for examples like larynx and lung cancer or other diseases which are site and/or age specific.

Note that the method proposed by Diggle and Rowlingson (1994) (DR), which conditions the analysis of a single disease on the joint distribution of cases and controls, cannot be used, with different $h_k(\boldsymbol{x})$ for each disease, as

$$\frac{\lambda_j(\boldsymbol{x})}{\sum_{k=1}^m \lambda_k(\boldsymbol{x})} = \frac{h_j(\boldsymbol{x})(1+f_j(\boldsymbol{x}))}{\sum_{k=1}^m h_k(\boldsymbol{x})(1+f_k(\boldsymbol{x}))}$$

and

$$\Pr(c(\boldsymbol{x})=1, t=j) = \frac{h_j(\boldsymbol{x})(1+f_j(\boldsymbol{x}))}{\sum_{k=1}^m h_k(\boldsymbol{x})(2+f_k(\boldsymbol{x}))}.$$

However, it should also be noted that if the DR model is taken *unconditionally* for a single disease, then the case event locations can be modelled via (7.9), with controls acting as the competing 'disease'.

An Alternative Formulation

An alternative formulation of this problem is to consider the special case where only control diseases are used to represent the background population 'at risk'. In that case we can consider the probability conditional on the binary labelling of a case of disease j at $\boldsymbol{x}$, which is

$$\frac{h_j(\boldsymbol{x})(1+f_j(\boldsymbol{x}))}{\sum_{k=1}^m [h_k(\boldsymbol{x}) + h_k(\boldsymbol{x})(1+f_k(\boldsymbol{x}))]} = \frac{h_j(\boldsymbol{x})(1+f_j(\boldsymbol{x}))}{\sum_{k=1}^m h_k(\boldsymbol{x})(2+f_k(\boldsymbol{x}))}.$$

Now, in this case, it is possible for the background function $h_j(\boldsymbol{x})$ to be 'conditioned out' but only if $h_j \equiv h_k \; \forall_k$.

When there is *a common control* for all diseases, then we can write

$$\Pr(c(\boldsymbol{x})=1; t=j) = \frac{1+f_j(\boldsymbol{x})}{2m+\sum_{k=1}^m f_k(\boldsymbol{x})},$$

$$\Pr(c(\boldsymbol{x})=0; t=j) = \frac{1}{2m+\sum_{k=1}^m f_k(\boldsymbol{x})}.$$

The conditional likelihood for the case-control realisations then becomes

$$L_3 = \prod_{k=1}^m \left[\prod_{\ell=1}^{n_k} \frac{1+f_k(\boldsymbol{x}_\ell)}{2m+\sum_{k=1}^m f_k(\boldsymbol{x}_\ell)}\right]\left[\prod_{d=1}^{c_k} \frac{1}{2m+\sum_{k=1}^m f_k(\boldsymbol{x}_\mathrm{d})}\right], \tag{7.12}$$

where ℓ denotes events of the kth group disease and d denotes locations of controls for kth disease, and n_k and c_k are the numbers of cases and controls for the kth disease. Note that, although the background factors out in this case the likelihoods for each disease/control set are not independent, and hence they must be examined jointly in any estimation procedure. The log likelihood from the above model is

$$\ell_3 = \sum_{k=1}^{m}\left[\sum_{\ell=1}^{n_k}\ln(1+f_k(\boldsymbol{x}_\ell)) - \sum_{\ell=1}^{n_k}\ln\left(2m+\sum_{k=1}^{m}f_k(\boldsymbol{x}_\ell)\right) - \sum_{d=1}^{c_k}\ln\left(2m+\sum_{k=1}^{m}f_k(\boldsymbol{x}_\mathrm{d})\right)\right].$$

Correlation Between Intensities

Cross-correlation between diseases in space may arise in a variety of situations. Common 'at-risk' population distributions can produce common elevations of incidence in a variety of diseases, e.g. bronchitis and pneumonia, larynx and respiratory cancer.

However, little appears to be known about the 'normal' spatial *cross*-correlation between disease types. For example, are there spatial conditions which produce patterns which are not predicted by age, sex or lifestyle strata? If so, this cross-correlation could require the inclusion of prior models which differ from the independence model of the previous section. Dependent point process models have been proposed for ordinary stationary point processes. In the absence of prior information on such cross-correlation, we have assumed that such modelling is not necessary and therefore have not included this function.

Prior Beliefs

We could extend the independent model analysis by assigning weights to the diseases of interest in relation to their perceived importance. For example, $\lambda(\boldsymbol{x})$ could be defined as

$$\lambda(\boldsymbol{x}) = \sum_{k=1}^{m} w_k\lambda_k(\boldsymbol{x}),$$

where w_k is a predefined 'importance' weight. In the case of the case/control formulation above, this leads to the likelihood

$$\prod_{k=1}^{m}\left[\prod_{\ell=1}^{n_k}\frac{w_k(1+f_k(\boldsymbol{x}_\ell))}{\sum_{k=1}^{m}w_k(2+f_k(\boldsymbol{x}_\ell))}\right]\left[\prod_{t=1}^{c_k}\frac{w_k}{\sum_{k=1}^{m}w_k(2+f_k(\boldsymbol{x}_t))}\right], \tag{7.13}$$

which has (7.12) as a special case when $w_i = 1\ \forall_i$. Alternatively, a subjectivist Bayesian analysis of importance could be employed. Because the results from a number of diseases or studies are being considered, it may be possible to consider the problem as an application of meta analysis. The assumption of additivity and independence is usually made in that approach. Again this area requires further work, especially as the assessment of particular diseases is often carried out in isolation from other diseases.

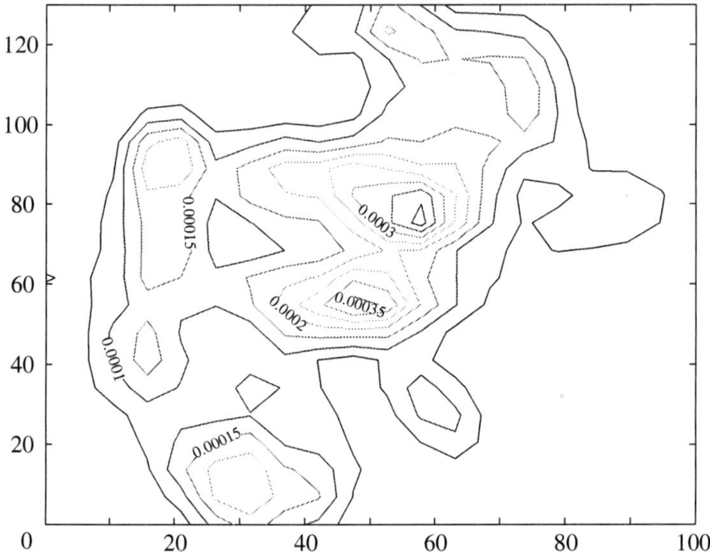

Figure 7.13 Arbroath: contour density map of the control realisation.

Data Example

Mortality from a range of diseases has been under investigation in a town in eastern Scotland for several years. The motivation for this examination was the existence of a steel foundry in the centre of the town. Previous work had linked residential proximity to steel foundries with an increase in several disease rates, but in particular respiratory cancer.

For the years 1966–1976 the numbers of deaths were obtained for five groups of disease. Respiratory, gastric and oesophageal cancers, and bronchitis were chosen because they can be sensitive to elevated levels of airborne environmental pollution. Coronary heart disease and the combination of cancers of the prostate, penis, breast, testes, cervix, uterus, colon and rectum were chosen as the control diseases. This set of lower-body cancers was chosen for its lack of known correlation with air pollution, while maintaining a similar age structure to the case diseases.

Figures 7.13, 7.14 and 7.15 show the surfaces produced by kernel density estimation for three groups of disease (control, gastric and oesophageal cancer and respiratory cancer). The smoothing constants for the estimates were chosen by likelihood cross-validation. The distributions of CHD and the control group of cancers are remarkably similar in their overall spatial expression and so the CHD map is not represented here.

Both show peaks to the north and south of the pollution source. The diseases most likely to show an association with the source, respiratory cancer and bronchitis, peak to the southwest and north of the source. Gastric and oesophageal cancers, which were also expected to show an association with the source, peak on an northeast–southwest axis. However, the pronounced peak only occurs to the northeast of the

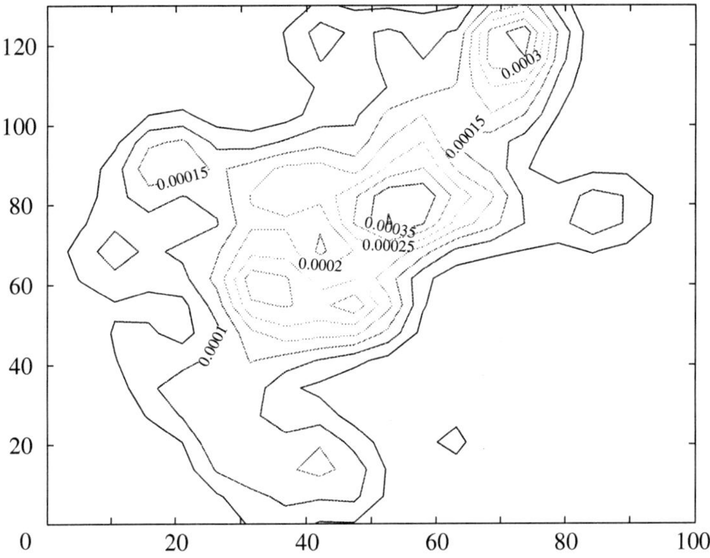

Figure 7.14 Arbroath example: gastric cancer contour density.

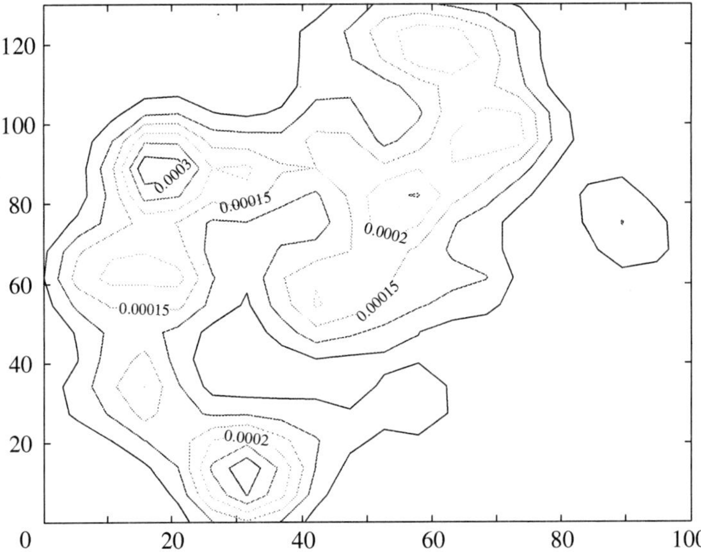

Figure 7.15 Arbroath study: respiratory cancer contour density.

foundry. Hence, while respiratory cancer and bronchitis have similar spatial forms, gastric and oesophageal cancer show different spatial forms.

For this data example, it is possible to examine $k = 3$ case diseases: respiratory cancer, bronchitis and gastric and oesophageal cancers. The control used in the analysis was lower-body cancers. These cancers have a comparable spatial distribution to CHD, and this provides support for their choice. Alternative choices, such as combined controls (CHD and lower-body cancers) or separate control analysis, have not been pursued here.

Our focus is on the application of the general dependence model (7.13) to the Arbroath example and on the effect of prior weighting systems on the analysis. The use of such a conditional logistic approach is justified as control realisations are available and a common control can be employed.

The model components which require definition in (7.13) are w_k and $f_k(\boldsymbol{x})$ $\forall k$.

Choices for w_k and $f_k(\boldsymbol{x})$

In the case of the prior weights, some latitude exists in the specification of constraints for individual w_k. It is usual to require $w_k \geqslant 0$ $\forall_k$, as the weights represent a relative ranking of contribution importance to health status. However, although it is often convenient and also easily interpretable, it is not required that $\sum_{k=1}^{m} w_k = 1$. In what follows we examine three weighting schemes, for w_1 (respiratory cancer), w_2 (bronchitis), w_3 (gastric and oesophageal cancer):

scheme (1) $w_1 = 1, w_2 = 1, w_3 = 1,$

scheme (2) $w_1 = 0.5, w_2 = 0.25, w_3 = 0.25,$

scheme (3) $w_1 = 0.1, w_2 = 0.3, w_3 = 0.6.$

The first scheme represents equal weighting for each disease, whereas the second represents a prior belief ranking which attributes greater importance to respiratory cancer, while the third scheme emphasises bronchitis and gastric and oesophageal cancer.

The model chosen for $f_k(\boldsymbol{x})$ was based on a simple distance-from-source decline model consisting of four parameters which can differ for each disease type,

$$f_k(\boldsymbol{x}) = \rho(1 + \alpha_1 \exp(-\alpha_2 d(\boldsymbol{x}) + \alpha_3 \log d(\boldsymbol{x}))),$$

where $d(\boldsymbol{x}) = \|\boldsymbol{x} - \boldsymbol{x}_0\|$.

A variety of distance and directional components could be included in these models. However, for the purposes of demonstration of the method we have included a log (distance) and distance effect which should capture monotone and peaked distance effects.

Computational Method

Model (7.13) consists of a likelihood, which can be maximised to yield conventional Maximum likelihood estimates and associated standard errors. However, in this application we employ a stochastic algorithm which allows exploration of the likelihood surface and provides standard errors derived directly from the surface, via simulation. This exploration avoids the problems which can arise with local maxima when large

Table 7.5 Modal parameter values for posterior marginal distributions under the weighting schemes.

(RC, respiratory cancer; G&OC, gastric and oesophageal cancer; B, bronchitis; sd, the empirical standard deviation of the realised values within the final converged sample.)

Scheme 1	RC	sd	G&OC	sd	B	sd
base rate (ρ)	0.3773	0.0129	0.3328	0.0130	0.7676	0.0204
link rate (α_1)	−0.0176	0.1027	−0.0176	0.0930	−0.0191	0.1168
distance: d (α_2)	0.0961	0.1266	0.1000	0.0731	0.1823	0.1807
log(d) (α_3)	0.0892	0.1134	−0.0247	0.1367	−0.0181	0.0942
Scheme 2	**RC**	**sd**	**G&OC**	**sd**	**B**	**sd**
base rate (ρ)	0.2551	0.0184	0.013	0.0019	0.0225	0.0335
link rate (α_1)	−0.0193	0.0735	5.8371	0.2997	−0.0189	0.1478
distance: d (α_2)	0.1214	0.1360	0.0325	0.0018	0.0740	0.0487
log(d) (α_3)	−0.0199	0.1652	1.496	0.0363	1.5562	0.1145
Scheme 3	**RC**	**sd**	**G&OC**	**sd**	**B**	**sd**
base rate (ρ)	1.2146	0.0688	0.8993	0.0371	0.1822	0.0073
link rate (α_1)	−0.0235	0.1599	−0.0194	0.1108	0.0468	0.0566
distance: d (α_2)	0.1685	0.1750	0.1358	0.1476	0.0168	0.0140
log(d) (α_3)	0.0841	0.1342	0.0923	0.1086	0.0923	0.1186

numbers of parameters are to be estimated and provides more information about the likelihood surface besides the maximum value.

The algorithm employed is a Metropolis–Hastings (M–H) MCMC sampler. The parameters included are assumed to have uniform distributions on suitable ranges and hence these are used as proposals for the M–H acceptance criteria. Convergence of the algorithm was checked using standard diagnostics.

Discussion

Table 7.5 displays the modal results of the sampler runs for each weighting system. Included in this table are the modal value of the final likelihood surface for each parameter component. In addition, the empirical standard deviation of the final converged sample is provided. It is used as a measure of variability but is not intended as an estimate of the variability of the modal estimate.

There appears to be considerable changes between the different weighting schemes. Respiratory cancer displays a stable pattern for certain parameters. The link rate (α_1), the distance parameter (α_2) and the log-distance parameter (α_3) all appear to have similar density estimates (not shown) and modal values across schemes. However, the base rate (ρ) changes considerably and displays a multimodal density in scheme 3. This may be related to ascribing a very low weight to this disease in this scheme.

In the case of bronchitis, the base rate appears to change markedly in scheme 3, whereas the α_3 parameter shows the strongest change in scheme 2. In the case of gastric and oesophageal cancer, there are other notable changes. Scheme 2 appears to alter all the modal values considerably. In addition, the standard deviations for this scheme are much altered.

The explanation for the change in the densities under these schemes lies in the ability of highly weighted diseases to dominate the total intensity. In addition, the weighting scheme can alter how much weight is given to specific parameters, e.g. the base rate. It is clear that, without prior judgement concerning weightings, equal weighting systems should be preferred. However, it is also important to be aware of the sensitivity of the final estimates to the weighting scheme chosen.

It is also clear from the analysis of results in Table 7.5 that many link and distance parameters have high variability. In scheme 1 only the base rate (ρ) appears to have low variability for any disease. This is also true for scheme 3. However, in scheme 2, both gastric and oesophageal cancer and bronchitis show low variability in distance parameters. Hence, under this scheme (which gives respiratory cancer a high weight) there appears to be some support for a distance-related effect.

The approach described above has the benefit that it has flexibility for the evaluation, in a single analysis, of multiple disease distributions which appear to show clustering around a putative source. The model described has four main advantages. First, we have shown that a flexible general framework for modelling multiple disease outcomes can be provided by competing risk modelling. In its simplest form it allows individual analysis of multiple diseases provided they are independently associated with the pollution source. Importantly, should the investigator predict multiple disease outcomes which are related, the model can be generalised to include weighting and cross-correlation between the diseases. In addition, a space-time extension is straightforward. The application of this model to the data derived from a small town highlights considerable differences in disease outcome. The three groups of diseases most likely to show an association with airborne pollution showed marked distance-related effects. Gastric and oesophageal cancer showed the most pronounced distance-related effects. The epidemiological data for this town mirror these findings. The similarity of the distribution of CHD and the group of 'other' cancers supports the use of these diseases as controls.

The Tract Count Situation

Define $\underline{n}$ as the $m \times J$ matrix of observed disease counts, where J is the number of disease types. Also, n_{ij} is the count of the jth disease in the ith tract, $\underline{n}_{\cdot j}$ is the $m \times 1$ column vector of counts of the jth disease, and $\underline{n}_{i\cdot}$ is the $1 \times J$ row vector of counts for the ith tract. Then the marginal totals are

$$\underline{n}_{iT} = \sum_{j=1}^{J} \underline{n}_{i\cdot}, \quad \underline{n}_{Tj} = \sum_{i=1}^{m} \underline{n}_{\cdot j} \quad \text{and} \quad N_{\mathrm{T}} = \sum_i \sum_j n_{ij}.$$

The intensity for the ith region can then be specified as

$$\Lambda_i = \int_{a_i} \lambda_T(\boldsymbol{u})\,\mathrm{d}\boldsymbol{u} = \int_{a_i} \sum_j \lambda_j(\boldsymbol{u})\,\mathrm{d}\boldsymbol{u}, \tag{7.14}$$

while we can also define the total intensity over the ith tract for the jth disease as $\Lambda_{ij} = \int_{a_i} \lambda_j(\boldsymbol{u})\,\mathrm{d}\boldsymbol{u}$. The underlying Poisson process assumptions for the total number of cases leads to a likelihood of the form:

$$L = \prod_{i=1}^{n} \{\lambda_T(\boldsymbol{x}_i)\} \exp\left\{-\sum_{l=1}^{m} \int_{a_l} \lambda_T(\boldsymbol{u})\,\mathrm{d}\boldsymbol{u}\right\}. \tag{7.15}$$

Conditional on the n events, the likelihood of the m vector of total disease counts $\{\underline{n}_{iT}\}$ is the multinomial form,

$$L = \prod_{l=1}^{m} q_l^{\underline{n}_{iT}},$$

where the conditional probability of a case in the ith tract is $q_i = \Lambda_i / \sum_{l=1}^{m} \Lambda_l$. Further conditional arguments leads to the likelihood for the realisation of $\{n_{ij}\} \mid m$, namely,

$$L = \prod_{i=1}^{m} \prod_{j=1}^{J} \left\{\frac{\Lambda_{ij}}{\sum_k \sum_l \Lambda_{kl}}\right\}^{n_{ij}}.$$

This leads to a log likelihood of the form,

$$l = \sum_{i=1}^{m} \sum_{j=1}^{J} n_{ij} \log \Lambda_{ij} - N_T \log \sum_{i=1}^{m} \sum_{j=1}^{J} \Lambda_{ij}. \tag{7.16}$$

Hence, the analysis of multiple disease counts within tracts can proceed from the above likelihood definition. Examination of the structure of the Λ_{ij} may allow simplifications of the likelihood as would the use of common disease backgrounds, as noted above. Further extensions could be conceived in which the components of the intensities have prior distributions and this area could be fruitfully exploited via Bayesian analysis. Approximate analysis of multiple disease maps has been attempted via multi-level modelling (Langford *et al.*, 1999b).

7.9.2 Space-Time Modelling

Finally, we have not considered the analysis of space-time processes in relation to pollution sources. If the times of events and exposure measurements are recorded, then the variety of possible models increases considerably. Traditionally, interest has focused on space-time clustering (Knox, 1964; Mantel, 1967; Chen *et al.*, 1984), although separate spatial and/or temporal clustering may have great importance. Diggle *et al.*

(1995) provide an edge-corrected space-time measure and apply it to incidence of legionnaire's disease in Glasgow (see also Bhopal *et al.*, 1992), and Lawson and Viel (1995) provide a different space-time testing method based on directional correlation.

One possible approach to modelling case event data is to examine the *conditional* intensity of a case event at $\{\boldsymbol{x}_i, t_i\}$ given the preceding event's spatio-temporal coordinates and construct a function of distance from the putative source, which includes this conditional specification. This is akin to the approach adopted by Lawson and Viel (1995). This could lead to a sequential test for association. The edge effects found in this procedure are considerable, as censoring at (possibly) random times can occur. These effects must be taken account of carefully.

In general, the equivalent competing risk models in survival analysis lead to similar likelihoods to those given above, but include a survivor function component with the dependence on time. In that case the probability of a disease event at x, in time period ∂t of type j, is

$$\lambda_j(x; t)\partial x \partial t,$$

and thus

$$L_t = \prod_{i=1}^{n} \lambda_j(x_i; t_i) \exp\left\{- \int_A \int_0^{t_0} \sum_{k=1}^{m} \lambda_k(u; v)\, \mathrm{d}u\, \mathrm{d}v\right\}$$

for uncensored event times, where t_0 is the study period time.

In this example, the intensity can be defined to have a space-time-dependent baseline and a distance dependence, for example:

$$\lambda_j(x, t) = h_0(x, t)(1 + \beta_j \|x - x_0\|).$$

This intensity specification could be extended to include case event history also, and could include covariates measured on individuals if available.

CHAPTER 8

Large Scale: Disease Mapping

8.1 INTRODUCTION

The representation and analysis of maps of disease incidence data are now established as a basic tool in the analysis of regional public health. The development of methods for mapping disease incidence has considerably progressed in recent years.

One of the earliest examples of disease mapping is the map of the addresses of cholera victims related to the locations of water supplies by John Snow in 1854. In that case, the street addresses of victims were recorded and their proximity to putative pollution sources (water supply pumps) was assessed.

The use made of maps of disease incidence are many and various. Disease maps can be used to assess the need for geographical variation in health resource allocation, or could be useful in research studies of the relation of incidence to explanatory variables. In the first case, the purpose of mapping is to produce a map 'clean' of any random noise and any artefacts of population variation. This can be achieved by a variety of means. In the second case, specific hypotheses concerning incidence are to be assessed and additional information included in the analysis (e.g. covariates). The first approach is close in approach to image processing, and the second approach can be regarded as a spatial-regression approach. This section focuses on the task of processing georeferenced disease incidence data to produce appropriate or 'true' estimates of the underlying risk over a given study area.

8.2 SIMPLE STATISTICAL REPRESENTATION

The representation of disease incidence data can vary from simple point object maps for cases, and pictorial representation of counts within tracts, to the mapping of estimates from complex models purporting to describe the structure of the disease events. In the following sections we describe the range of mapping methods from simple representation to model based forms.

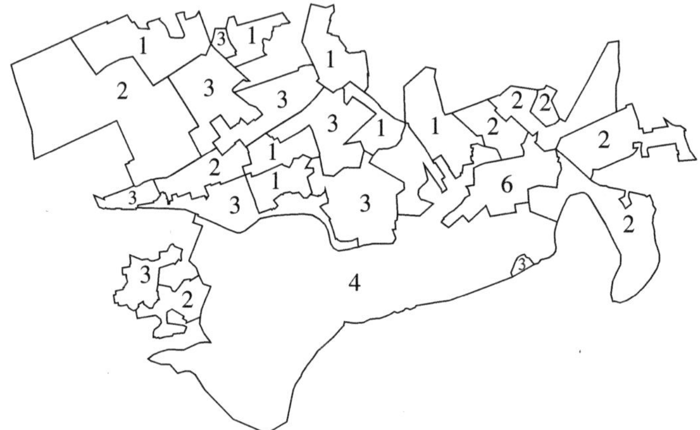

Figure 8.1 Falkirk: central Scotland: counts of respiratory cancer within census tracts.

8.2.1 Crude Rates

The simplest possible mapping form is the depiction of disease rates at specific sets of locations. For case events, this is a map of case event locations. For counts within tracts, this is a pictorial representation of the number of events in the tracts plotted at a suitable set of locations (e.g. tract centroids) (see Figure 8.1). The locations of case events within a spatially heterogeneous population can display a small amount of information concerning the overall pattern of disease events within a window. Ross and Davis (1990) provide an example of such an analysis of leukaemia cluster data. However, any interpretation of the structure of these events is severely limited by the lack of information concerning the spatial distribution of the background population which might be 'at risk' from the disease of concern. This population also has a spatial distribution and failure to take account of this spatial variation severely limits the ability to interpret the resulting case event map. In essence, areas of high density of 'at-risk' population would tend to yield high incidence of case events and so without taking account of this distribution, areas of high disease intensity could be spuriously found.

In the case of counts of cases of disease within tracts, similar considerations apply when crude count maps are constructed. Here, variation in population density also affects the spatial incidence of disease. However, it is also important to consider how a count of disease could be depicted in a mapped representation. Counts within tracts are totals (or averages) of events from the whole tract region. If tracts are irregular, then a decision must be made to either 'locate' the count at some tract location (e.g. tract centroid, however defined) with suitable symbolisation, or to represent the count as a fill colour or shade over the whole tract. In the former case the choice of location will affect interpretation. In the latter case, symbolisation choice could distort interpretation also, although an attempt to represent the whole tract may be attractive.

In general, methods which attempt to incorporate the effect of background 'at-risk' population are to be preferred. These are discussed in the next section.

8.2.2 Standardised Mortality/Morbidity Ratios, Standardisation and Relative Risk Surfaces

To assess the status of an area with respect to disease incidence it is convenient to attempt to first assess what disease incidence should be locally 'expected' in the area and then to compare the observed incidence with the 'expected' incidence. This approach has been traditionally used for the analysis of counts within tracts and can also be applied to case event maps. In the following sections, many of the results derived in Chapter 4 and Sections 4.3.5, 5.1.2 and 5.1.3 are discussed in the context of disease mapping.

Case Events

Case events can be mapped as a map of point event locations. For the purposes of assessment of differences in local disease risk, it is appropriate to convert these locations into a continuous surface describing the spatial variation in *intensity* of the cases. Once this surface is computed, then a measure of local variation is available at any spatial location within the observation window. Denote the intensity surface as $\lambda(\boldsymbol{x})$, where $\boldsymbol{x}$ is a spatial location. This surface can be formally defined as the first-order intensity of a point process on $\mathbb{R}^2$. The surface can be estimated by a variety of methods including density estimation (Härdle, 1991). To provide an estimate of the 'at-risk' population at spatial locations, it is necessary to first choose a measure which will represent the intensity of cases 'expected' at such locations. Define this measure as $g(\boldsymbol{x})$. Two possibilities can be explored. First, it is possible to obtain rates for the case disease from either the whole study window or a larger enclosing region. Usually, these rates are available only aggregated into larger regions (e.g. census tracts). The rates are obtained for a range of subpopulation categories which are thought to affect the case disease incidence. For example, the age and sex structure of the population or the deprivation status of the area (Carstairs, 1981) could affect the amount of population 'at risk' from the case disease. The use of such external rates is often called external standardisation (Inskip *et al.*, 1983). Rates computed within census tracts will be smoother than those based on density estimation of case events. An alternative method of assessing the 'at-risk' population structure is to use a case event map of a disease which represents the background population but is not affected by the aetiological processes of interest in the case disease. For example, the spatial distribution of CHD (ICD codes 410–414), could provide a *control* representation for respiratory cancer (ICD code 162) when the latter is the case disease in a study of air pollution effects, as CHD is less closely related to air pollution insult. While exact matching of diseases in this way will always be difficult, there is an advantage in the use of control diseases in case event examples. If a realisation of the control disease is available in the form of a point event map, then it is possible to also compute an estimate of the first-order intensity of the control disease. This estimate can then be used to compare case intensity with background intensity.

The comparison of estimates of $\lambda(\boldsymbol{x})$ and $g(\boldsymbol{x})$ can be made in a variety of ways. First, it is possible to map the ratio form:

$$R(\boldsymbol{x}) = \frac{\hat{\lambda}(\boldsymbol{x})}{\hat{g}(\boldsymbol{x})}. \tag{8.1}$$

Note that $g(\boldsymbol{x})$ can be estimated from census tract standardised rates instead. Care must be taken to consider the effects of study/observation window edges on the interpretation of such a ratio. Some edge-effect compensation should be considered when there is a considerable influence of window edges in the final interpretation of the map.

Apart from ratio forms it is also possible to map transformations of ratios (e.g. $\log R(\boldsymbol{x})$) or to map

$$D(\boldsymbol{x}) = \hat{\lambda}(\boldsymbol{x}) - \hat{g}(\boldsymbol{x}). \tag{8.2}$$

In all the above approaches to the mapping of case event data some smoothing or interpolation of the event or control data has to be made. The optimal approach to this operation depends on the method used for estimation of each component of the map. Optimal methods for smoothing constant choice are known for intensity/density estimation and kernel smoothing and these are discussed further in Section 8.2.3.

Tract Counts

As in the analysis of case events, it is usual to assess maps of count data by comparison of the observed counts, to those counts 'expected' to arise given the tracts' 'at-risk' population structure. Traditionally, the ratio of observed to expected counts within tracts is called a standardised mortality/morbidity ratio (SMR) and this ratio is an estimate of *relative risk* within each tract (i.e. the ratio describes the risk of being in the disease group rather than the background group). The justification for the use of SMRs can be supported by the analysis of likelihood models with multiplicative expected risk (as described in Section 5.1.3). In Section 8.3.1, we explore further the connection between likelihood models and tract-based estimators of risk.

Define n_i as the observed count of the case disease in the mth tract, and e_i as the expected count within the same tract. Then the SMR is defined as

$$R_i = \frac{n_i}{e_i}. \tag{8.3}$$

The alternative measure of relation between observed and expected counts, which is related to an additive risk model, is the difference:

$$D_i = n_i - e_i. \tag{8.4}$$

In both cases, the comments made above about mapping counts within tracts apply. In this case it must be decided whether to express the R_i or D_i as fill patterns in each region or across regions, or to locate the result at some specified tract location, such as the centroid. If it is decided that these measures should be regarded as continuous across regions, then some further interpolation of R_i or D_i must be made.

8.2.3 Interpolation

In many of the mapping approaches mentioned above, use must be made of interpolation methods to provide estimates of a surface measure at locations where there are no observations. For example, we may wish to map contours of a set of tract counts if we believe the counts to represent a continuously varying risk surface. For the purposes of contouring, a grid of surface interpolant values must be provided. Smoothing of SMRs has been advocated by Breslow and Day (1987). Those authors employ kernel smoothing to interpolate the surface (in a temporal application). The advantage of such smoothing is that the method preserves the positivity condition of SMRs: the method does not produce negative interpolants (which are invalid), unlike kriging methods. Other interpolation methods also suffer from this problem. Many mapping packages utilise interpolation methods to provide gridded data for further contour and perspective view plotting. However, often the methods used are not clearly defined or based on mathematical interpolants (e.g. the Akima interpolator).

Note that the above comments also apply directly to case event density estimation. The use of kernel density estimation is recommended, with edge correction as appropriate. For ratio estimation, Kelsall and Diggle (1995b) recommend the joint estimation of a common smoothing parameter for numerator and denominator of $R(\boldsymbol{x})$ when a control disease realisation is available.

8.2.4 Exploratory Mapping Methods

The above discussion concerning the construction of disease maps applies directly to purely exploratory analysis of disease spatial patterns. For example, the construction of ratios or differences of case and background measures and transformations thereof can be examined in an exploratory approach to disease mapping. This form of mapping is useful for highlighting areas of incidence requiring further consideration. Contour plots or surface views of such mapped data can be derived. However, inspection of maps of simple ratios or differences cannot provide accurate assessment of the statistical significance of, for example, areas of elevated disease risk. Comments concerning the psychological interpretation of mapped patterns also apply here (see Section 5.1.1 and Chapter 3).

8.3 BASIC MODELS

In Section 8.2, we discussed the use of primarily *descriptive* methods in the construction of disease maps. These methods do not introduce any particular model structure or constraint into the mapping process. This can be advantageous when at an early or exploratory stage in the analysis of disease data, but when more substantive hypotheses and/or greater amounts of prior information are available concerning the problem, then it may be advantageous to consider a model-based approach to disease map construction. In what follows we consider first likelihood models for the individual case responses and then discuss the inclusion of extra information in the form of random effects.

8.3.1 Likelihood Models

Denote a realisation of m case events within a window $W = T \cup A$ as $\boldsymbol{x}_i, i = 1, \ldots, m$. In addition, define the count of cases of disease within the mth tract of an arbitrarily regionalised tract map as n_i.

Case Event Data

Usually, the basic model for case event data is derived from the following assumptions:

(1) individuals within the study population behave independently with respect to disease propensity, after allowance is made for observed or unobserved confounding variables;

(3) the underlying 'at-risk' population has a continuous spatial distribution, within specified boundary vertices;

(3) the case events are unique, in that they occur as single spatially separate events.

Assumption 1 above allows the events to be modelled via a likelihood approach, which is valid conditional on the outcomes of confounder variables. Further, assumption 2, if valid, allows the likelihood to be constructed with a background continuous modulating function $\{g(\boldsymbol{x})\}$ representing the 'at-risk' population. The uniqueness of case event locations is a requirement of point process theory (orderliness (Daley and Vere-Jones, 1988)), which allows the application of Poisson process models in this analysis.

Given the above assumptions, it is possible to specify that the case events arise as a realisation of a Poisson point process, modulated by $g(\boldsymbol{x})$, with first-order intensity:

$$\lambda(\boldsymbol{x}) = \rho g(\boldsymbol{x}) f(\boldsymbol{x}; \boldsymbol{\theta}). \tag{8.5}$$

In this definition, $f(\cdot)$ represents a function of confounder variables as well as location. The confounder variables can be widely defined, however. For example, a number of random effects could be included as well as observed covariates, as could functions of other locations. The likelihood associated with this is given by

$$L = \prod_i [\lambda(\boldsymbol{x}_i\}] \exp\left\{-\int_W \lambda(\boldsymbol{u})\, \mathrm{d}\boldsymbol{u}\right\}. \tag{8.6}$$

For suitably specified $f(\cdot)$, a variety of models can be derived. In the case of disease mapping, where only the background is to be removed without further model assumptions, then a reasonable approach to intensity parametrisation is $\lambda(\boldsymbol{x}) = \rho g(\boldsymbol{x}) f(\boldsymbol{x})$. The preceding definition can be used as an informal justification for the use of intensity ratios $(\hat{\lambda}(\boldsymbol{x})/\hat{g}(\boldsymbol{x}))$, in the mapping of case event data. Hence, such ratios represent the local 'extraction' of 'at-risk' background, under a multiplicative hazard model. Under a pure additive model, on the other hand, differencing the two estimated rates would be supported.

Tract Count Data

In the case of observed counts of disease within tracts, then given the above Poisson process assumptions it can be assumed that the counts are Poisson distributed with, for each tract, a different expectation: $\int_{a_i} \lambda(\boldsymbol{u})\,\mathrm{d}\boldsymbol{u}$, where a_i denotes the extent of the ith tract. The log likelihood based on a Poisson distribution is then, bar a constant only depending on the data, given by

$$l = \sum_{i=1}^{m} \left\{ n_i \log \int_{a_i} \lambda(\boldsymbol{u})\,\mathrm{d}\boldsymbol{u} - \int_{a_i} \lambda(\boldsymbol{u})\,\mathrm{d}\boldsymbol{u} \right\}. \tag{8.7}$$

Often, a parametrisation in (8.7) is assumed where, as in the case event example, the intensity is defined as a simple multiplicative function of the background $g(\boldsymbol{x})$. An assumption is often made at this point, that the integration over the mth tract area leads to a constant term which is not spatially dependent, i.e. any conditioning on $\int_W \lambda(\boldsymbol{u})\,\mathrm{d}\boldsymbol{u}$, the total integral over the study region, is disregarded. This assumption (the decoupling approximation) leads to considerable simplifications, but at a cost. Often, neither the spatial nature of the integral is considered nor the fact that any assumption of constancy must include the tract area within the integral approximation, are considered. The effect of such an approximation *should* be considered in any application example, but is seldom found in the existing literature.

The approximation of constant intensity, i.e. the assumption of a step function over the whole study window, leads to

$$\lambda_i = \rho |a_i| \hat{g}_i f_i.$$

Assuming that $\hat{g}_i$ can be estimated from the expected rates for the disease within each tract (e_i) (or counts of a control disease), then it can be shown that the local tract-specific estimate of f_i is given by

$$\hat{f}_i = \frac{n_i}{\rho |a_i| \hat{g}_i}. \tag{8.8}$$

Of course, ρ can be estimated via maximisation of (8.7) and the resulting substitution into (8.8) leads to

$$\hat{f}_i = \frac{n_i \sum_{i=1}^{m} |a_i| \hat{g}_i \hat{f}_i}{(\sum_{i=1}^{m} n_i) |a_i| \hat{g}_i}.$$

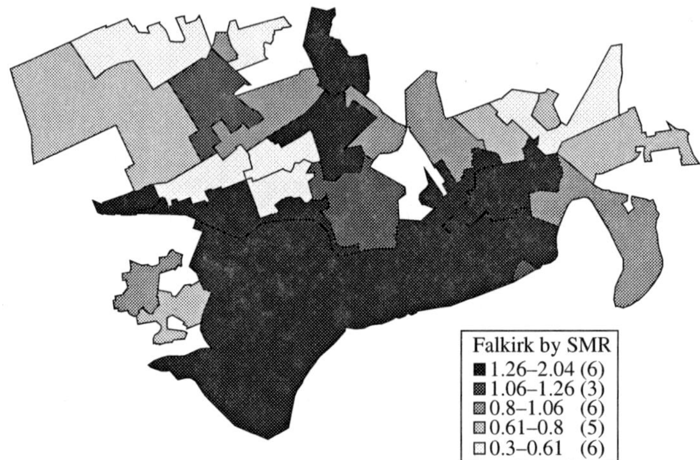

Figure 8.2 The SMR thematic map for the Falkirk example. Reproduced from Lawson and Cressie (2000) with permission from Elsevier Science.

This leads to a solution for f_i of

$$\hat{f}_i = \frac{n_i}{|a_i|\hat{g}_i},$$

which is just the standardised mortality ratio for the ith tract weighted by $1/|a_i|$. Note that the assumption that $|a_i| = 1 \; \forall \; m$ leads to the conventional estimate of tract relative risk, namely the SMR. Of course, ignoring the spatial configuration of tracts to this extent could lead to considerable bias in the resulting map. Figure 8.2 displays the SMR map of relative risks for the Falkirk example. Note the comparison with the crude map (Figure 8.1), having accounted for the population background.

The mapping of 'extracted' intensities for case events or modified SMRs for tract counts is based on the view that once the 'at-risk' background is extracted from the observed data, then the resulting distribution of risk represents a 'clean' map of the ground truth. Of course, as the background function $g(\boldsymbol{x})$ must usually be estimated then some latitude in the resulting map will occur by inclusion of different estimators of $g(\boldsymbol{x})$. For example, for tract count data, the use of external standardisation alone to estimate the expected counts within tracts may provide a different map from that provided by a combination of external standardisation and measures of tract-specific deprivation (e.g. deprivation indices). If any confounding variables are available and can be included within the estimate of the 'at-risk' background, then these should be considered for inclusion within the $g(\boldsymbol{x})$ function. Examples of confounding variables could be found from national census data, particularly relating to socio-economic measures. These measures are often defined as 'deprivation' indicators, or could relate to lifestyle choices. For example, the local rate of car ownership or percentage unemployed within a census tract or other small area could provide a surrogate measure for increased risk, due to correlations between these variables and poor housing, smoking lifestyles and ill health. Hence, if it is possible to include such variables in the $g(\boldsymbol{x})$

estimation, then any resulting map will display a close representation of the 'true' underlying risk surface.

When it is not possible to include such variables within $g(\boldsymbol{x})$, it is sometimes possible to adapt a mapping method to include covariables of this type by inclusion within $f(\boldsymbol{x})$ itself. Kelsall and Diggle (1998) have proposed a general method for the inclusion of covariates within a generalised additive model for relative risk.

8.3.2 Random Effects and Bayesian Models

In the above sections some simple approaches to mapping intensities and counts within tracts have been described. These methods assume that once all known and observable confounding variables are included within the $g(\boldsymbol{x})$ estimation then the resulting map will be clean of all artefacts and hence depicts the true excess risk surface. However, it is often the case that unobserved effects could be thought to exist within the observed data and that these effects should also be included within the analysis. These effects are often termed *random* effects, and their analysis has provided a large literature both in statistical methodology and in epidemiological applications (Manton *et al.*, 1981; Searle *et al.*, 1992; Tsutakawa, 1988; Marshall, 1991a; Lawson *et al.*, 1996a; Breslow and Clayton, 1993; Clayton, 1991). Within the literature on disease mapping there has been a considerable growth in recent years in modelling random effects of various kinds. In the mapping context, a random effect could take a variety of forms. In its simplest form a random effect is an extra quantity of variation (or variance component) which is estimable within the map and which can be ascribed a defined probabilistic structure. This component can affect individuals or can be associated with tracts or covariables. For example, individuals vary in susceptibility to disease and hence individuals who become cases could have a random component relating to different susceptibility. This is sometimes known as frailty. Another example is the interpolation of a spatial covariable to the locations of case events or tract centroids. In that case some error will be included in the interpolation process, and could be included within the resulting analysis of case or count events. The locations of case events could also not be known precisely or subject to some random shift. This form of spatial random effect may be related to uncertain residential exposure. (However, this type of uncertainty may be better modelled by a more complex integrated intensity model, which no longer provides an independent observation model.) Finally, within any predefined spatial unit, such as tracts or regions, it may be expected that there could be components of variation attributable to these different spatial units. These components could have different forms depending on the degree of prior knowledge concerning the nature of this extra variation. For example, when observed counts thought to be governed by a Poisson distribution display greater variation than expected (i.e. variance greater than mean), this is sometimes described as overdispersion. This overdispersion can occur due to various causes. Often, it arises when clustering occurs in the counts at a particular scale, but it can also occur when considerable numbers of cells have zero counts (sparseness). This can arise when rare diseases are mapped. In spatial applications, it is further important to distinguish two basic forms of extra variation. First, as in the aspatial case, a form of independent and spatially uncorrelated extra variation can be assumed. In addition, there could also be correlated heterogeneity. Essentially, this form of extra variation implies that there exists spatial autocorrelation between spatial units. This autocorrelation could arise for a variety of reasons. First, the disease of concern could be naturally clustered in its spatial distribution at the scale of observation. Many infectious diseases display such spatial clustering, a number of apparently non-infectious diseases also cluster. Second, autocorrelation can be induced in spatial disease patterns by the existence of unobserved environmental or frailty effects. Hence, the extra variation observed in any application could arise from confounding variables which have not been included in the analysis. In disease mapping examples, this could easily arise when simple mapping methods are used (such as SMRs) combined with crude age–sex standardisation of rates.

In the above discussion of heterogeneity, it is assumed that a global measure of heterogeneity applies to a mapped pattern. That is, any extra variation in the pattern can be captured by including a general heterogeneity term in the mapping model. However, often spatially specific heterogeneity may arise where it is important to consider local effects as well as, or instead of, general heterogeneity. To differentiate these two approaches we use the term *specific* and *non-specific*. Specific heterogeneity implies that spatial locations are to be modelled locally, e.g. clusters of disease are to be detected on the map. Whereas 'non-specific' describes the global approach to such modelling, which does not address the question of the location of effects. In the above definition, it is tacitly assumed that the locations of clusters of disease can be regarded as random effects themselves. Hence, there are strong parallels between image processing tasks and the tasks of disease mapping. Modelling specific heterogeneity is an object recognition task, while non-specific heterogeneity is a segmentation task (Ripley, 1988, Chapter 5).

Random effects can take a variety of forms and suitable methods must be employed to provide correctly estimated maps under models including these effects. In this section, we discuss simple approaches to this problem both from a frequentist and a Bayesian viewpoint.

A Frequentist Approach

Usually, a random effect is assumed to have a defining distribution. For example, a common assumption made when examining tract counts is that $n_i \sim \text{Poisson}(\lambda_i)$ independently, and that $\lambda_i \sim G(\alpha, \beta)$. This latter distribution is often assumed for the Poisson parameter and provides for a measure of overdispersion relative to the Poisson distribution itself, depending on the α, β values used. The likelihood for observed counts is now given by the product of a Poisson likelihood and a gamma distribution. At this stage a choice must be made concerning how the random intensities are to be estimated or otherwise handled. One approach to this problem is to average over the values of λ_i to yield what is often called the *marginal* likelihood. Having averaged over this density it is then possible to apply standard methods such as maximum likelihood. This is usually known as marginal maximum likelihood (Bock and Aitken, 1981). In this approach the parameters of the gamma distribution are estimated from the integrated likelihood. A further development of this approach is to convert the product density to a form where a mixture of components based on mass points of the parameter distribution is derived. This approach is essentially non-parametric and does not require the complete specification of the parameter distribution (Aitken, 1996a). This approach is discussed further in Section 8.4.

Although the example specified here concerns tract counts, the method described above can equally be applied to case event data, by inclusion of a random component in the intensity specification. Here a complication arises due to the requirement to evaluate a spatial integral involving the random effect. However, a number of approximation methods can be employed.

A Bayesian Approach

It is natural to consider modelling random effects within a Bayesian framework. First, random effects naturally have prior distributions and the product density discussed above is a joint posterior distribution for the data and parameters of interest. Hence, applications of full Bayes and empirical Bayes methods have developed naturally in the field of disease mapping. The prior distribution(s) for the ($\boldsymbol{\theta}$, say) parameters has (have) hyperparameters (in the Poisson-gamma example above, these were α, β). These hyperparameters can also have hyperprior distributions. The distributions chosen for these parameters depend on the application. In the full Bayesian approach, inference is based on samples of parameters ($\boldsymbol{\theta}$) taken from the joint posterior distribution. However, as in the frequentist approach above, it is possible to adopt an intermediate approach where the hyperparameters are estimated and further inference is made conditional on the estimated hyperparameters. In the tract count example, this would involve the estimation of α and β, followed by inference on the estimated posterior distribution (Carlin and Louis, 1996, pp. 67–68).

Few examples exist of simple Bayesian approaches to the analysis of case event data in the disease mapping context. The approach of Lawson *et al.* (1996a) can be used with simple prior distributions for parameters and the authors also provide approximate EB estimators based on Dirichlet tile area integral approximations. Diggle *et al.* (1998) also examined a Bayesian formulation where a Gaussian prior distribution with parametrised covariance was employed. More advanced models are discussed in Section 8.4. For count data, a number of examples exist where independent Poisson distributed counts (with constant tract rate, λ_i) are associated with prior distributions of a variety of complexity. The earliest examples of such a Bayesian mapping approach are the examples of Manton *et al.* (1981) and Tsutakawa (1988). Clayton and Kaldor (1987) also developed a Bayesian analysis of a Poisson likelihood model where n_i has expectation $\theta_i e_i$, and found that with a prior distribution given by $\theta_i \sim G(\alpha, \beta)$, the posterior expectation of θ_i is

$$\frac{n_i + \alpha}{e_i + \beta}. \tag{8.9}$$

Estimates of the hyperparameters were obtained from considering the negative binomial likelihood which is the unconditional distribution of $\{\theta_i\}$. Hence, it would be possible to directly map the θ_i estimates as posterior means.

On the other hand, the distribution of θ_i conditional on n_i is $G(n_i + \alpha, e_i + \beta)$ and a full Bayesian approach would require the sampling of θ_i from this distribution possibly with suitable sample summarisation (e.g. empirical average of θ_i, etc.). Other approaches and variants in the analysis of simple mapping models have been proposed by Tsutakawa (1988) and Devine and Louis (1994). Linear Bayes methods for smoothing relative risks have been proposed by Marshall (1991a). These local and global estimators are based on the form:

$$\hat{\theta}_i = h + C\left(\frac{n_i}{e_i} - h\right), \tag{8.10}$$

where

$$h = \frac{\sum n_i}{\sum e_i}, \qquad \bar{e} = \sum \frac{e_i}{m},$$

$$C = \frac{\kappa - h/\bar{e}}{\kappa - h/\bar{e} + h/e_i}, \qquad \kappa = \sum_i e_i\left(\frac{n_i}{e_i} - h\right)^2 \Big/ \sum e_i.$$

Figure 8.3 displays the Falkirk LB estimator. Figure 8.4 displays the map of EB estimates for the Falkirk example. These example approaches, of course, do not recognise the spatial structure of the estimates by ignoring the tract geometries and other effects mentioned above.

In the next section, more sophisticated models for the prior structure of the parameters of the map are discussed.

8.4 ADVANCED METHODS

The methods of the last section make simple assumptions about the structure of the mapping problem, and, indeed, often make simplifying assumptions about the nature of prior distributions employed. In the next section, more sophisticated assumptions concerning the nature of random effects are made and a number of methods appropriate for modelling such effects are proposed. Before considering more complex prior models, it is useful to consider some non-parametric methods which can be used with only limited prior knowledge.

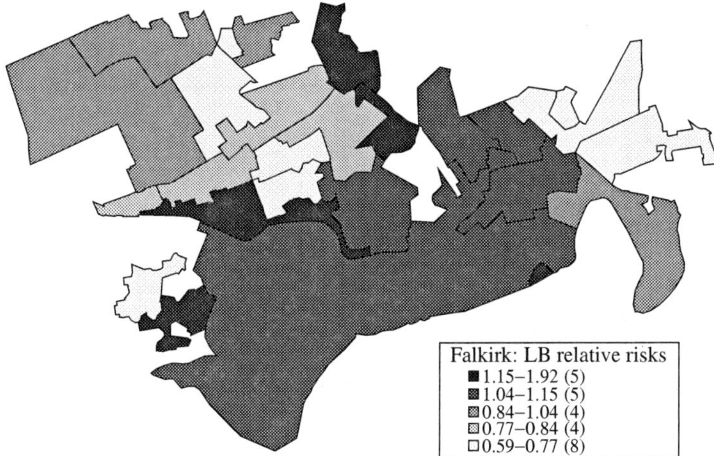

Figure 8.3 Falkirk example: linear Bayes relative risks.

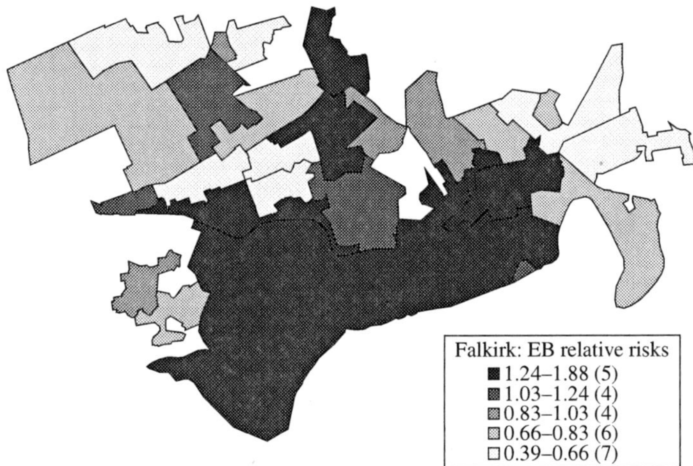

Figure 8.4 Empirical Bayes (gamma-Poisson) relative risk map of the Falkirk example.

8.4.1 Non-Parametric Methods

It is possible to consider a variety of non-parametric methods for the analysis of disease maps, while maintaining a degree of parametrisation within the model. One possibility is to consider the EB formulation given above, in which the parameter of interest is averaged over its parameter space,

$$\int f(n_i \mid \theta_i) g(\theta_i)\, \mathrm{d}\theta_i = \int f(n_i \mid \theta_i)\, \mathrm{d}G(\theta_i), \tag{8.11}$$

where f is the data density and g is a prior distribution. We assume that f is an appropriate data density and that g is a completely unspecified prior density. Carlin and Louis (1996) note that the Robbins estimator, a non-parametric estimator of a Poisson intensity, can be derived from the above definition.

Assume a Poisson density for f with expectation θ_i. Then the Bayesian estimate of θ_i, $\hat{\theta}_i$ say, given by the posterior expectation, is

$$(n_i + 1)m_G(n_i + 1)/m_G(n_i),$$

where $m_G(n_i)$ is the marginal distribution of n_i. For this simple case, a simple estimate of m_G is also available. A possible extension of this case is to the situation where θ_i is modified to accommodate an observed expected rate (e_i). In that case we replace θ_i with $\theta_i e_i$ and an approximate empirical Bayesian estimate of θ_i can be derived as

$$\hat{\theta}_i = \left(\frac{n_i + 1}{e_i}\right)\frac{m_G(n_i + 1)}{m_G(n_i)}.$$

In this case, the marginal distributions can also be estimated as empirical probabilities from the realisation of counts. This method appears to associate the estimate of the relative risk in each cell with the proportion of cells with higher $(n_i + 1)$ counts. However, this estimator performs poorly in many situations and Carlin and Louis (1996) discuss some of its associated problems. One way to avoid the problems inherent in the above estimator is to estimate $G(\theta)$ non-parametrically via non-parametric maximum likelihood (NPML) (Aitken, 1996a; Carlin and Louis, 1996). In that approach, the problem in (8.11) is replaced by a finite mixture sum with a finite number of mass points corresponding to discrete values of G. The application of NPML to prior distributions which include spatial correlation has not been attempted so far but could provide a useful *semi-parametric* approach to modelling with unobserved correlated heterogeneity.

8.4.2 Incorporating Spatially Correlated Heterogeneity

It is possible to formulate a non-Bayesian model for disease incidence which includes spatial correlation (for example Ferrandiz *et al.*, 1995). A recent proposal has suggested the use of gamma-Poisson random field models in the context of modelling tract count data (Wolpert and Ickstadt, 1998). While this provides a natural extension to Poisson likelihood models, the models do not provide for scale aggregation between case event and count realisations and so their use may be limited to large-scale mapping problems where tract geometries play a lesser role (see, for example, comments on the decoupling problem by Hjort (1998), Diggle (1993), Sections 8.3.1, 5.2 and Chapter 4).

On the other hand, it is quite natural to consider a two-stage hierarchy for incidence where events are independently distributed, conditional on knowledge of the other stage in the hierarchy where parameters may be spatially correlated. This has intuitive appeal where some unobserved environmental heterogeneity is thought to be present, and hence could induce spatial correlation in expected rates within small areas. Besag *et al.* (1991b) first proposed a model where the second level in the hierarchy included three different components: trend, uncorrelated and correlated heterogeneity. Their Bayesian model (the BYM model) was applied to tract count data, where it was supposed that there could be unobserved effects which could be modelled via random effects.

The approach adopted for modelling correlated heterogeneity structure is to parametrise the relative risk for the ith tract as

$$\theta_i = \exp\{t_i + u_i + v_i\}, \tag{8.12}$$

where t_i is a spatial trend term, u_i is a spatially correlated heterogeneity term and v_i is an uncorrelated heterogeneity term. In the example that follows we do not include a trend term, but this could be used in other examples, and, of course, it could include regression terms which are functions of spatial variables or covariates. Prior distributions for the u and v terms were specified by Besag and co-workers. The intrinsic autoregressions improper difference prior distribution developed from the lattice models of Kunsch (1987) was used, where the definition of spatial distribution in terms of differences allows the use of a singular normal joint distribution. Hence, the prior for $\{u\}$ is defined as

$$p(u \mid r) \propto \frac{1}{r^{m/2}} \exp\left\{-\frac{1}{2r}\sum_i \sum_{j\in\delta_i}(u_i - u_j)^2\right\}, \tag{8.13}$$

where ∂_i is a neighbourhood of the ith tract. The neighbourhood ∂_i was assumed to be defined to the first neighbour only. More general weighting systems could be used with the difference function, of course, where distance between tracts or length of common boundary, were incorporated. The uncorrelated heterogeneity (v_i) is defined to have a conventional Gaussian prior:

$$p(\boldsymbol{v}) \propto \sigma^{-m/2} \exp\left\{-\frac{1}{2\sigma}\sum_{i=1}^{m} v_i^2\right\}. \tag{8.14}$$

Both r and σ are assumed to have improper inverse exponential hyperpriors:

$$\text{prior}(r, \sigma) \propto \mathrm{e}^{-\epsilon/2r}\mathrm{e}^{-\epsilon/2\sigma}, \qquad \sigma, r > 0, \tag{8.15}$$

where ϵ was taken as 0.001. These prior distributions penalise the absorbing state at zero, but provide considerable indifference over a large range. Alternative hyperpriors for these parameters which are now commonly used are in the gamma and inverse gamma family, which can be defined to penalise at zero but yield considerable uniformity over a wide range. In addition, these types of hyperpriors can also provide peaked distributions if required.

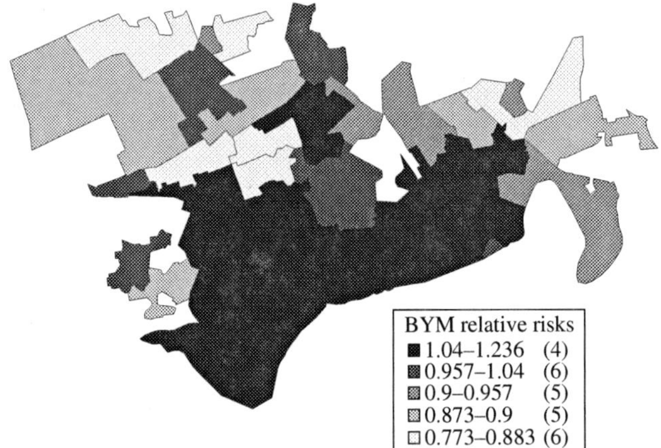

Figure 8.5 Full Bayesian model (BYM) posterior relative risk expectation map: Falkirk example.

The full posterior distribution for the original formulation where a Poisson likelihood is assumed for the tract counts is given by

$$P(u, v, r, \sigma \mid n_i) = \prod_{i=1}^{m} \{\exp(-e_i\theta_i)(e_i\theta_i)^{n_i}/n_i!\} \times \frac{1}{r^{m/2}} \exp\left\{-\frac{1}{2r}\sum_i \sum_{j\in\delta_i}(u_i - u_j)^2\right\} \times \sigma^{-m/2} \exp\left\{-\frac{1}{2\sigma}\sum_{i=1}^{m} v_i^2\right\} \times \text{prior}(r, \sigma).$$

This posterior distribution can be sampled using MCMC algorithms such as the Gibbs or Metropolis–Hastings samplers. A Gibbs sampler was used in the original example, as conditional distributions for the parameters were available in that formulation.

An advantage of the intrinsic Gaussian formulation is that the conditional moments are defined as functions of the number of neighbours,

$$E(u_i \mid \cdots) = \overline{u_i} \quad \text{and} \quad \text{var}(u_i \mid \cdots) = r/n_{ni}, \tag{8.16}$$

where n_{ni} is the number of neighbours of the ith tract.

Figure 8.5 displays the map of posterior relative risk expectations for the full Bayesian model for the Falkirk example.

The map is considerably smoother than the EB version due to the spatial correlation in the model formulation. Figure 8.6 displays the Bayesian residual map derived from the final converged MCMC sample.

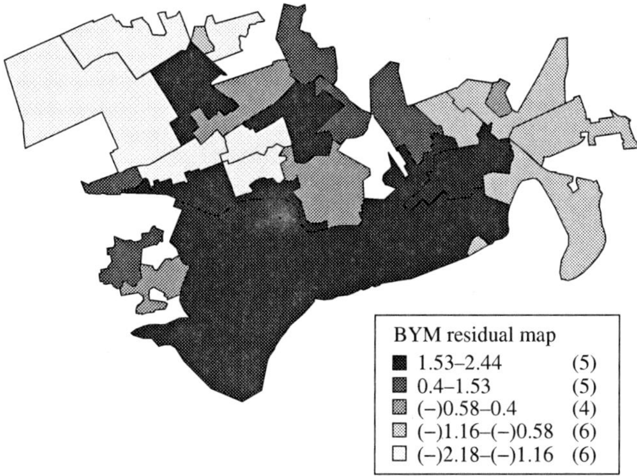

Figure 8.6 Crude Bayesian residual map for the Falkirk example under the BYM model.

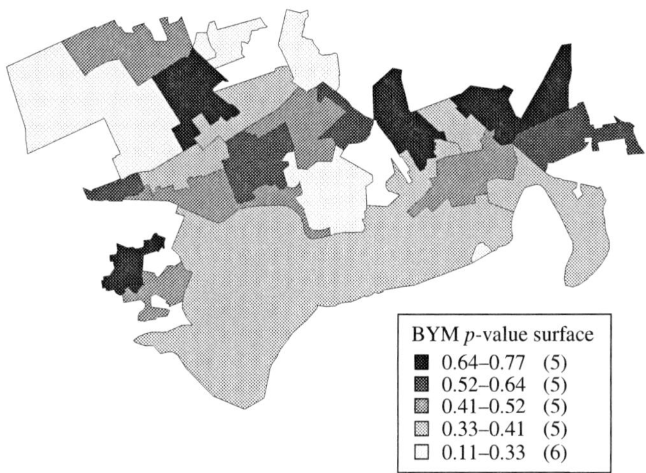

Figure 8.7 Simulation envelope p-surface for the ranking of Bayesian residuals for the Falkirk example.

There appears to be clear differentiation of high and low areas. However, none of the residuals are extreme given the simulation envelope p-value surface for this example. Figure 8.7 displays this surface.

This type of model has been extended to case event cluster modelling, where the weights are specified as functions of distance to other points within a fixed distance neighbourhood (see Section 6). Other examples of applications of the model are given by Ghosh *et al.* (1998), Clayton and Bernardinelli (1992) and Best *et al.* (1998), amongst others.

Alternative models for spatial correlation prior structure have been proposed by Clayton and Kaldor (1987) and extended by Stern and Cressie (1999). However, these can produce conditioning on neighbour *totals* rather than averages, and hence may not take into account the number of neighbours in the neighbourhood. In addition, a full multivariate normal prior distribution has been proposed, where a parametrised covariance structure was used, first by Lawson (1994b), and subsequently in a fully Bayesian context (Lawson *et al.*, 1996a; Diggle *et al.*, 1998). The advantage of such a specification is the ability to model a variety of components in the covariance (e.g. scales of covariation). However, full $m \times m$ covariance matrices must be inverted and sampled within posterior sampling algorithms. This has a considerably greater (though not prohibitive) computational cost than sampling with the intrinsic autoregression prior specification. If the only requirement of the autocorrelation prior is to capture correlated heterogeneity (as, for example, a background effect), then it would appear that the intrinsic formulation provides a simple and computationally cheap solution.

8.5 APPROXIMATE METHODS

While a full Bayesian modelling approach can be implemented relatively easily given the availability of posterior sampling algorithms, a variety of methods have also been developed which seek to approximate components of the posterior distribution of relative risks. These approximate methods vary from quadratic approximations of the Poisson likelihood, through log-normal algorithmic approximations found in multilevel modelling (Langford *et al.*, 1999a, 1999b), to asymptotic approximations using quasi-likelihood methods (generalised linear mixed models) (Breslow and Clayton, 1993; Yasui and Lele, 1997; McNab and Dean, 2000). These approximations can provide relatively simple estimation methods, while some measure of the appropriateness of the approximating assumptions should always be made. For example, the Laplace approximation applied to a spatial tract count example implies that increasing domain asymptotics must be employed, which may not be appropriate when conditioning on the spatial window. In addition, quasi-likelihood methods can lead to biases in the estimation of parameters (see Biggeri *et al.* (1999) for a discussion).

8.6 EVALUATION OF MODEL PERFORMANCE

To a limited degree, assessment of the behaviour of a variety of models for relative risks has taken place. Clayton and Kaldor (1987) made an early comparison of a variety of different relative-risk estimation methods. They found that for the SMR, EB, full Bayes with autocorrelation and non-parametric EB, all methods produced the same *ranking* of tract relative risks (i.e. the ordering of magnitude of risk was maintained for all tracts). This may be related to the fact that posterior expectation is used (see Conlon and Louis, 1999). Sensitivity of Bayesian models to prior specification, has been considered by Yasui *et al.* (2000), Eberley and Carlin (2000), Best *et al.* (1998) and Pascutto *et al.* (2000), and previously by Bernardinelli *et al.* (1995a).

A variety of results have been reported from these studies. Considerable sensitivity to weighting systems employed in the specification of the spatial correlation prior is to be expected, and this effect has been confirmed. Recommendations for prior model selection include the use of scaled priors to provide calibrated relative risks. Sensitivity of scale parameters in the random-effect priors to hyperprior specification has also been noted. In addition, prior sensitivity of covariate effect parameters has been observed. From this work there appears to be no general conclusions to draw except that sensitivity exists and '*great care must be taken when prior distributions are postulated*' (Pascutto *et al.*, 2000). None of these studies assess edge effects on maps, which also, *a priori*, must have a significant effect when, for example, spatial correlation priors are invoked. This effect has been demonstrated by Lawson *et al.* (1999b) on a mapped example (see Section 5.5.5). The problem is accentuated when small study windows are used or study regions with many boundary tracts (Ghosh *et al.*, 1998) and will be sensitive to the choice of edge correction model utilised.

A simulation-based evaluation of a wide range of estimation methods for relative risks has been attempted (Lawson *et al.*, 2000a). In that study, a large number of 'true' relative risk models were simulated for a large county map of Eastern Germany. The true models chosen for this examination ranged from simple constant risk models to complex Bayesian random-effect models, including trend and different types of heterogeneity (correlated and uncorrelated). In addition, mixture models of different types were examined. Realisations of counts in the county map were generated, and the authors examined both goodness-of-fit to the realised counts and to the true relative risk model. The models chosen were selected to represent the range of possible underlying risk that might be encountered. Thus, while basic trend models were present, random-effect and mixture models with trend were also examined. In addition, specific clusters were introduced into some random-effect models. The true models were grouped into broad classes: fixed-effect models with trend; random-effect models with either trend, uncorrelated or correlated heterogeneity; mixture models with a variety of components (such as trend, and random effects); models with specific cluster terms and selections of random effects and trend; and finally Poisson-gamma distribution models with a variety of fixed parameters. A range of methods were applied to the realisations from the true models, including smoothing methods (non-parametric regression), empirical Bayes, full Bayes and linear Bayes methods. The results of this fitting exercise were wide ranging. The overall conclusions of the work were the following.

1. The BYM model (as originally specified, without trend components) is the most robust and fitted well across a range of true models, even when the true model included trend. This model performed relatively badly for certain true mixture models, however.

2. The Poisson-gamma model and global linear Bayes models of Marshall (1991a) followed closely to the BYM model but also performed badly with some true mixture alternatives.

3. All models performed relatively badly when structured and unstructured heterogeneity was present.

4. Marginal mixture models perform badly overall when relative risk comparisons are made, and in some cases, are not optimal for true mixture models.

5. The global linear Bayes models of Marshall perform better overall than the local linear Bayes version.

6. Smoothing methods perform very badly in recovering true relative risks, in particular, the Kelsall and Diggle method applied to counts.

7. The BYM model provides greatest robustness against misspecification, and models not including spatially correlated heterogeneity (structured) are less robust (gamma-Poisson and linear Bayes methods).

In general, these results suggest that the use of Bayesian models which do not include both unstructured overdispersion and structured heterogeneity may induce considerable residual spatial correlation which remains unexplained. Even when trend components or other covariables are included in an analysis, it is important to include both heterogeneity components.

8.7 HYPOTHESIS TESTING IN DISEASE MAPPING

In most published disease mapping accounts an approach based on modelling of mapped rates is assumed. While such an approach has many advantages, not least of which is the flexibility to examine a variety of models, it is sometimes the case that basic features of the map are to be examined and hence only single or small sets of parameters are to be considered. In that case, it may be relatively straightforward to carry out a statistical test. If the focus of the study is to provide a map which is free of statistical artefacts (such as noise), then it is not strictly appropriate to carry out tests, as the focus implies *estimation* of rates. However, if the focus lies on the assessment of some feature such as correlated heterogeneity (autocorrelation) or overdispersion, then it is possible to carry out tests for such effects. Tests for correlated heterogeneity were discussed in Section 6. However, there are many other types of test which could be considered here.

We consider a map to be composed of *first-order* (trend) effects and *second-order* covariance and variance effects. The latter effects will here also include overdispersion. The first-order effects are also sometimes called trend surface effects. These effects are represented by long-range variation over the map. As such they represent different extremes of possible spatial variation. The second-order effects represent short-range variation, and, at the shortest range, instantaneous variance, and hence can include such features as overdispersion.

8.7.1 First-Order Effects

The modelling of first-order or trend effects and associated tests in the disease mapping context has been considered by Lawson and Harrington (1996). Here we draw a distinction between the analysis of general spatial trend and analysis of specific hypotheses concerning *ecological* variables (as are common in the analysis of putative sources of hazard), even if these variables have spatial expression or have spatial surrogates. The analysis of the latter is discussed in Section 10 and at greater length under the special case of putative sources of hazard (Section 7).

The testing of hypotheses concerning simple spatial trend are usually carried out under some defined parametric model. In the simplest case this will usually consist of an independent likelihood-based model for the case events or tract counts. When it is appropriate to assume such a model, then it is straightforward to carry out tests for simple spatial trend. We assume that the spatial trend variables (e.g. the (x, y) locations of cases, tract centroid coordinates, etc.) are measured at the locations of data observations. Given this condition, then inclusion of such variables leads to a regression-type model and conventional likelihood ratio (LR), score and Wald tests can be derived for such a situation. For the tract count case, Lawson (1993c) has examined a variety of likelihood-based tests for spatial effects. Assuming the multinomial log-likelihood,

$$l = \sum_i \left\{ n_i \log \int_{a_i} \lambda(\boldsymbol{u}) \,\mathrm{d}\boldsymbol{u} \right\} - (n_i) \log \sum_i \int_{a_i} \lambda(\boldsymbol{u}) \,\mathrm{d}\boldsymbol{u},$$

then it is possible to derive score, LR or Wald tests for particular specifications of $\lambda(\boldsymbol{u})$. These tests have no special *spatial* features and are standard likelihood-based tests for regression parameters. For the specification,

$$\lambda(\boldsymbol{x}) = g(\boldsymbol{x})m(F(\boldsymbol{x})\alpha),$$

where α is a p-dimensional vector, we can derive the score vector as

$$U = \sum_{j=1}^{m} n_j \frac{m_j\{g(\boldsymbol{x})m'(F(\boldsymbol{x})\alpha)\}}{m_j\{g(\boldsymbol{x})m(F(\boldsymbol{x})\alpha)\}} - \left(\sum_{j=1}^{m} n_j\right) \frac{\sum_{j=1}^{m} m_j\{g(\boldsymbol{x})m'(F(\boldsymbol{x})\alpha)\}}{\sum_{j=1}^{m} m_j\{g(\boldsymbol{x})m(F(\boldsymbol{x})\alpha)\}}, \tag{8.17}$$

where $m_j = \int_{a_j} \lambda(\boldsymbol{u}) \,\mathrm{d}\boldsymbol{u}$, and m' denotes differentiation with respect to the relevant parameter(s), and we assume that integral differentiation is possible. For simple specifications of F, the design matrix of spatial variables, (8.17) can have relatively simple forms. For example, if we make the tract approximation, $\lambda(\boldsymbol{u}) \equiv \lambda_j = g_j m(F_j\alpha)$, within the jth tract, then (8.17) becomes

$$U = \sum_{j=1}^{m} n_j \frac{m'(F_j\alpha)}{m(F_j\alpha)} - \left(\sum_{j=1}^{m} n_j\right) \frac{\sum_{j=1}^{m} |a_j| g_j m'(F_j\alpha)}{\sum_{j=1}^{m} |a_j| g_j m(F_j\alpha)},$$

where a_j is the jth tract extent. This can lead to simple test statistics. For example, the score test for a one-dimensional spatial trend (in $\boldsymbol{x}_j$ say), with $m(F_j\alpha) = 1 + \exp(\alpha\boldsymbol{x}_j)$, an additive relative risk, would be based on

$$U = \sum_{j=1}^{m} n_j \boldsymbol{x}_j \frac{\exp(\alpha\boldsymbol{x}_j)}{1+\exp(\alpha\boldsymbol{x}_j)} - \left(\sum_{j=1}^{m} n_j\right) \frac{\sum_{j=1}^{m} |a_j| g_j \boldsymbol{x}_j \exp(\alpha\boldsymbol{x}_j)}{\sum_{j=1}^{m} |a_j| g_j \{1+\exp(\alpha\boldsymbol{x}_j)\}},$$

which under the null hypothesis, $H_0 : \alpha = 0$, is

$$U = \frac{1}{2} \sum_{j=1}^{m} n_j \boldsymbol{x}_j - \left(\sum_{j=1}^{m} n_j\right) \frac{\sum_{j=1}^{m} |a_j| g_j \boldsymbol{x}_j}{2 \sum_{j=1}^{m} |a_j| g_j}.$$

This score vector is just a comparison of average values of the counts with those expected based on the region areas and the underlying population. Note that, bar the factor $\frac{1}{2}$, this score vector is the same as that derived for a purely multiplicative risk model, i.e. $m(F_j\alpha) = \exp(F_j\alpha)$. Normalisation of these vectors by the appropriate information matrix will lead to different test statistic forms.

For the case event situation, a variety of tests can be considered in a similar fashion to the tract count case. With reference to the likelihood (8.6) and intensity specification given by $\lambda(\boldsymbol{x}) = \rho g(\boldsymbol{x}) f(\boldsymbol{x}; \boldsymbol{\theta})$, it is possible to derive tests specific to $\boldsymbol{\theta}$ parameters suitably defined in the $f(\boldsymbol{x}; \boldsymbol{\theta})$ function. A general score vector with jth component, for the natural parametrisation $f(\boldsymbol{x}; \boldsymbol{\theta}) = \exp\{F(\boldsymbol{x})\alpha\}$, with $F(\boldsymbol{x})$ and α defined as above, is given by

$$\sum_{i}^{m} F_{ij} - c_1 \int F_j g(\boldsymbol{u}) \exp\{F(\boldsymbol{u})\alpha\} \, \mathrm{d}\boldsymbol{u},$$

where $c_1 = m / \int g(\boldsymbol{u}) \exp\{F(\boldsymbol{u})\alpha\} \, \mathrm{d}\boldsymbol{u}$ and F_j denotes the jth variable in F, the $(m \times p)$ design matrix (Lawson, 1994a). In this formulation $g(\boldsymbol{u})$ must be estimated, and in previous analyses a plug-in estimate has been obtained from the population background (Lawson, 1993b). Such score tests can be evaluated using Monte Carlo test critical regions.

In the situation where it is believed that uncorrelated or correlated heterogeneity exists in the map, then this must be treated as a nuisance effect and incorporated under the null hypothesis. Usually, in a non-Bayesian setting, this would require estimation of the heterogeneity under the null model, and subsequent testing of first-order effects, conditional on the estimated heterogeneity (Cox and Hinkley, 1974). Proposals for such tests have been made, where Laplace approximations or quadratic approximations are employed (Lawson and Harrington, 1996). The tests can be employed in either the tract count or case event situation.

In a formal Bayesian approach, hypothesis tests would not be used, and instead interval estimation would usually be employed.

8.7.2 Second-Order and Variance Effects

Testing hypotheses concerning second-order effects involve the assessment of correlated heterogeneity, while variance effects concern extra-variation in the incidence of disease. In the case of correlated heterogeneity, testing involves the assessment spatial correlation within the disease incidence, given the population background. Essentially, this form of testing overlaps with the area of non-focused clustering and general cluster testing. However, as in the case of first-order effects, the existence of *other* effects in the map should be considered and these can also be estimated under the null hypothesis. If first-order (trend) effects or other covariate effects exist, then these should be estimated in that way. Hence, it may be useful to adopt a two-stage approach to testing for correlated heterogeneity:

stage 1 estimate trend, covariate and extra-variation within a model with no spatial correlation;

stage 2 test for spatial correlation, including the estimated nuisance effects substituted within the correlation test statistic.

It may be possible to construct a test statistic of this kind. However, no exact test statistics currently exist in this case. Tests for autocorrelation for count data often do incorporate the population background estimate but often do not include the facility to estimate covariates or extra-variation. Tests such as the quadratic form of Whittemore and co-workers (Whittemore *et al.*, 1987) and its extensions (Tango, 1995) do not allow incorporation of estimated covariate parameters or extra-variation. Note that the use of Moran's I statistic for assessment of autocorrelation, even in population modified form (Oden, 1995; Assuncao and Reis, 1999), does not provide for estimation of nuisance effects as background, and hence is unlikely to be at all informative in this situation.

Another approximate procedure is to fit a parametric model in stage 1 above, and then test for correlation in the residuals from the fitted model. There is a large literature on the topic of testing for spatial correlation amongst residuals (Cliff and Ord, 1981). In particular, Moran's I statistic provides one such measure, although a Monte Carlo assessment of the test statistic is recommended. This procedure mimics the iterative estimation procedures of REML and generalised least squares.

8.8 SPACE-TIME DISEASE MAPPING

As in other application areas, it is possible to consider the analysis of disease maps which have an associated temporal dimension. The sequential analysis of georeferenced case events will be discussed in the following chapter (Chapter 9). The two most common formats for observations are

(1) georeferenced case events which have associated a time of diagnosis/registration/onset, i.e. we observe within a fixed time period T, m cases at locations $\{x_i, t_i\}$, $i = 1, \ldots, m$;

(2) counts of cases of disease within tracts are available for a sequence of T time periods, i.e. we observe a binning of case events within $m \times T$ space-time units: $n_{it}, i = 1, \ldots, m, t = 1, \ldots, T$.

In the case event situation, few examples exist of mapping analysis. However, it is possible to specify a model to describe the first-order intensity of the space-time process (as in the spatial case). The intensity specification at time t can be specified as

$$\lambda(\boldsymbol{x}, t) = \rho g(\boldsymbol{x}, t) f_1(\boldsymbol{x}; \theta_x) f_2(t; \theta_t) f_3(\boldsymbol{x}, t; \theta_{xt}), \tag{8.18}$$

where ρ is a constant background rate (in space $\times$ time units), $g(\boldsymbol{x}, t)$ is a modulation function describing the spatio-temporal 'at-risk' population background in the study region, f_k are appropriately defined functions of space, time and space-time, and θ_x, θ_t, θ_{xt} are parameters relating to the spatial, temporal and spatio-temporal components of the model.

Here each component of the f_k can represent a *full* model for the component, i.e. f_1 can include spatial trend, covariate and covariance terms, and f_2 can contain similar terms for the temporal effects, while f_3 can contain *interaction* terms between the components in space and time. Note that this final term can include *separate* spatial structures relating to interactions which are not included in f_1 or f_2. The exact specification of each of these components will depend on the application, but the separation of these three components is helpful in the formulation of components.

The above intensity specification can be used as a basis for the development of likelihood and Bayesian models for case events, if it can be assumed that the events form a modulated Poisson process in space-time, then a likelihood can be specified as in the spatial case.

Note that the above case event intensity specification can be applied in the space-time case where small-area counts are observed within fixed time periods $\{l_t\}$, $t = 1, \ldots, T$, by noting that

$$E\{n_{it}\} = \int_{l_t} \int_{a_i} \lambda(\boldsymbol{u}, t)\, \mathrm{d}\boldsymbol{u}\, \mathrm{d}t,$$

under the usual assumption of Poisson process regionalisation. In addition, the counts are independent conditional on the intensity given, and this expectation can be used within a likelihood modelling framework or within Bayesian model extensions. In previous published work in this area, cited above, the expected count is assumed to have constant risk within a given small-area/time unit, which is an approximation to the continuous intensity defined for the underlying case events. The appropriateness of such an approximation should be considered in any given application (see also Chapter 10). If such an approximation is valid, then it is straightforward to derive the minimal and maximal relative risk estimates under the Poisson likelihood model assuming $E\{n_{ij}\} = \lambda_{ij} = e_{ij}\theta_{ij}$, where e_{ij} is the expected rate in the required region/period. The maximal model estimate is $\hat{\theta}_{ij} = n_{ij}/e_{ij}$, the space-time equivalent of the SMR, while the minimal model estimate is

$$\hat{\theta} = \frac{\sum_i \sum_j n_{ij}}{\sum_i \sum_j e_{ij}}.$$

Smooth space-time maps, e.g. empirical Bayes or full Bayes relative risk estimates, will usually lie between these two extremes. If the full integral intensity is used, then these estimates have the sums in their denominators replaced by integrals over space-time units.

Development of count data modelling based on tract/period data has recently seen considerable development. The first example of such modelling was by Bernardinelli *et al.* (1995b). In their approach, they assumed a model for the log relative risk of the form,

$$\log(\theta_{ij}) = \mu + \phi_i + \beta t_j + \delta_i t_j, \tag{8.19}$$

where μ is an intercept (overall rate), ϕ_i is an area (tract) random effect, βt_j is a linear trend term in time t_j, δ_i an interaction random effect between area and time. Suitable prior distributions were assumed for the parameters in this model and posterior sampling of the relevant parameters was performed via Gibbs Sampling. Note in this formulation there is no spatial trend, only a simple linear time trend and no temporal random effect. The components in (8.18) above allow a range of effects in each of the spatial and temporal components, however, and this model could be extended in a variety of directions.

Waller *et al.* (1997) and Xia and Carlin (1998) (see also Carlin and Louis (1996)) subsequently proposed a different model where the log relative risk is parametrised as

$$\log(\theta_{ijkl}) = \phi_i^{(j)} + \delta_i^{(j)} + \text{fixed covariate terms } (kl),$$

where $\phi_i^{(j)}$ and $\delta_i^{(j)}$ are uncorrelated and correlated heterogeneity terms which can vary in time. This model was further developed by Xia and Carlin (1998), who also examined a smoking covariate which has associated sampling error and spatial correlation. Their model was defined as

$$\log(\theta_{ijkl}) = \mu + \zeta t_j + \phi_{ij} + \rho p_i + \text{fixed covariate terms } (kl),$$

where an intercept term μ is included with a spatial random effect nested within time $\{\phi_{ij}\}$, a linear time trend ζt_j, and p_i is a smoking variable measured within the tract unit. In these model formulations no spatial trend is admitted and all time-based random effects are assumed to be subsumed within the ϕ_{ij} terms.

To allow for the possibility of time-dependent effects in the covariates included (race and age), Knorr-Held and Besag (1998) formulated a different model for the same data set (88 county Ohio lung cancer mortality, 1968–1988). Employing a binomial likelihood for the number at risk $\{n_{ijkl}\}$ with probability π_{ijkl}, for the counts, and using a logit link to the linear predictor, they proposed

$$\eta_{ijkl} = \ln\{\pi_{ijkl}/(1 - \pi_{ijkl})\},$$

where

$$\eta_{ijkl} = \alpha_j + \beta_{kj} + \gamma_{lj} + \delta z_i + \theta_i + \phi_i. \tag{8.20}$$

The terms defined are α_j, a time-based random intercept; β_{kj}, a kth age group effect at time j; γ_{lj}, a gender $\times$ race effect for combination l at the jth time; a fixed covariate effect term δz_i, where the z_i is an urbanisation index; and θ_i, ϕ_i are correlated and uncorrelated heterogeneity terms which are not time-dependent. No time trend or spatial trend terms are used, and these effects will (partly) be subsumed within the heterogeneity terms and the $\alpha_j + \beta_{kj} + \gamma_{lj}$ terms.

More recent examples of spatio-temporal modelling include extensions of mixture models (Boehning *et al.*, 2000), which examine time periods separately without interaction, and the use of a variant of a full multivariate normal spatial prior distribution for the spatial random effects (Sun *et al.*, 2000). Other developments include the extension of the Knorr-Held and Besag model to include different forms of random interaction terms (Knorr-Held, 2000), and the use of covariates at different levels of aggregation (Zhu and Carlin, 2000).

Overall, there are a variety of forms which can be adopted for spatio-temporal parametrisation of the log relative risk, and it is not clear as yet which of the models so far proposed will be most generally useful. Many of the above examples exclude spatial and/or temporal trend modelling, although some examples absorb these effects within more general random effects. Allowing for temporal trend via random walk intercept prior distributions provides a relatively non-parametric approach to temporal shifting, while it is clear that covariate interactions with time should also be incorporated. Interactions between purely spatial and temporal components of the models have not been examined to any extent, and this may provide a fruitful avenue for further developments. If the goal of the analysis of spatio-temporal disease variation is to provide a parsimonious *description* of the relative risk variation, then it would seem to be reasonable to include spatial and temporal trend components in any analysis (besides those defined via random effects).

Finally, it is relevant to note that there are many possible variants of the two basic data formats which may arise, partly due to mixtures of spatial aggregation levels, but also to changes in the temporal measurement units. For example, it may be possible that the spatial distribution of case event data is only available within fixed time periods, and so a hybrid form of analysis may be required where the evolution of case event maps is to be modelled. Equally, it may be the case that repeated measurements are made on case events over time so that attached to each case location is a covariate (possibly time-dependent) which is available over different time periods. In that case a form of spatio-longitudinal analysis might be considered. A special case of this might be the analysis of time-to-endpoint for georeferenced cases of disease (e.g. death/recovery/remission). This could be regarded as a spatial survival analysis (Henderson, 2000).

In general, spatio-temporal disease mapping is largely in its infancy and is likely to be a fruitful area for future developments.

8.9 DISEASE MAPPING: A GERMAN CASE STUDY

From a public health point of view the investigation of the regional distribution of lip cancer mortality may be fruitful for a number of reasons. First, there may be clear urban–rural differences in lip cancer risk, due to differences in occupational status and exposure to sunlight (Tomatis *et al.*, 1990), thus the mortality of lip cancer is closely related to increased sunlight exposure and hence outdoor occupations. Thus identification of high-risk areas in disease maps could provide evidence of factors which are unknown in the aetiology, or could mirror the distribution of known explanatory variables such as the proportion of the local population employed in farming, fishing or forestry.

The association of skin cancers with air pollution via ambient carcinogen concentration in air is also an issue. A recent review by Katsouyanni and Pershagen (1997) summarised the evidence that ambient air pollution may have an effect on cancer risk. However, due to the difficulties in exposure assessment the effect of air pollution on cancers is still controversial. Thus, identification of high-risk areas in disease maps may be a starting point for further analytic studies.

Finally, there are several protective agents, such as selenium or antioxidants like vitamins E or A, under discussion (Blot, 1997). Thus identification of high-risk areas could be a starting point for intervention trials, introducing chemoprevention using minerals and/or vitamins. And, of course, the identification of low-risk areas could provide hypotheses for unknown protective factors.

As a result, the implications from disease maps of lip cancer mortality are manifold. The common denominator of the ideas above is to display the heterogeneity of disease risk in maps. Here, the case study presents and compares the results of several methods for disease mapping using mortality data from the former East Germany region (now eastern Germany) for the period 1980–1989. The total number of deaths during this 10-year period was 2291.

Lip cancer has been examined within other study regions, most notably the Scottish lip cancer example (Stern and Cressie, 1999; Clayton and Kaldor, 1987; Breslow and Clayton, 1993; Best *et al.*, 1998). However, that example has considerable edge effects and the geometry of the subareas is highly variable. The east German example provides a more regular map, avoiding some of these problems.

8.9.1 The Data

The establishment of population-based cancer registries is still under development in Germany. Only mortality data are routinely available. Thus for this analysis, mortality data for lip cancer are used.

When constructing disease maps, one of the first steps is the choice of the spatial resolution. Frequently, the spatial resolution is limited by the availability of the data. In Germany there is unfortunately no central database accessible as a source for small-area health data. Data even on a spatial resolution of the 'Landkreise' (local region) are not routinely available. Such data can only be obtained by directly addressing the census bureaus (Statistische Landesämter) of the 16 states of Germany. As a result the collection of health data on a small-area level such as the Landkreise is quite tedious and expensive. For the former DDR (eastern Germany), registration of deaths due to lip cancer in 220 regions is complete for the period 1980–1989.

Once the spatial resolution has been defined an appropriate estimator of relative risk must be considered. A frequently used measure of relative risk is the standardised mortality ratio $\hat{\theta}_i = n_i/e_i$, where the expected cases e_i are calculated based on a reference population. For our data, we used the age-specific lip cancer mortality rates from eastern Germany for the study period as reference population. The necessary population data of the individual area were taken from the database 'Statistik regional' (Bundesamt, 1997).

Here we can use the $\hat{\theta}_i$ of the individual region as an estimate for the relative risk of that area compared to the whole country.

8.9.2 Simple Methods

Once the spatial resolution and the epidemiological measure are defined a suitable mapping method has to be chosen. A common approach for the construction of thematic maps in epidemiology is the choropleth method (Howe, 1963). This method implies categorising each area and then shading or colouring the individual regions accordingly (see Chapter 3).

One of the traditional approaches of categorisation is based on the percentiles of the SMR distribution. Most cancer atlases use this approach usually based on quartiles, quintiles or sixtiles (Walter and Birnie, 1991). Figure 8.8 shows the map of lip cancer mortality based on the quintiles of the SMR distribution.

There is clearly high variability in the data, with relative risk estimates ranging from 0 to 3.82. This would indicate a relative risk which is up to four times higher in high-risk areas or over six times lower in low-risk areas. But in the worst case, this variability reflects only random fluctuations due to different population size and corresponding small counts.

These maps can suffer from the presence of artefacts which are unobserved in the data. Again, population size is a possible confounder, in this example large areas tend to have significant results. Unobserved heterogeneities can be present and may need to be accounted for in the analysis. In addition, the proportion of the areas employed in agriculture, fisheries and forestry (AFF) may also be an explanatory variable. Figure 8.9 displays the distribution of this variable in this example. It is clear that there is a north–south gradient, with higher proportions in the north of the area.

8.9.3 The Empirical Bayes Approach

The Parametric Empirical Bayes Approach

To circumvent the above mentioned problems, random-effect models are frequently used. Several parametric distributions like the gamma or log-normal distribution have

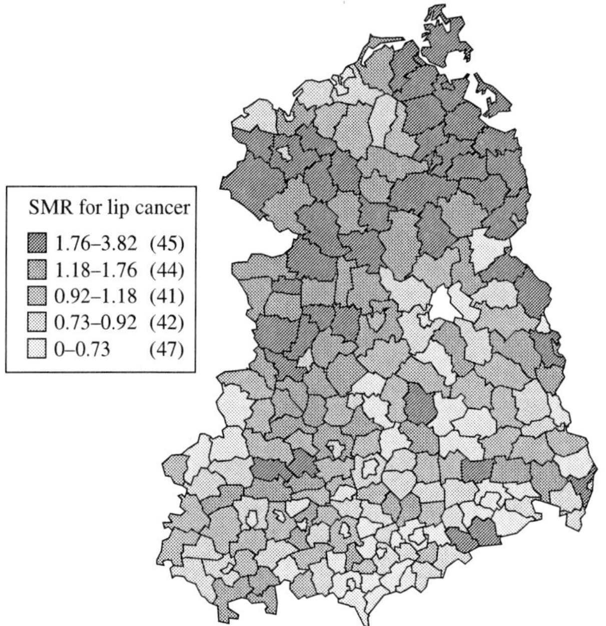

Figure 8.8 Eastern Germany region: lip cancer standardised mortality ratio (SMR) for 220 local regions.

been suggested for the prior distribution of the relative risk: $g(\theta)$, for details see Section 8.3.2 and a recent review by Mollie (1999). The parameters of the prior distribution can be estimated from the data, in this case the θ_i are assumed to be gamma distributed with $\theta_i \sim \Gamma(\alpha, \nu)$ and the hyper-parameters α and ν are estimated from the data. The posterior expectation of the relative risk of the individual area as

$$\hat{\theta}_{eb,i} = \frac{n_i + \hat{\nu}}{e_i + \hat{\alpha}}.$$

Such estimators are displayed in Figure 8.4 for the Falkirk example and are not considered further here.

8.9.4 Full Bayesian Analysis

In this section we demonstrate the use of a fully Bayesian modelling approach to the analysis of the German lip cancer data. Using the notation of the previous sections, we define the Poisson likelihood for a realisation $\{n_i\}$, $i = 1, \ldots, m$, of counts in m small areas as

$$L = \prod_{i=1}^{m} \mathrm{e}^{-\lambda_i} (\lambda_i)^{n_i} / n_i!.$$

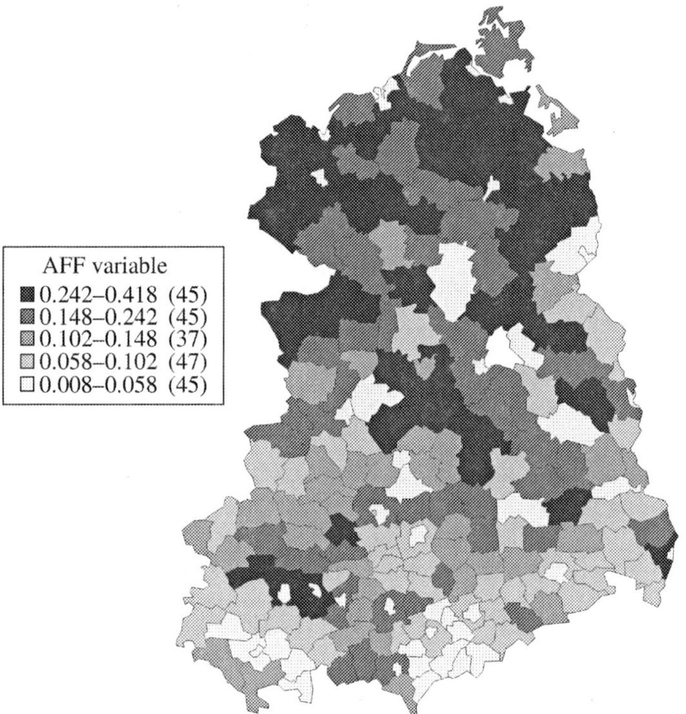

Figure 8.9 AFF variable: eastern Germany example.

Here,

$$\lambda_i = e_i \exp\{t_i + u_i + v_i\},$$

where e_i is the expected rate for the ith small area, and we have a log-linear link between the Poisson expectation and terms t_i, u_i, v_i. These model terms represent different types of variation which could be considered in the model. The first term represents trend in the rates across the study region and can be thought of as *long-range* variation. In our example, we do not include trend variation, although it is straightforward to do so in any particular application. The second and third terms (u_i, v_i) represent types of random effect or heterogeneity, which can be included if there is thought to be any extra random structure in the counts which may remain unexplained by the other model components. This extra structure could be due to inherent extra variation not captured by the Poisson likelihood model (see Section 8.3.2). In addition, there could also exist autocorrelated variation which is often termed correlated heterogeneity. In our model we represent correlated heterogeneity by u_i and uncorrelated by v_i. Because we wish to apply a fully Bayesian analysis to the data set, we assume that all parameters in our model have prior distributions. In fact, the heterogeneity terms are random effects, and as we have no other external support for

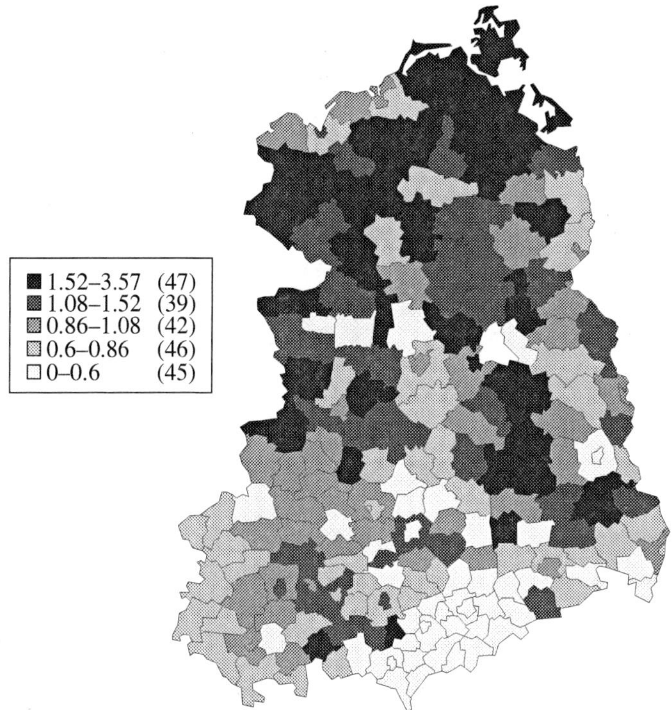

Figure 8.10 Posterior expected relative risks for the BYM model for the German lip cancer example.

their estimation (than the data set) we need to make distributional assumptions to allow us to properly distinguish their form.

The prior distributions employed here are those specified by Besag and co-workers. The correlated random effect has an intrinsic singular Gaussian prior distribution,

$$p_i(u_i \mid \cdots) \propto \frac{1}{\sqrt{\beta}} \exp\left\{ - \sum_{j \in \partial_i} w_{ij}(u_i - u_j)^2 \right\}, \tag{8.21}$$

where $w_{ij} = 1/2\beta \ \forall \ i, j$. The neighbourhood ∂_i is assumed to be the areas with common boundary with the ith area. The uncorrelated heterogeneity (v_i) is defined to have a Gaussian prior distribution:

$$p(\boldsymbol{v}) \propto \sigma^{-m/2} \exp\left\{ -\frac{1}{2\sigma} \sum_{i=1}^{m} v_i^2 \right\}. \tag{8.22}$$

These prior distributions have parameters which must also be considered to have hyperprior distributions. Both β and σ are assumed to have improper inverse exponential hyperpriors,

$$\text{prior}(\beta, \sigma) \propto \mathrm{e}^{-\epsilon/2\beta} \mathrm{e}^{-\epsilon/2\sigma}, \qquad \sigma, r > 0, \tag{8.23}$$

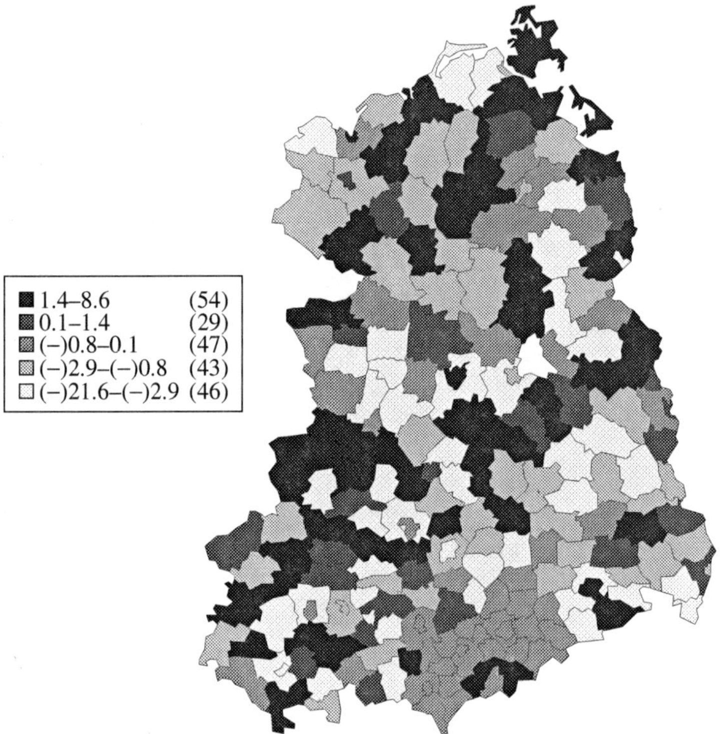

Figure 8.11 Bayesian residuals from the BYM model for the German lip cancer example.

where ϵ is taken as 0.001. These prior distributions penalise the absorbing state at zero, but provide considerable indifference over a large range.

Once the prior distributions are specified, we must consider the evaluation of the full posterior distribution (P_0), which combines the Poisson likelihood and all the prior distributions. To sample parameter values from P_0 we employ a Markov chain Monte Carlo (MCMC) method. We have employed a Metropolis–Hastings algorithm to sample all parameters. This algorithm allows for the iterative evaluation of proposed new parameters via the use of posterior ratios. Convergence of the algorithm was assessed by the Geweke criteria, based on log-posterior monitoring, and chains with separate start values were examined. Cowles and Carlin (1996) and Brooks (1998) discuss the variety of methods available for convergence checking of this algorithm.

Our analysis of the lip cancer mortality data has led to the production of a posterior expected relative risk map (Figure 8.10). This map represents a summary of the final converged relative risks for the data set from the sampling algorithm.

The resulting map shows some marked features. First, the inclusion of a correlation term has smoothed the map and produced many patches of similar risk level. This is commonly found when autocorrelation is included in such analysis. The main

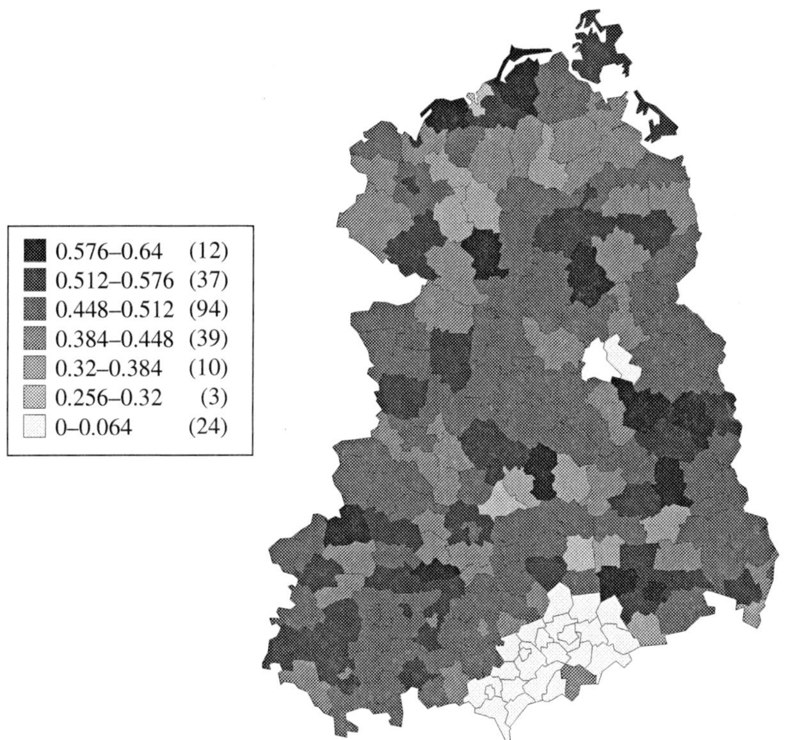

Figure 8.12 Simulation envelope p-value surface for the rank of the Bayesian residuals: German lip cancer example.

features displayed on the map relating to differences in lip cancer incidence are (i) a large concentration of elevated risk in the northwestern area of the study region, (ii) a noticeable north–south gradient, with elevated risks in the northern region.

The residual analysis from the Bayesian model fit suggests that there is considerable variation in residuals both in magnitude and sign. The crude residual map (Figure 8.11) displays a general patchwork with little spatial aggregation although there may be a suggestion of a concentration of high positive residuals in the north of the study area. This may reflect the possible north–south gradient which was also reflected in the AFF variable map (Figure 8.9). These results are also reflected in the rank residual p-value surface (Figure 8.12) which shows few areas with values in the upper extreme range (more than 0.95). However, there are marked areas with extreme low values and these are mainly in the southern region of the map. This may suggest that the large negative residuals found in this area are indeed extreme and may further support the north–south gradient which is not explicitly modelled here.

CHAPTER 9

Large Scale: Surveillance

The Centers for Disease Control (CDC) defines public health surveillance as

> the ongoing, systematic collection, analysis, and interpretation of health data essential to the planning, implementation, and evaluation of public health practice, closely integrated with the timely dissemination of these data to those who need to know. The final link of the surveillance chain is the application of these data to prevention and control. A surveillance system includes a functional capacity for data collection, analysis, and dissemination linked to public health programs.
>
> (Thacker and Berkelman, 1992; Thacker, 1994)

It is clear from this that a broad definition of surveillance is implied and that it relates to a wide range of monitoring methods related to health. From a statistical point of view it is relevant to consider how statistical methods can be developed or employed to aid the task of surveillance of populations. Clearly, many techniques within spatial statistics, previously mentioned here, may be useful in this task. However, it is also clear that both a temporal element must be included in the analysis, where changes in disease distribution are possible, and also that consideration must be given to how such methods can be implemented within a general surveillance framework.

An idea related to surveillance is that of screening. The use of screening to provide prospective criteria for the early detection of disease onset (Greenberg *et al.*, 1996) is well established in such areas as cervical or mammarian cancer. This involves testing of individuals at specific time points to attempt to assess if onset of a condition is likely or imminent. In general, screening could be applied to populations as well as individuals, in that specific changes in the general incidence of a disease may trigger public health interventions. This intervention would usually be designed to reorient the allocation of health resources to attempt to improve the health status of the population under study. However, screening is usually associated with individual assessment or monitoring, while surveillance is usually carried out at an aggregate population level.

In this chapter the use and development of statistical methods for geographical disease surveillance will be considered. Reference will also be made, where appropriate, to temporal aspects of surveillance which have seen greater development to date. Some consideration of the possibilities for spatio-temporal disease surveillance will also be considered.

Surveillance has an implicit temporal dimension, i.e. populations are often monitored over time to assess whether changes have occurred within the population which may warrant action.

In the next section, some ideas commonly used in statistical process control (SPC) are introduced and their relevance to disease surveillance is considered.

9.1 PROCESS CONTROL METHODOLOGY

A number of methods have been developed for the detection of changes in populations over time. These methods are characterised by the estimation of *changepoints* in a sequence of disease events or a time-series of population rates (Lai, 1995), or the determination of or application of *control limits* to the behaviour of a system. In this area there are some simple methods available to assist in the assessment of change or 'in control' behaviour. Some of these methods are derived from SPC, which was developed for the monitoring of industrial processes over time, and could be applied within a disease surveillance programme, with due care. For example, it is well known that the temporal variation in count data can be monitored by using a Poisson control chart (C chart), upon which specific limits can be plotted, beyond which corrective action should be taken. Besterfield (1990) specifies upper and lower control limits for the *average* count as

$$\text{UCL} = \bar{c} + 3\sqrt{\bar{c}}, \qquad \text{LCL} = \bar{c} - 3\sqrt{\bar{c}},$$

where $\bar{c} = \sum_{j=1}^{g} c_j/g$, and g is the number of items sampled. Of course, this is a standard control chart definition and makes a number of assumptions. This is a 3-σ normal approximation pivotal interval based on *independent* count data. An exact interval can be constructed for independent Poisson counts. However, if the counts were correlated even under the null hypothesis, then some allowance must be made for this correlation in the chart. A further issue, when such methods are to be used within disease monitoring, is the issue of how to incorporate any changes in the background 'at-risk' population which may arise. One possibility in the temporal domain is to employ relative risk estimates (e.g. SMRs), and to use an appropriate sampling distribution to provide appropriate control limits. A simple possibility might be to employ a log transformation of the SMR (possibly with a correction factor) and to assume an approximate Gaussian sampling distribution. However, the SMR at a given time point is a saturated estimate and to avoid instabilities related to the ratio form it may be better to monitor sample *averages* of SMRs (or transformations of averages) over time periods. The incorporation of correlation or correlated heterogeneity may also be important to consider. For large aggregation scales, time-series methods have been employed which allow temporal dependence (Farrington and Beale, 1998).

In addition, special types of chart (*cusum* charts) have been developed specifically to detect changes in pattern over time (changepoints). These are constructed by cumulative recording of events over time, the accumulation being found to be sensitive to changepoint in the process under consideration. Some recent work in the application of these ideas in medical surveillance and monitoring is by Frisen and co-workers (Frisen and Mare, 1991; Frisen, 1992). While these methods may have appeal, special adaptations of the methods need to be developed to deal with the spatial and spatio-temporal nature of geographical surveillance.

For data in the form of case events, a number of methods have been developed in the temporal domain. The sets monitoring technique of Chen (1993, 1997) is a recent example. This uses the idea that the interval between cases is assumed to be exponentially distributed with mean $\varphi = 1/\lambda$, where λ is the rate of monthly case diagnoses. Observed intervals are compared to φ as they arise. An alarm is signalled if the last n intervals are shorter than a critical length. Extensions to this idea can also be made in the direction of *cusums*, except in this case they would be cumulative interval lengths which could be monitored. A cusum method for counts, in an industrial process control context, has been proposed by Lucas (1985) and Montgomery (1991). A review of surveillance methods in the temporal domain, with an emphasis on infectious disease monitoring, has been provided by Farrington and Beale (1998).

In the spatial case, there is a wide range of methods which can be applied to a *single* realisation of case events within a fixed time frame/period. Many of the methods described in the sections above concerning disease mapping /clustering or ecological analysis could be applied as surveillance tools. For example, general clustering tests could be applied, or residuals from disease maps fitted in each time period could be examined. The types of question which might be appropriate to answer with these methods are ones such as the following. Is there evidence of unusual variation in incidence in the map? Is there evidence of 'unusual' clustering on the map? Is there a spatial trend on the map related to, for example, a putative source?

However, when the question relates to a spatio-temporal pattern or change in pattern, then there are few methods currently available which are designed for this purpose.

9.2 SPATIAL MONITORING

In this section, we consider two situations where monitoring or surveillance is carried out. First, we examine the situation of a *fixed* time period or frame where all cases of a disease are recorded. Second, the examination of an evolving time frame is considered. In the first situation, a time period, $\mathcal{T}$ say, and a spatial window or frame W are specified.

9.2.1 Fixed Spatial and Temporal Frame

Case Events

For m case events within the frame, the location of each event is recorded in space-time coordinates $\{\boldsymbol{x}_i, t_i\}$, $i = 1, \ldots, m$. First, it is important to consider the simple situation where the $\{t_i\}$ are unknown. When locations are only known, then a spatial realisation is only available and the spatial structure can be examined for spatial effects only, for example, spatial clusters/clustering, association with putative sources, etc. In principle, any relevant spatial testing or modelling procedure, described in previous chapters, could be applied, and their choice would depend on the specific hypotheses to be assessed. For example, it might be of public health concern to monitor clustering of disease within the space-time frame chosen, and so a cluster model or general clustering test might be performed. This form of surveillance does not explicitly include any temporal comparison, although it is possible that, for the same spatial frame, different time frames might be informally compared.

When the spatial and temporal coordinates of case events are available, then a temporal component of analysis can be included. Here, it is assumed that a sequential analysis is precluded, and that the complete realisation of events within the space-time frame is to be considered. The inclusion of a temporal component considerably widens the scope and potential focus of the surveillance task.

First, it is possible to consider general models for the spatio-temporal variation in disease, and to estimate spatial, temporal and spatio-temporal aspects of these models for the complete realisation of events. The intensity of such a model could be, in its general form, as in (8.18),

$$\lambda(\boldsymbol{x}, t) = \rho g(\boldsymbol{x}, t) f_1(\boldsymbol{x}; \theta_x) f_2(t; \theta_t) f_3(\boldsymbol{x}, t; \theta_{xt}).$$

If our focus in the surveillance task is to assess spatio-temporal features of the realisation, then focus can be made on the θ_{xt}, although it may be of interest to focus on purely temporal and spatial aspects as well. In the case where spatio-temporal clustering is of interest, then $f_3(\boldsymbol{x}, t; \theta_{xt})$ can be structured to include cluster term(s) and the other components can be regarded as nuisance terms. For purely temporal effects, a wide variety of methods have been proposed. Methods based on simple temporal trend models, or more complex point process models, can be proposed which could include cluster function terms which allow the estimation of temporal clusters, as well as trends. Clearly, for the temporal case, the estimation of model parameters for the current time frame may allow the prediction of temporal effects in future time frames, and so this approach provides a link with dynamic sequential modelling of temporal effects. In general, the estimation of temporal effects would have to be made jointly with other components.

For purely spatial effects, the estimation of parameters in θ_x would need to be carried out jointly with other components, as in the other cases.

Tract Counts

For tract counts within fixed spatial regions, a similar approach may be employed with the adoption of the integrated intensity,

$$E\{n_{ij}\} = \int_{l_j} \int_{a_i} \lambda(\boldsymbol{x}, t)\, \mathrm{d}\boldsymbol{x}\, \mathrm{d}t,$$

for the time frame $\mathcal{T}$ within which there are fixed time periods $\{l_j\}$, $j = 1, \ldots, \mathcal{T}$. Here, we assume that modelling of the complete realisation of counts within the time frame $\mathcal{T}$ is to be undertaken. Again, similar considerations apply when focusing on different components of the intensity. In the spatio-temporal case we may be concerned with clustering or interaction of spatial and temporal random effects, and these would have to be estimated jointly with other components. With a purely temporal focus, it is possible to employ Poisson regression with the decoupling approximation to estimate temporal trend and covariate effects, but this would usually involve estimation of the spatial and spatio-temporal effects as nuisance, and it is better to jointly estimate these components. Similar considerations apply when a spatial focus is required.

While it is possible to adopt a purely parametric approach to surveillance, as described above, it is also possible that an approach which does not make many assumptions may be favoured. This might be particularly true where little is known about the aetiology of the disease under consideration, and a non-parametric approach might be suitable. In that case, the methods adopted depend on the focus of the enquiry. For example, if the purpose is to examine the space-time variation in disease to, say, isolate areas of elevated risk (possible clusters), then smoothing techniques may be best suited to this approach. Non-parametric density estimation or kernel regression could be employed. The approach of Kelsall and Diggle (1995b) and Lawson and Williams (1993) to the estimation of relative risk surfaces could be extended to the space-time framework. This approach could lead to the construction of p-value surfaces. The main drawback of these methods is that they do not employ probability models for the data likelihood and so may not correctly represent the underlying true risk. This has been found in simulation studies which evaluated a variety of purely spatial methods (Lawson *et al.*, 2000a). Based on these results, EB methods of smoothing based on relatively simple probability models for the random variation may be preferred. Alternatively, the relative risk generalised additive models (GAMs) of Kelsall and Diggle (1998) may be extended.

9.2.2 Fixed Spatial Frame and Dynamic Temporal Frame

We consider two basic scenarios depending on whether monitoring continues until the time of the next event (be it a case event with known location in space-time or a case event known only to reside within a particular census tract), or monitoring is carried out within specific sequential time periods. In the former, the occurrence of a new event activates the examination of the map. In the latter case, the end of a time period allows the retrospective evaluation of the map. This latter situation is the simplest method of surveillance which can be carried out easily with routinely collected health data. For example, the yearly recordings of mortality counts within small areas is commonly available in many countries.

Case Events

Time to next event monitoring When locations of cases in space-time are available, it is possible to consider how a 'time-to-event' monitoring system could be developed. In the case of strictly temporal monitoring, an early example of a sequential method for examining point events was proposed by Bartholomew (1956). The method assumes that events in time follow a heterogeneous Poisson process and a sequential test is derived for detecting an increasing or decreasing trend with a constant rate null hypothesis. The method could be applied, with a little extra effort, to a monitoring exercise where it is required that changes in the temporal component of a space-time model be monitored. More recently, Chen (1978) and Chen *et al.* (1993) have proposed a method of temporal surveillance based on the assumption that times between events have a simple exponential distribution with fixed mean μ. A method of detecting sequences of short times was developed. The key parameters are (n, τ), where an aberrance (cluster alarm) is declared if the intervals between $n + 1$ consecutive events are all less than τ. The false detection probability is given by

$$(1 - \mathrm{e}^{-\tau/\mu})^n.$$

The analysis is undertaken whenever an event occurs. Some assumptions made in this approach may need to be checked in any application. For example, the exponential interval distribution is derived from a stationary Poisson process assumption for the case events. However, over certain time periods there may be considerable variation in μ as well as possible non-stationarity and/or unobserved heterogeneities. Mirroring the assumptions made for spatial case event intensities, it would be a basic assumption of the case event temporal distribution that

$$\lambda(t) = g(t) f(t),$$

where it may be possible to assume that $g(t) \equiv g$, a constant for certain time periods. In that case $n \sim \text{Poisson}(\int_0^T g(u) f(u)\, \mathrm{d}u)$ within a time period T.

In the case of a spatio-temporal monitoring procedure, it is possible to adopt a sequential test for some simple likelihood-based models. For example, if the joint space-time intensity of an event at $\{\boldsymbol{x}, t\}$ is specified as $\lambda(\boldsymbol{x}, t; \theta)$, where θ could be possibly multidimensional, then the likelihood ratio for a simple comparison of $H_0 : \theta = \theta_0$ against $H_1 : \theta = \theta_1$, where n events have occurred (i.e. $i = 1, \ldots, n$) is given by

$$Q = \prod_{i=1}^{n} \left\{ \frac{\lambda(\boldsymbol{x}_i, t_i; \theta_1)}{\lambda(\boldsymbol{x}_i, t_i; \theta_0)} \right\} \exp\{-\Lambda_{\theta_1} + \Lambda_{\theta_0}\}, \tag{9.1}$$

where $\Lambda_\theta = \int_0^{t_n} \int_W \lambda(\boldsymbol{x}, t; \theta)\, \mathrm{d}\boldsymbol{x}\, \mathrm{d}t$, and t_n is the time of the nth event. Sequential limits (a, b say) can be evaluated as $a < Q < b$ as usually defined for sequential probability ratio tests (SPRTs) (see Rao (1973, Chapter 7) and Frisen and Mare (1991)). In this case, sampling continues and Q updated until either $Q \leqslant a$ and then accept H_0 or $Q \geqslant b$ and accept H_1. Variants of this approach could be constructed where conditionally specified first-order intensities are employed, or where composite hypotheses are allowed (Siegmund, 1985).

It is also possible to construct tests which are sequential but exploit MCMC methods whereby the null distribution of the test is the equilibrium distribution of the chain, and the chain is run from the current observed data in specified directions towards the equilibrium distribution. For example, to test for spatio-temporal correlation in case events, a test statistic could be calculated from the existing data, and a birth–death algorithm could be employed which has as its equilibrium distribution complete spatio-temporal randomness (conditional on nuisance parameters). Besag and Clifford (1991) have discussed the sequential implementation of such procedures.

Clearly, any extensions of these procedures to models where prior distributions are admitted would require the deployment of Bayesian methodology. In this area a number of possible approaches might be fruitful. For the detection of changes in overall pattern in space-time, Bayes factors could be examined. In the case of spatio-temporal models it may be possible to examine two different situations: (1) use the predictive distribution of future events to examine the distribution of the next case to arise, or (2) to compare a model for the current realisation of cases with a model fitted to the current realisation and the new case. The first option may require a formulation which is akin to the updating methods of Kong *et al.* (1994) and Berzuini *et al.* (1997) originally applied to fixed time frame examples.

Particular hypotheses found in spatio-temporal studies may require the development of specific models or test procedures, however. For example, while it may be of benefit to examine global clustering via sequential or other methods, it may also be important to devise methods which examine the local variation in clustering in subsections of space or time. To this end, models or tests which monitor localised aggregations of events (which may be aggregated to assess global features) may be a fruitful avenue for further development.

Fixed time period monitoring The evolution of mapped case event data in fixed time periods can be regarded as a special case of the above situation where the spatial distribution of cases is to be examined/compared between time slices. In this situation, it is possible to consider the examination of the cumulative realisation of events (up to the current period), either by sequential examination of the cumulative effects of time progression or by a comparison of the current complete realisation to the previous complete realisation of events. In addition, it would be possible to construct a sequential procedure which would detect changes to the spatio-temporal distribution of events by addition of each time frame. The methods discussed in the above section could be adapted to this situation also.

Tract Counts

Time to next event monitoring Rogerson (1997) has proposed a method of monitoring where a cusum of standardised deviation from expectation are computed whenever a new case arises within a tract count. This method relies upon the computation of a global clustering measure (in the paper, Tango's general clustering test C_G is used) and its comparison with the expected value conditional on the measure computed at the time of the previous case event. The statistic used is of the form,

$$Z_i = \frac{C_{G,i} - E(C_{G,i} \mid C_{G,i-1})}{\sigma_{C_{G,i}|C_{G,i-1}}},$$

where the subscript i denotes the current event and $i-1$ denotes the previous event, and $\sigma_{C_{G,i}|C_{G,i-1}}$ is the standard error of the difference. The conditional expectation is defined by computing a function of the clustering measure with a single case added to the $i-1$th counts in each of the m tracts in turn. The $\{Z_i\}$ will not be normally distributed and the author recommends that batches of these measures be averaged. Process control methods are used to monitor these batch means. In principle, this method could be used with a range of possible general tests for spatial pattern as long as the expectations and variances could be computed within Z_i. The method can also be specified for surveillance around putative sources of hazard.

There are a number of limitations to this approach to space-time surveillance, however. First, there is no explicit mechanism in the procedure for incorporation of changes in expected counts or in the spatial covariance matrix (assumed to be fixed) within C_G. Features of these parameters could evolve with time also. Secondly, there is no explicit measurement made of the time to the new event and temporal effects are not modelled. Consideration of the correlation induced in the $\{Z_i\}$ by this approach should also be made. In addition, the approach is defined for global measures of spatial structure, and, as mentioned above, it may be more appropriate to design a monitoring procedure for localised detection of changes whether these be clusters or individual areas of excess risk.

Note that a testing procedure akin to equation (9.1) could be proposed for the tract count case also, where the Poisson process likelihood is replaced by a Poisson count likelihood and a sequential sampling procedure could be employed.

Fixed time period monitoring Clearly, updating algorithms could be applied in this situation, and the imputation methods, possibly based on SIR (sampling-importance resampling (Carlin and Louis, 1996, pp. 157–159)), could be used to provide faster updating of model parameters. Methods similar to those discussed for case events could be developed. Some methods have been considered already for fixed lattice data (Jarpe, 1998).

9.3 CONCLUSIONS

As is clear from the speculative nature of much within this chapter, there is considerable scope for development of new methods within the general area of surveillance. While it is possible to employ many methods already developed outwith the surveillance context, within surveillance systems, there is a need to develop spatial methods which are sensitive to the sequential nature of the surveillance task. This could be via updating algorithms or through the sequential methods previously discussed. Ultimately, it would be useful to develop methods which could be employed easily or routinely within a public health surveillance context. This development may need both the development of methods, their dissemination and the incorporation of methods into a suitable surveillance system as tools which can be used by public health analysts.

CHAPTER 10

Ecological Analysis

10.1 INTRODUCTION

Ecological analysis is closely associated with disease mapping. The focus of ecological studies is the relationship between measured covariables and geographical disease incidence. Usually, hypotheses concerning aetiological factors and disease risk are to be examined. The aetiological relationship may have a spatial expression, because spatial distribution avoids the temporal censoring inherent in cohort studies. An early ecological study with a spatial structure was the British Regional Heart Study reported by Cook and Pocock (1983). In that work, disease counts in regions were related to regional averaged explanatory variables, via a regression model including spatial autocorrelation. Richardson (1992) provides a review of some of the issues found in geographical ecological studies. See also the general discussion of Biggeri *et al.* (1999) and Plummer and Clayton (1996).

Additionally, ecological studies are often associated with changes in the resolution level of the measurements made on covariables. For example, event location data may be available for the case disease but only expected death rates in census tracts may be available for use in characterising the 'at-risk' population. In that case, the expected deaths are available at a lower level of resolution than the cases.

Associated with these changes of resolution and comparison of risk factor covariables and disease outcome are the issues of *ecological* and *atomistic* fallacy. These two issues tend to affect the main data types found in geographical disease studies, namely tract counts and case event locations.

The ecological fallacy arises when an attempt is made to ascribe to individuals the average properties of large groups of population. The atomistic fallacy arises when an individual's disease experience is used to impute average characteristics for a population group. Both of these problems arise when *different* resolution levels are used in a study of relationships, and are not tied to the two extremes of case events and tract counts. It should be borne in mind that in *any* regression or correlation exercise some attempt is usually made to assess the relationship between measurements at different resolutions, although in classical regression the observations are usually made on the same subject.

The problem, known as the *ecological fallacy* (also named *ecological bias*), was first pointed out by Robinson (1950), who demonstrated that the total correlation between two variables as measured at an ecological level can be expressed as the sum of a within-group and a between-group component. This was later extended to linear model regression relations by Duncan *et al.* (1961). The sources of ecological bias have been investigated by many authors (see, for example, Greenland (1992), Greenland and Robins (1994) and Steel and Holt (1996)).

In addition to the individual level sources (misspecification, within-group confounding, no additive effects, misclassification), special attention has been given to the bias due to the grouping of individuals. In particular Greenland and Morgenstern (1989) analysed how grouping influences associations of exposure factors to disease, they pointed out that ecological bias may also arise from confounding by group and effect modification by group. Consider some groups indexed by i and let p_i be the proportion of exposed subjects (a dichotomous variable), r_{0i} the individual rate in unexposed subjects and r_{1i} the individual rate in exposed subjects in the ith group. The crude rate in the ith group is given by

$$\begin{aligned} r_{+i} &= r_{0i}(1 - p_i) + r_{1i} p_i \\ &= r_{0i} + D_i p_i, \end{aligned}$$

where $D_i = r_{1i} - r_{0i}$ is the individual rate difference. Consider a population linear regression model of average disease level on the average exposure level in groups,

$$r_{+i} = \alpha + \beta p_i + e_i,$$

then $1 + \beta/\alpha$ is termed the ecological rate ratio. Greenland and Morgenstern demonstrated that the ecological regression coefficient β can be viewed as the expected rate difference at individual level plus two bias terms. The mathematical relationship is given by

$$\beta = E(D_i) + \frac{\mathrm{cov}(p_i; r_{0i})}{\mathrm{var}(p_i)} + \frac{\mathrm{cov}([p_i - E(p_i)]p_i; D_i)}{\mathrm{var}(p_i)}.$$

The first bias component,

$$\frac{\mathrm{cov}(p_i; r_{0i})}{\mathrm{var}(p_i)},$$

is present when the unexposed rate is associated with the level of exposure in the group, and it may be viewed as a bias term due to confounding by group. It is plausible that such confounding acts because some external factor causing the disease is associated with groups having higher level of exposure factor. The second bias component,

$$\frac{\mathrm{cov}([p_i - E(p_i)]p_i; D_i)}{\mathrm{var}(p_i)},$$

is present when the risk difference in a group is associated with the level of exposure, and it may be viewed as a bias term due to effect modification by group. Based on this result, one commits ecological fallacy if one assumes that ecological rate ratio $1+\beta/\alpha$ is only determined by the individual rate difference effect, when, in fact, it may also be caused by the two bias components effect. Several strategies can be adopted to deal with the potential pitfalls of ecological modelling. First, one could try to estimate the joint distribution of outcome and explanatory variables within areas using a sample drawn from the populations investigated, and use the information collected to adjust the ecological regression coefficient and standard errors. This approach has been proposed by Plummer and Clayton (1996) and Prentice and Sheppard (1995). The reader should note that this derivation does not include spatial effects and it can also be viewed as an example of a mixed design with individual and ecological variables. (Langford *et al.* (1999a) and Lawson and Williams (1994) provide examples of multiple level exposure risk modelling.) When sampling within areas is not feasible, a second strategy could be to adjust for the correlation between area prevalence of the exposure variable and baseline rate of disease, provided no effect modification occurs. If the level of aggregation is sufficiently thin, a regression model for autocorrelated data would result in a sort of stratification by spatial closeness, where the baseline rates would be expected not to vary. A justification of this approach in terms of a hidden spatially structured confounder has been made (Clayton *et al.*, 1993). Indeed, where the spatial variation of the risk factor is similar to that of the disease, geographical location may act as a confounder.

There are a number of effects of these fallacies on statistical methods. First, care must be taken in the interpretation of the estimated relationships, derived from changes in resolution level. It is possible that estimated ecological relationships are markedly different from those estimated from individual data. Second, special models may be required to deal specifically with such changes. For example, random effects might be employed to allow for the effect of changes in resolution. Frailty models can be used in the atomistic case (Clayton, 1991). Plummer and Clayton (1996) discussed specific models where the linkage between resolution levels is explicit. Lawson and Williams (1994) proposed a hybrid likelihood model for different resolution levels between case events and expected death rates in tracts. Note that the analysis of putative sources of health hazard is a special case of ecological analysis where a specific small set of explanatory variables, such as distance, direction, and functions of distance around a putative source, are used to explain the disease incidence. Third, the issue of measurement error in covariables can arise in such studies. This can occur naturally when a covariable can only be measured with error or could arise due to the necessity of interpolation of covariables to locations of interest. For example, deprivation indices (Carstairs, 1981) are now routinely available for census tracts in the UK. However, these may have associated measurement error due to uncertainty in the population characterisation in each tract. This error should be incorporated in any study associating deprivation indices and disease incidence. Another source of error, which is related to measurement error in covariables, is the error which may arise within the *expected* rates used to represent the population at risk. This is sometimes known as the 'denominator' problem, as such rates often form the denominator within a relative risk ratio estimator. There may be substantial error inherent in such rates, which are usually available only at census tract level and often at fixed time points. The errors relate to the difficulty in estimating the population characteristics within any region accurately. Often, expected rates are available only at fixed time points (e.g. census years) and any comparison of population at risk at such a time point with other times may be prone to some error. Migration of population coupled with ascertainment errors may lead to such problems. A considerable effort has been expended to study and quantify such changes in population within demographic and social studies (Boyle and Halfacree, 1998). The topic of small-area estimation deals specifically with this issue (Ghosh and Rao, 1994).

Often, within spatial epidemiology the assumption is made that the expected rates are fixed quantities, and subsequent analysis is based on conditioning on these rates. One possible approach to this problem is to try to estimate directly the change in area population using models for migration and other factors. Another possibility is to include a random component within the model for the incidence, which reflects uncertainty in the expected rates. This can be included within a hierarchical Bayesian formulation (Best and Wakefield, 1999). If other random effects are included within the model, there will be an issue concerning identifiability of the expected rate random effect, unless either a condition is placed on the effect or external data support is available.

Another common example of such error is found when covariables are only measured at locations other than those of the disease measurement. For example, pollution levels are often measured in networks, and these networks do not usually relate directly to health data measurement units. Usually, it is required to know or estimate the pollution level at, or in the vicinity of, the disease measurement, i.e. at or near a case event address or within a census tract. To do this, *interpolation* of measurements is required. Interpolation methods are characterised by smoothing operations which include some propagation of error to the site of interest. In a spatial setting, it might be appropriate to use kriging or, possibly, non-parametric kernel smoothers to provide such interpolation. Lawson and Williams (1994) provide an example of such interpolation of expected deaths to case event locations using kernel methods. In general, such error propagation can be seen as an extra element within a hierarchical Bayesian modelling approach, and a number of examples of this approach have been reported. Two-stage EB methods, utilising kriging estimators, are outlined by Donnelly *et al.* (1994) and Donnelly (1995), while full Bayes methods via Gibbs sampling have also been proposed by Pascutto *et al.* (1996).

Finally, specific *spatial* concerns can arise in ecological studies which should be noted. For example, edge effects can occur when data external to the study region is not observed (censored), and also when the model or estimation method assumed for the data depends on neighbourhoods. For example, the effect of edge censoring on the estimation of general autocorrelation over the whole study region may be limited, especially if there is a large area internal to the region. However, if tract-specific relative risks are to be estimated, then there could be considerable edge effects (within edge tracts at least). If the estimation method required the *local* estimation, based on a finite neighbourhood of the tract in question, then (1) if external tracts are not measured, then censoring will occur and bias may result in the edge tract relative risk estimate, or (2) even if external tracts are not present, as in an island, the estimation method may require that neighbourhoods be used in the estimation process. In the case of edge tracts, these have fewer expected neighbours and this can both effect the bias and variance of edge tract estimates. An example of problems which might arise in this way are described in Section 2.5. Bernardinelli and co-workers have described a study of diabetes incidence in relation to malaria prevalence (Pascutto *et al.*, 1996; Bernardinelli *et al.*, 1995a, 1995b). The model employed in that study uses a variance estimator which depends on the *number* of neighbours of a tract. As the number of neighbours is stochastically smaller in edge regions, then the resulting variances are likely to be higher there. Confounded with this effect is the fact that high malarial incidence occurs mainly in low-lying regions close to coasts (edges), and hence mainly in regions with high variance. The effect of this uncertainty in the model-fitting process is worthy of further investigation, as it could have an impact on the resulting estimators.

Another spatial concern, which has been stressed by many authors, is the need in ecological studies to include spatial correlation within any model of the spatial variation of incidence (Clayton *et al.*, 1993). There are many reasons for this requirement. First, unobserved covariates or unknown aetiological factors could be present in a study region, and hence their presence could induce such correlation. This could be apparent when residuals examination is performed as a diagnostic check on model accuracy. Often, these effects can disappear when suitable explanatory variables are added to a model. However, it is clearly important that any fitted model should have a criterion of goodness-of-fit that (standardised) residuals from the model should display little spatial correlation. Otherwise, the model has left unexplained structure in the data. Unfortunately, many recent analyses, particularly hierarchical Bayesian examples (for example Ghosh *et al.*, 1998) do not provide such analysis. Whether the inclusion of a random spatial correlation/heterogeneity term is required to provide, for example, improved standard error estimates or to account for random differences in rates based on tract geometries is debatable, and must depend on the purpose of the study. In general, it would appear that if the aim of the study is to provide good estimates of regression parameters in ecological studies, then there is a need to model the residual correlation structure. It can also be important to include both unstructured and structured (correlated) heterogeneity in the same analysis (Besag *et al.*, 1991b).

10.2 SMALL-SCALE MODELLING ISSUES

Changes of scale can also impact upon the need to include random effects within any analysis. Clayton and co-workers argue for the inclusion of spatial autocorrelation within any ecological analysis due to the inevitable effect of unobserved explanatory variables (Clayton *et al.*, 1993). Indeed, any change in aggregation level may require the addition of a fixed or random effect to compensate for extra variation induced by, for example, differences in region geometries and unobserved environmental factors operating at different scales.

At small spatial scales it is important to also consider how models for case events can be aggregated to tract counts and thereby reduce the bias induced by approximation at the aggregate level. If we define the case event intensity as $\lambda(\boldsymbol{x}) = g(\boldsymbol{x})f(\boldsymbol{x})$, then within the ith tract the expected count, under the usual Poisson process assumptions, is given by

$$E(n_i \mid \theta) = \lambda_i = \int_{a_i} g(\boldsymbol{u})f(\boldsymbol{u})\,\mathrm{d}\boldsymbol{u}.$$

If we assume that both $g(\boldsymbol{u})$ and $f(\boldsymbol{u})$ are the intensities of spatial Poisson processes, then it is reasonable to define their spatial covariance at an arbitrary point $\boldsymbol{x}$ as

$$\operatorname{cov}(g(\boldsymbol{x}), f(\boldsymbol{x})) = |a_i|^{-1}\left\{\int g(\boldsymbol{u})f(\boldsymbol{u})\,\mathrm{d}\boldsymbol{u} - |a_i|^{-1}\int g(\boldsymbol{u})\,\mathrm{d}\boldsymbol{u}\int f(\boldsymbol{u})\,\mathrm{d}\boldsymbol{u}\right\}.$$

Here it is assumed that $g(\boldsymbol{u})$ is constant within any area, i.e. $\int_{a_i} g(\boldsymbol{u})\,\mathrm{d}\boldsymbol{u} = \boldsymbol{g}_i|a_i|$, and is substituted into the covariance. This term describes the *spatial ecological bias* due to aggregation/averaging to tract level. This bias is only zero when, in the trivial case, there is no linear association between population and risk. Clearly, this is not appropriate under the usual definition of the relation between excess risk and background. This point has been made repeatedly by a variety of authors (Diggle, 1993; Diggle and Elliott, 1995; Lawson and Waller, 1996; Lawson and Cressie, 2000) (see also Section 5.2). Essentially, this *decoupling* occurs whenever a constant risk model is assumed to hold within small areas, and is a fundamental feature of much Bayesian modelling in this area. Hence, the assumption of a Poisson distribution for disjoint tract counts with $E(n_i \mid e_i, \theta_i) = e_i\theta_i$ yields a decoupled model which provides biased aggregation from point event to count. As many analyses begin with this assumption, and extend the model, often via random effects, then these analyses are approximate and can only hope to recover from this approximation if the random effects associated with the tracts can account for the disregard for the tract geometry and spatial variation within tracts. At small spatial scales this effect could be marked, and it is important to be able to directly account for tract geometries in any aggregated model. Dean and Balshaw (1997) have examined, in the temporal case, the effect of using aggregated counts as compared to event times within a non-homogeneous (heterogeneous) Poisson process formulation. They found that first-order effects (treatments) can be well (efficiently) estimated, but in general the overall process intensity was poorly estimated. Clearly, with random-effect models this may also hold true if there is reasonable linearity in the model. However, where unobserved covariates arise which could confound with underlying nonlinearity, then there may be efficiency loss within aggregation.

10.2.1 Hypothesis Tests

It is possible to carry out hypothesis tests for particular effects within small-scale ecological analysis, and many of the considerations for such tests applied in disease mapping also apply in this situation. Consider a general model of the form,

$$E(n_i \mid \cdots) = \int_{a_i} g(\boldsymbol{u})f(\boldsymbol{u})\,\mathrm{d}\boldsymbol{u},$$

where $f(\boldsymbol{u})$ may consist of both spatially dependent covariates and tract-specific covariates. We can denote this set-up by

$$f(\boldsymbol{u}) = \rho m\{F_1(\boldsymbol{u})\alpha + F_2\beta + \gamma(\boldsymbol{u}) + \delta(\boldsymbol{u})\}, \tag{10.1}$$

where $m\{\cdot\}$ is a suitable link function, F_1 is a design matrix of spatially dependent covariates (e.g. pollution field values, distances, etc.), F_2 is a design matrix of tract-specific covariates (e.g. census indicators, deprivation indices, etc.), α and β are parameter vectors, and $\gamma(\boldsymbol{u})$, $\delta(\boldsymbol{u})$ are spatial heterogeneity processes. Hypothesis tests in ecological analysis will often be concerned with making inference on some features of the parameter vectors α and β with other factor effects regarded as nuisance. Hence, it is feasible that the heterogeneity processes and other nuisance parameters could be estimated and a test performed with these estimates 'plugged-in'. So far, there has been no attempt to perform such testing in the general formulation above. However, as noted in Section 8.7, some approximate tests have been proposed which employ likelihood, posterior and decoupling approximations (Lawson and Harrington, 1996). One fruitful area of potential development would be the use of generalised Monte Carlo significance tests (Besag and Clifford, 1991), which could be used within Markov chain sampling algorithms.

10.3 LARGE-SCALE MODELLING ISSUES

Ecological analysis carried out at large spatial scales carries some particular restrictions which do not emerge to the same extent in studies in small areas, such as census tracts. By large spatial scale it is assumed that the study region may consist of, for example, all municipalities within a country, or countries within a continent. That is, the scale of study will encompass numbers of urban and rural areas and have dimensions measured in, at least, hundreds of kilometres. The main problems which arise in such studies are related to the grouping of population into large and spatially extensive regions and their association with measured covariables, which are often also aggregated or averaged over large areas.

First, the characteristics of the spatial structure of any disease incidence at large scales may not mirror that found at lower spatial scales. For example, a disease may be found to cluster within areas of say 2 km radius (i.e. the cluster span is 4 km), but when municipalities have counts aggregated the effect of such clustering could disappear due to the *smoothing* effect of aggregation. Hence, the effect of scale change is to change the model components to suit the aggregation level found. In addition, if no aggregation is found associated with scale change, then extra model components may be required to model this scale dependence. This could mean that new long-range or short-range effects may need to be considered. Second, connected with the above comments is the concern that the population characteristics can change considerably over larger regions and so, as well as greater smoothing due to aggregation, there could also be greater heterogeneity between areas of the map. This could lead to the necessary inclusion of long-range trend components in any model for the disease incidence, as well as scale-dependent effects. There should be a clear distinction made here between increasing the size of a study window, and thereby obtaining greater information on disease incidence over a larger area, as opposed to the aggregation of incidence into counts at a larger spatial scale within the expanded window, with the concomitant loss of detailed information concerning the small-scale structure. In the first case, a rich model structure with scale-dependent components may be considered, whereas in the latter case only a model structure appropriate for the level of aggregation can be employed. Cressie (1996) has suggested that a 'geography' variable be included within the explanatory variables to provide a scale-dependent component in any analysis. He considered a binary factorial fixed effect for a two-scale problem, and derived a variety of results for the case of a Gaussian field model. This type of effect could also be considered within a hierarchical model for disease incidence. Multilevel modelling can be applied to multiscale problems, and an example of this is given by Langford *et al.* (1999a). Further, the Bayesian modelling of *misaligned* data where relative risks within small spatial subsets of tracts are to be estimated represents another approach to scale change (Mugglin and Carlin, 1998).

Finally, the relationship between the disease incidence and explanatory variables may change depending on the scale of the study region. For example, the case address locations of a rare disease may be obtained and it is the purpose of the analysis to assess the relationship between the spatial distribution of the disease and measured air pollution concentration over the whole study region. The pollution levels are measured on a grid of monitoring stations. Denote these as z_k^*, $k = 1, \ldots, g$. The stations are irregularly distributed across the region and do not correspond with the case address locations. To make inferences concerning the relation between disease incidence and local pollution, some interpolation of the pollution measurements must be made. Often, the interpolated value of pollution at the case location is required. That is, we must find $\hat{z}^*(\boldsymbol{x}_i)\ \forall\ m$. The smoothing of z^* will usually depend on parameters and hence an added level of error will be included when the interpolated values are used. If analysis is based purely on the interpolated values without reference to this source of error, then a conditional form of model will result. However, it is possible to include this error in a hierarchical model for the disease incidence which treats the smoothing parameters as extra model parameters which can be estimated or sampled. For example, in the case event situation we could specify the hierarchy as

$$
\begin{aligned}
[\boldsymbol{x}_i \mid \beta, \alpha, \kappa, r] &\sim \text{PP}\{m(G\beta + F_z\alpha)\}, \\
[F_z \mid z^*] &\sim N\{z^*, \sigma_z\}, \\
[z^* \mid \kappa, r] &\sim \text{MVN}\{\mu_z, K(\kappa, r)\}, \\
[\kappa] &\sim \text{Gamma}(\varsigma, \tau), \\
[r] &\sim \text{Gamma}(\upsilon, \phi), \\
[\beta] &\sim N(\beta_0, \omega_\beta), \\
[\alpha] &\sim N(\alpha_0, \omega_\alpha),
\end{aligned}
$$

$$[\sigma_z] \sim \text{Gamma}(\pi, \varpi),$$

where $K(\kappa, r)$ is a parametrised covariance matrix depending on a variance (κ) and a covariance range (r) parameter, G is a design matrix of non-spatial covariates, and F_z is a design matrix of functions of the covariate z^* and the other spatial covariables. Zidek *et al.* (1999) have considered a similar specification for a Poisson count model.

Modelling of disease incidence in large-scale ecological analysis has to reflect the scale of analysis of the study and may require the use of special random-effect components to incorporate differing levels of aggregation in covariates, as exemplified in the example cited above. One particular effect of increased spatial scale is that, if the subregion size also increases (i.e. aggregation occurs), then it may be possible to invoke infill asymptotic results (Cressie, 1993) which allow some model simplification. The first asymptotic result of relevance is the convergence in distribution of the tract counts to a Gaussian distribution. The assumption of a Gaussian data likelihood for large-scale ecological analyses has been made by Cook and Pocock (1983) and subsequently by Richardson *et al.* (1992). The assumption of asymptotic normality of the subregion counts can be justified by the central limit theorem applied to a Poisson distribution. The result implies that the subregion counts will have a normal distribution with mean and variance fixed as the integral over the subregion of the underlying Poisson process intensity, i.e.

$$[\boldsymbol{x}_i \mid \alpha] \sim \text{PP}\{m(F_z\alpha)\},$$

$$[n_i \mid \alpha] \sim \text{Poisson}\left\{\int_{a_i} m(F_z\alpha)\,\mathrm{d}\boldsymbol{x}\right\}$$

leads to

$$N\left(\int_{a_i} m(F_z\alpha)\,\mathrm{d}\boldsymbol{x}, \int_{a_i} m(F_z\alpha)\,\mathrm{d}\boldsymbol{x}\right).$$

Note that to be consistent with an underlying (modulated) Poisson process, the normal approximation must have its mean equal to its variance and each subregion has different means and variances. This could be a very restrictive assumption, as uncoupling of the mean–variance relationship may be one of the attractive features of the use of a two-parameter asymptotic distribution. Also, if it is initially assumed that a normal distribution is valid for subregion counts, then any uncoupled variance will not be consistent with an underlying Poisson process. This would also apply if a two-stage model were to be assumed for the case events. For example, the assumption that the intensity of the case event process were itself the realisation of a spatial stochastic process (a Cox process) would lead *conditionally* to the same Poisson process and the same regionalised result. It may be tempting at this point to consider a standard spatial Gaussian process formulation for the subregion counts. This model assumes that the count realisation comes from a multivariate normal distribution with a defined variance-covariance matrix. An alternative would be to assume the standard geostatistical model where a normal likelihood is assumed for the counts, and where the expected values in each subregion have an MVN prior distribution. This could lead to kriging-type estimators for the expectations if standard geostatistical methods are followed (Wackernagel, 1995). Both of these approaches allow the uncoupling of the variance of the count distribution. While this approach to large-scale modelling cannot map onto a lower-scale model, it does have the advantage that it allows the incorporation of a variety of additional model features. A general quadratic normal approximation to a variety of likelihood models which allows the incorporation of such features is possible. Clayton and Kaldor (1987) first proposed the use of such an approximation with a Poisson distribution. This allows for uncoupling of the mean and variance. Note that normal approximations to likelihoods are likely to be reasonably good with infill asymptotics and indeed the likelihood may dominate any prior distributions which are assumed.

10.3.1 Hypothesis Tests

The use of hypothesis testing to assess particular aspects of ecological relations at a large spatial scale follows directly from the basic models used, and the concerns and issues relating to small-scale analysis also apply here. If the normal approximation is assumed as defined above, then hypothesis tests for elements of the vector α follow as for a normal error regression analysis with an integral expectation. Hypothesis tests for any non-spatial components, where the spatial parameters are nuisance parameters would have to be constructed in the usual way, with α estimated under the null hypothesis, or integral averaging would have to be employed. A Bayesian approach could include prior distributions for the relevant parameters and the appropriate posterior ratios or predictive Bayesian information criterion (BIC) measures could be constructed. As opposed to modelling, few, if any, examples exist of such hypothesis testing at large spatial scales.

10.4 A SIMPLE EXAMPLE: SUDDEN INFANT DEATH IN NORTH CAROLINA

Cressie and Chan (1989) presented an analysis of counts of sudden infant death (SID) in the 100 counties of North Carolina, USA, for the period 1974–1978 (see also Cressie (1993)). It is thought that the counts of SID are related to deprivation gradients in the state. The original analysis addressed this issue, while here we provide an example of spatial modelling based on a constant state-wide expected rate (2.06/1000 live births). In this example, the regions (counties) are irregular and they display considerable spatial structure. The SID SMRs appear to be high in the northwest, northeast and the south (Figure 10.1). For modelling purposes, we have assumed a Poisson data likelihood with intensity,

$$E(n_i) = e_i \exp\{\eta_i\},$$

where e_i is the expected count, n_i is the SID count for the ith county and the saturated estimate is $\tilde{\eta}_i = \log(n_i/e_i)$. Table 10.1 displays the results for the best subset model

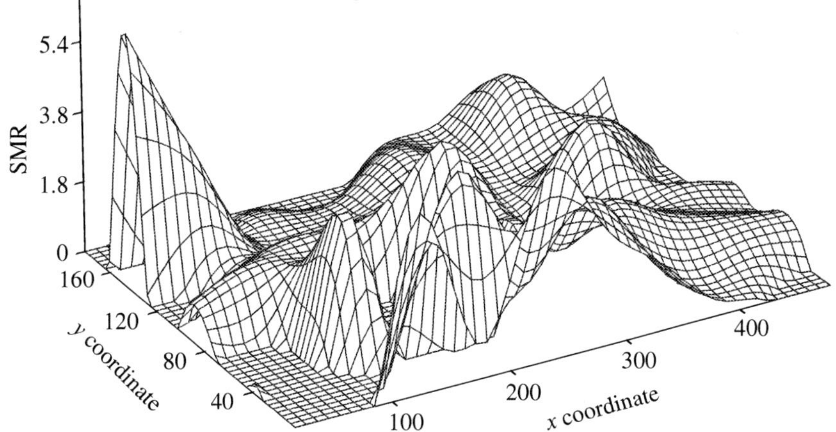

Figure 10.1 North Carolina SIDs example: SMR relative risk surface.

Table 10.1 SIDs North Carolina: results for the best subset BIC model.

parameter	MAP estimate	MAP standard error	M–H modal estimate	M–H standard error†
1	−1.0867	3.8419	−1.216	0.921
x	28.780	6.2697	20.572	8.915
y	17.677	6.6576	14.232	4.782
x^2	8.3156	8.8170	2.159	2.019
y^2	−26.603	4.9683	−24.782	5.293
σ^2	1.0008	0.3557*	1.8647	0.012 2
R	0.2008	0.0354*	0.001 51	0.001 39
log(posterior)	−116.151		−104.2	
ABIC	242.30		218.4	

*s.e. estimated from REML likelihood curvature.
†s.e. estimated from final 100 converged iterations.

for a set of five spatial variables $(1, x, y, x^2, y^2)$. Here the SID variation is thought to relate to the long spatial range described by these variables. In this example, the log-relative risk parameter is assumed to have a spatial Gaussian prior distribution including an exponential model spatial covariance (with variance σ^2 and covariance range R) as described in Sections 5.2.4 and 8.4. Two approaches to estimation of posterior features have been examined here: a MAP estimation approach using a quadratic likelihood approximation, and a full MCMC approach using a Metropolis–Hastings sampler algorithm. A comparison of these estimation methods has been made, based on the BIC criterion. The M–H algorithm was checked for convergence using conventional diagnostic checks (Robert and Casella, 1999) and convergence occurred within 5000 iterations.

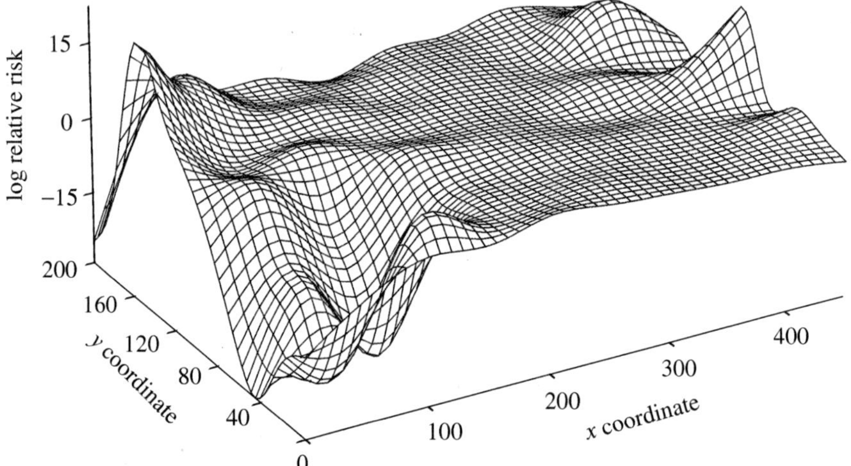

Figure 10.2 North Carolina SIDs example: modal estimate relative risk surface.

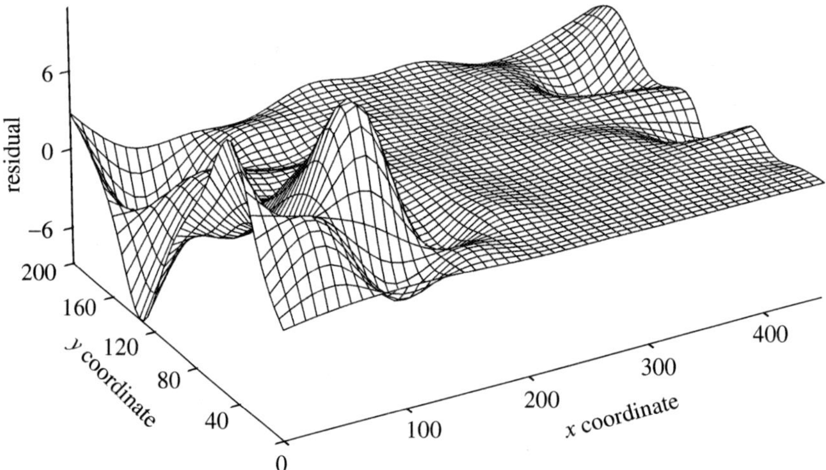

Figure 10.3 North Carolina SIDs example: crude residual surface.

The results suggest that there is a linear (x–y) component and also a quadratic term in the SID surface (y^2). The main difference between MAP and MCMC modal estimates here is the lack of spatial correlation found in the M–H result. Otherwise the two approaches give similar results. The log relative risk estimates under the best MAP model are displayed in Figure 10.2. The residual surface for the MAP estimates (Figure 10.3) shows considerable unexplained structure in the northeast and northwest counties, and hence the model is not completely successful in accounting for the spatial structure over the whole study region. Note that Cressie (1993) also found considerable residual structure in such areas after fitting the deprivation model.

10.5 A CASE STUDY: MALARIA AND IDDM

This case study in ecological analysis is a brief synthesis of a series of papers by Bernardinelli and co-workers, concerning the relation of malaria to insulin dependent diabetes mellitus (IDDM) (Clayton and Bernardinelli, 1992; Bernardinelli *et al.*, 1995b, 1997, 1999; Pascutto *et al.*, 1996).

There is scientific interest in studying the association between IDDM and malaria, since they are both associated with the human leukocyte antigens (HLA) system. The association between IDDM and the HLA system, known to be involved in controlling immunological responses, has long been established.

Malaria is the most important natural selective factor on human populations that has been discovered to date. These elements support the hypothesis that in areas of high endemicity, malaria operates the genetic selection responsible for the influence on the susceptibility to autoimmune diseases. In Sardinia, malaria is known to have selection for some serious hereditary diseases such as b-thalassemia, Cooley's disease and favism, the latter caused by glucose-6-phosphate dehydrogenase (G6PD) enzyme deficiency.

Sardinia is therefore a particularly suitable place for investigating the association between IDDM and malaria. IDDM incidence in Sardinia is quite atypical of other Mediterranean countries. Sardinia has the second highest incidence in Europe (33.2 per 100 000 person years) after Finland (40 per 100 000). A study carried out on the cumulative prevalence of IDDM in 18-year-old military conscripts born in the period 1936–1971 showed that the risk for IDDM began increasing with the male birth cohort of 1950 and that the increasing trend is much higher than the one observed in Europe.

Population genetic studies suggest that, in the plains of Sardinia where malaria had been endemic, some genetic traits were selected to provide greater resistance to the haemolysing action of Plasmodium. In the hilly and mountainous areas, where malaria was almost absent, this adaptation did not occur. Bernardinelli and co-workers obtained the incidence of IDDM from a case registry operated in Sardinia since 1989. The incidence data referred to the period 1989–1992 and cover the population aged 0–29 years. The number of IDDM cases within the 366 communes of Sardinia was available. Also considered was the number of malaria cases (z_i) in the communes for the period 1938–1940, and populations (n_i) from the 1936 census per commune were also available. The prevalence of malaria $\{z_i/n_i\}$ between 1938 and 1940 was considered as a covariate in the model for IDDM incidence.

In their modelling approach, Bernardinelli and co-workers assumed a Poisson likelihood regression model for the IDDM counts, but also found extra-Poisson variation and included a random-effect term to allow for this effect,

$$n_i \sim \text{Poisson}(\rho_i e_i), \qquad (10.2)$$

where ρ_i is the area specific relative risk. A log link was assumed for ρ_i, i.e.

$$\log \rho_i = \alpha_i + \beta x_i.$$

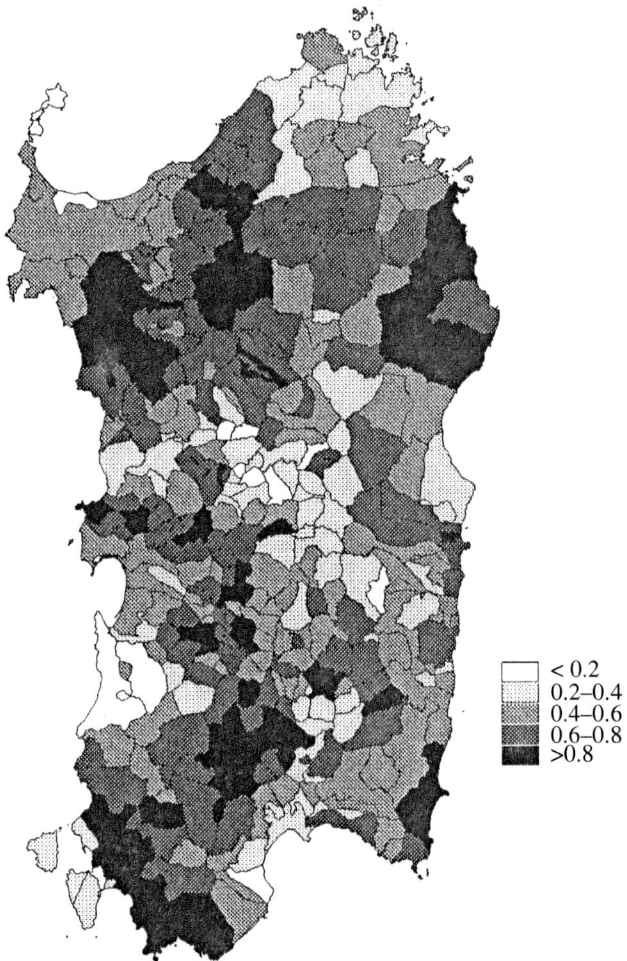

Figure 10.4 Bayesian estimates of long-term malaria prevalence in Sardinia: proportion of the population affected θ_i. Reproduced with permission from Bernardinelli *et al.* (1999).

It was assumed that the covariate x_i is related to the number of malaria cases by a logit link,

$$\log\left(\frac{\theta_i}{1-\theta_i}\right) \sim N(x_i, 2.25), \tag{10.3}$$

where θ_i is the binomial probability of a malaria case, i.e.

$$z_i \sim \text{Binomial}(n_i, \theta_i). \tag{10.4}$$

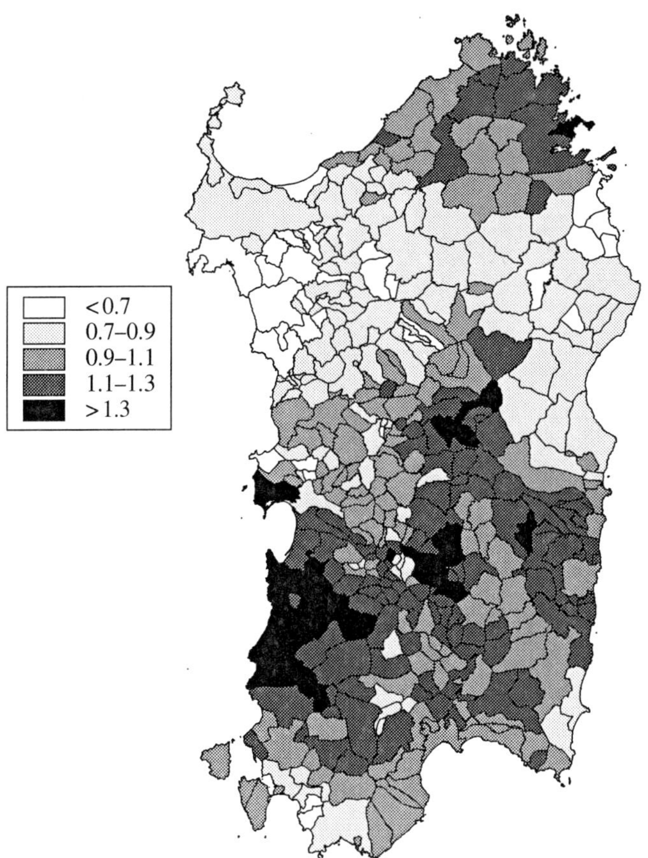

Figure 10.5 Bayesian estimates of the relative risk of IDDM ρ_i. Reproduced with permission from Bernardinelli *et al.* (1999).

The intercept parameter α_i is assumed to have a conditional intrinsic Gaussian prior distribution with a single parameter governing its mean and variance. Their specification does not include separate components for types of heterogeneity.

This specification (10.3) leads to wider standard errors in the parameter estimates of the regression fit. They noted that the malaria prevalence may include extra noise/error and that effect being explicitly modelled. They note that, in practice, ecological covariates can rarely be observed directly. Available data may be either imperfect measurements of, or proxies for, the true covariate. Sometimes, epidemiological data concerning another disease may be used as a proxy variable. For example, to study the geographical variation of heart disease mortality, an important covariate would be the proportion of smokers living in each area. Such data on smoking would generally not be available, so the prevalence of lung cancer recorded by the cancer registry for each area might be a useful proxy. The simplest approach to this problem would be to estimate the true covariate from the proxy for each area independently, using the proxy estimate in the ecological regression. When the proxy variable is an accurate measure of the true covariate, this approach would be reasonable. However, when the correspondence between the two is not so close, this approach has several disadvantages: 'not accounting for measurement error causes the point estimate of the regression coefficient to be underestimated and its precision overestimated.'

The results of the geographical study of the lagged effect of malaria prevalence and IDDM suggested a significant negative association between long-term malaria endemicity and diabetes. This suggests that people who live in areas where malaria has been particularly frequent have a lesser risk of IDDM than those who lived in a low prevalence area in 1938. Diabetes risk is considerably lower in the low-lying regions than in the hills and mountains. Malaria endemicity in the low-lying areas could have prevented the onset of IDDM via stronger selection processes. The 95% credible interval for the correlation between malaria and IDDM is [−0.812, −0.182] with a point estimate of nearly −0.6. This interval is wide but there is some support for a negative relationship. Figures 10.4 and 10.5 display the results of the analysis described.

CHAPTER 11

Infectious Disease Modelling

11.1 INTRODUCTION

The development of models for the behaviour of infectious diseases and epidemic spread has, until recently, been focused on theoretical stochastic models, often confined to the temporal dynamics only. These models have often been developed under simplified assumptions, to allow ease of mathematical development and manipulation (Anderson and May, 1992). However, the types of assumption made are often unrealistic in application to routinely available epidemic data, and it is unfortunate that few attempts have been made, first, to address the quality of routinely available data and, second, to build methods of analysis which allow the modelling of such data. Becker (1989, 1995) has noted that there has been little development of methods specifically designed for the analysis of real epidemic data and, in particular, for the analysis of populations where the individuals have heterogeneous risk of infection, which are by far the most common form of population found in real applications. In addition, Becker noted that few attempts have been made to model the space-time behaviour of infectious disease within heterogeneous populations. More recently, empirical studies of the correlation structure and contact rates of country-wide populations have been published (Bolker and Grenfell, 1996; Keeling *et al.*, 1997; Rhodes and Anderson, 1996). In that work, large-scale analyses of epidemic progressions were considered, with some analysis of heterogeneity of population by subgroups.

Here we aim to address both the incorporation of heterogeneous population and the modelling of spatio-temporal spread of the disease. To do this we borrow some ideas from the recent developments in the modelling of non-infectious diseases (Lawson and Leimich, 2000). In particular, in studies of non-infectious disease, it is commonplace to incorporate population heterogeneity within models for disease distribution. We term the heterogeneous population the 'at-risk' background. This corresponds with the usual definition of the susceptible population, i.e. the population of susceptibles are those who are 'at risk' at any specified point in space-time of getting infected with the disease of concern. In addition, the formulation of models for the space-time behaviour of non-infectious disease relies on the specification of components which depend directly on, or are modified by, this function of susceptibles. This parallels the development of models for infectious disease (Becker, 1989, Chapter 6). In addition, the connection between the modelling of *clusters* of disease where the aetiology is unknown or uncertain (e.g. leukaemias) leads to the consideration of infectious agents and hence overlaps with infectious disease modelling. While modelling of disease clusters per se can be achieved without recourse to models for infectious behaviour, it is reasonable to assume that spatial and temporal clustering can be modelled explicitly via a form of contact probability field which will lead to clustering in space-time. This field can be derived from purely descriptive models for spatial clusters of disease (see, for example, Chapter 6). In the next section, this connection is developed for infectious disease data. The development follows closely on Lawson and Leimich (2000).

11.2 MODEL DEVELOPMENT

In what follows it is assumed that a realisation of n disease events occurs within a fixed spatial and temporal window. We denote these windows as U and T, respectively. The disease events are cases of infection and hence $\{\boldsymbol{x}_i, t_i\}$, $i = 1, \ldots, n$, represents the locations and infection times of all the cases. Now at any specified time t_* there will be a finite number of infectives who have the potential to convert susceptibles to infected cases. Denote the set of infectives at t_* as $I(t_*) : \{\boldsymbol{x}_{I_j}, t_{I_j}\}$, $j = 1, \ldots, n_{t_*}$. We assume that the probability of any susceptible being infected is related to the set $I(\cdot)$, and hence we construct our model around dependence on the current infective set at any time. In previous work on such models in the temporal domain, the basic assumption is made that the incidence of infection is a simple product of susceptible number and infective number. However, to make the dependence specific for spatial and temporal locations, it is convenient to specify a more detailed model of this association. First, we specify the form of the susceptible population. As this population will be spatially and temporally variable, we introduce a three-dimensional field representation $S(\boldsymbol{x}, t)$ which represents the degree of local susceptibility in the population at $(\boldsymbol{x}, t)$. This specification of the susceptible population can be seen as a general method which can make allowance for discrete susceptible locations (e.g. houses) or more continuous backgrounds (e.g. urban areas). In the case of discrete locations, $S(\boldsymbol{x}, t)$ will have a series of spikes at those locations. This definition of the susceptibility function mirrors the use of such a function for non-infectious diseases. In that case, $S(\boldsymbol{x}, t)$ is often estimated from standardised rates for the community, given the local population (age–sex) structure (Inskip *et al.*, 1983). In studies of infectious spread where the infection arises within a large population, $S(\boldsymbol{x}, t)$ could be estimated non-parametrically via density estimation (Silverman, 1986).

First, we assume that we can model the disease process at any time, given knowledge of the current state of the infective population. To do this, we assume that the first-order intensity of cases can capture the model structure adequately, and hence the incidence of cases, conditional on the current $I(\cdot)$, can be modelled via a modulated heterogeneous Poisson process with first-order intensity:

$$\lambda(\boldsymbol{x}, t) = \rho S(\boldsymbol{x}, t) b_t(\boldsymbol{x}, t), \tag{11.1}$$

where

$$b_t(\boldsymbol{x}, t) = \sum_{j=1}^{n(t)} h(\boldsymbol{x} - \boldsymbol{x}_{I_j})g(t - t_{I_j}), \tag{11.2}$$

where $S(\boldsymbol{x}, t)$ is the local density of susceptibles at $(\boldsymbol{x}, t)$, ρ is the overall density (space $\times$ time units), h is a spatial cluster function which relates the location of a susceptible to any current infective location, $n(t)$ is the current number of infectives (just before time t). The g function is a cluster function depending on the temporal position (t) in relation to the time of infectivity of the known infectives (t_{I_j}). This can be structured to model special temporal infectivity periods (e.g. prodromal duration in measles). The h, g functions will usually have a distance decay form, i.e. they may produce lower intensity the further away a potential case is from the location and time of the infective events. The temporal function can include an infectivity period and other forms. This specification of the first-order intensity relates the local density of susceptibles to their spatial and temporal distance from currently infective people. While this form of intensity definition considers the epidemic to be described by a space-time interaction term $(b_t(\boldsymbol{x}, t))$, it is possible to generalise the intensity specification to include separate spatial and temporal components which purely specify spatial or temporal effects. This could allow the incorporation of parameters describing transmission rates in time and space separately and to model, for example, spatial transmission between selected social groups. Our focus in what follows is, essentially, the susceptible-infected-removed (SIR) model, where susceptibles can become infective and cannot become susceptible again. However, the approach can easily be extended to more complex epidemics which include re-infection dynamics. In addition, it should be noted that the general modelling framework proposed here can easily be extended to allow the kind of temporal nonlinear dynamics which can characterise longer-term time-series of epidemics (e.g. measles (Rhodes and Anderson, 1996)). This extension can be achieved by the inclusion of correlated prior distributions for the components of $\lambda(\boldsymbol{x}, t)$, while maintaining the likelihood framework, albeit extended to a Bayesian formulation.

Here, we apply the basic model described above with spatio-temporal interaction only. The justification for this approach is discussed in Section 11.5.

11.3 MODELLING SPECIAL CASES

In a later section we will consider some modifications to this model, in an application to a German measles epidemic, reported by Pfeilsticker (1863) and recently revisited by Oesterle (1990), Aaby *et al.* (1995) and Becker and Wang (1998). However, before discussing these specific modifications, it is worthwhile considering a special case of this model and the resulting simplifications.

11.3.1 Proportional Hazards Interpretation

Given the temporal nature of this problem, in which events occur at observed time points, it is interesting to pursue the connection between this modelling approach and conventional survival analysis. In the proportional hazards model, a risk set is observed over time and any failures (disease cases) are assessed conditional on the risk set R specified just prior to the failure time of the individual of concern. A similar development can be pursued here. If we regard (11.1) as the hazard function for a disease case, then we can specify the probability of an infection within $R(t)$ within a small time increment δt approximately as

$$\sum_{R(t)} \lambda(\boldsymbol{x}, t)\delta\boldsymbol{x}\delta t,$$

where $\delta\boldsymbol{x}$ is a small area around $\boldsymbol{x}$. Hence, we can also specify a conditional probability of a particular individual at $\boldsymbol{x}_i$ becoming infected as

$$\frac{\lambda(\boldsymbol{x}_i, t)\delta\boldsymbol{x}\delta t}{\sum_{R(t)} \lambda(\boldsymbol{x}, t)\delta\boldsymbol{x}\delta t}.$$

If it is assumed that the δ terms cancel, we can take the product of these conditional probabilities evaluated at the case infection times to give a conditional likelihood,

$$L = \prod_i \frac{\lambda(\boldsymbol{x}_i, t_i)}{\sum_{j \in R(t_i-)} \lambda(\boldsymbol{x}_j, t_i)}, \tag{11.3}$$

where $R(t_i-)$ denotes the risk set just prior to infection time t_i. In general, the background susceptible function will *not* factor out of this likelihood and so there is still a requirement to estimate the susceptible function directly. Note that direct maximisation of (11.3) is possible and this could avoid the evaluation of integrals over spatial and temporal domains required by the Poisson process likelihood formulation. Of course, the conditional nature of this formulation does not account for the full information available on the parameters in $\lambda(\boldsymbol{x}, t)$, as this ignores the observed times of case infection. However, usually the 'baseline' hazard, in this case the susceptibility function, does not factor out of the likelihood and must be estimated during the analysis, and for complete epidemics there will be no censored individuals and so there is likely to be little loss of information in these situations.

11.3.2 Subgroup Modifications

If we now consider an epidemic where the population is split into different susceptibility classes, etc., then we can easily modify the above model to accommodate these differences. Define m classes, $l = 1, \ldots, m$, where the class denotes a different population subgroup of susceptibles, and define $\boldsymbol{S}$ as a row vector of groups with differing susceptibility

$$\boldsymbol{S} : [s_1(\boldsymbol{x}, t), s_2(\boldsymbol{x}, t), \ldots, s_m(\boldsymbol{x}, t)].$$

Also define a column vector of cluster function terms which relate a current group to infectives in another group, i.e. we now consider the population to be split into groups with differing susceptibilities. Each group could have, at any time, susceptibles and infectives within it. Define

$$H = \begin{cases} \sum h_{11}g_{11} + \cdots + \sum h_{1m}g_{1m}, \\ \sum h_{21}g_{21} + \cdots + \sum h_{2m}g_{2m}, \\ \vdots \\ \sum h_{m1}g_{m1} + \cdots + \sum h_{mm}g_{mm}, \end{cases}$$

where h and g denote the cluster function terms defined above but where $(\boldsymbol{x}, t)$ refer to location in space-time of the first subscripted group and $\boldsymbol{x}_{t_j}$ and t_{t_j} refer to the infective locations in space and time of the second subscripted group. The summation $\sum$ being over the infectives in the second subscripted group. The ith row of $\boldsymbol{H}$ represents the total contribution of infectives from all groups to the 'epidemic potential' of a susceptible in the ith group.

Now the total intensity is given by

$$\boldsymbol{SH} = \sum_i s_i(\boldsymbol{x}, t)\left\{\sum_j \sum_l h_{ij}g_{ij}\right\}, \tag{11.4}$$

where the inner summation ($\sum_l$) is over the infectives within the jth group, and the intensity for an individual case in the ith group is

$$s_i(\boldsymbol{x}, t)\left\{\sum_j \sum_l h_{ij}g_{ij}\right\}.$$

11.4 CLUSTER FUNCTION SPECIFICATION

In what follows we consider in more detail the definition of the cluster functions h and g. These functions determine the contact relationships between potential cases and the existing infected population.

11.4.1 Spatial Dependence

The spatial dependence function $h(u)$ can take a variety of forms depending on the choice of contact distribution specified. The simplest forms are those which assume that u is a simple distance measure relating a case residence $(\boldsymbol{x})$ to the residences of infectives $(\boldsymbol{x}_{I_j})$. In that case the definition of h can reduce to a function of distance between residences. Here the inter-residence distance is assumed to form a surrogate for exposure. This may be reasonable for certain types of disease, where contact occurs via 'local' behaviour. Where special contact patterns are important (e.g. with Aids), inter-residence distance may not be a useful surrogate.

A typical spatial dependence cluster function is defined in Section 11.5.2.

11.4.2 Temporal Dependence

The spatial interaction discussed above is directly modified by the temporal cluster function in (11.1). This modification implies that even when strong spatial association is present, if weak temporal association is present, there will be a reduced probability of infection. This appears to be a realistic assumption for most infectious diseases. Often, it is useful to consider a model for the temporal infection process in an individual and to base a $g(\cdot)$ function on this specification. A typical profile of infection can be broken into three stages: a period of incubation, an infectious period, and a final period. Often, the final period is represented by *removal* of the susceptible from the population, if the disease is such that after infection there is little or no probability of contracting the disease again. This type of model is often referred to as an SIR model.

A typical specification for $g(\cdot)$ is then

$$g(t - t_I) = \begin{cases} f_1(t) & \text{if } t < t_{I_0}, \\ f_2(t) & \text{if } t_{I_0} \leqslant t < t_{I_1}, \\ f_3(t) & \text{if } t \geqslant t_{I_1}, \end{cases}$$

where the f_i functions apply to different periods and t_{I_0} and t_{I_1} are the start and end times of the infectious period. Figure 11.3 displays a typical form of this function.

11.5 DATA EXAMPLE

The spread of a measles epidemic is considered here, and was first described by Pfeilsticker (1863) and Oesterle (1990). For general issues relating to Measles epidemics, see, for example, Cliff *et al.* (1998). This measles epidemic occurred within a small isolated village, Hagelloch, Germany, in 1861, effectively a closed community. The data set is unusually complete, as Pfeilsticker meticulously recorded the progress of the epidemic. On a daily basis the household and name of the family members affected was recorded, including the start, development and disappearance of the various symptoms, body temperature, and any complications or deaths. There is a complete record of all susceptibles. Oesterle mapped the locations of susceptibles and cases in space, and established the most likely infector for each susceptible that became infected.

The population of the village at the time of the epidemic comprised 577 inhabitants. There were 200 children up to the age of 15, who were born after the previous measles epidemic or escaped infection as infants. Twelve of these can be regarded as not susceptible as they were immigrants who had had measles before, infants aged six months or less (carrying placental immunity), or were kept in isolation. The remaining 188 susceptible children were infected.

In this example, the temporal transmission rate was previously found to be relatively constant, and most interest lies in the spatio-temporal interaction of the disease spread. In this situation it is natural to consider a spatio-temporal interaction model for the data, such as (11.1). This specification allows the examination of how spatial

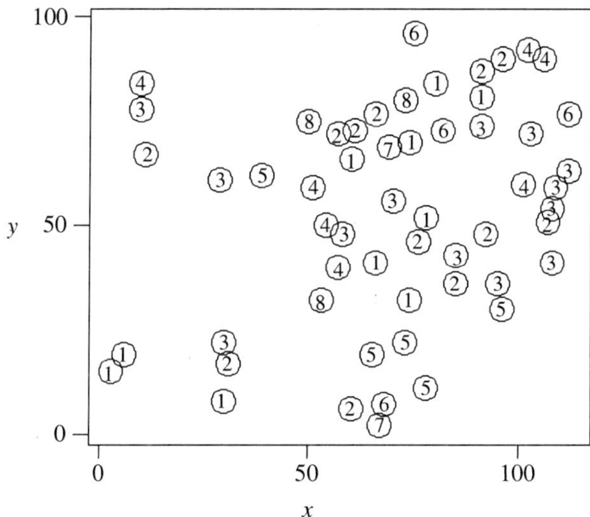

Figure 11.1 Map of Hagelloch, showing the number of susceptibles in each household before the start of the epidemic. Reproduced with permission from Lawson and Leimich (2000).

aggregation relates to temporal clustering of the cases, and hence can describe the existence of aggregation interaction.

In what follows, we employ the general proportional hazards model (11.1), (11.3) to this data set. This model requires the specification of the first-order intensity in (11.1).

11.5.1 Distribution of Susceptibles $S(\boldsymbol{x}, t)$

The number of susceptibles at location $\boldsymbol{x}$ at time t, $S(\boldsymbol{x}, t)$ is known from the data (see Figure 11.1). Time in the model is discrete, as observations were made daily, hence we examine the risk sets for these time periods. The grid of locations (Oesterle, 1990), which was approximately 100×100 units, was scaled to 1×1. To obtain a continuous surface representing the local density of susceptibles, the data at each time t were replaced by a bivariate Gaussian kernel density estimate $\hat{S}(\boldsymbol{x}, t)$. As there is no reason, *a priori*, to assume that a different smoothing constant is required for each dimension, we have assumed that a common smoothing parameter can be employed. The common smoothing parameter was calculated as in Silverman (1986), $0.96\sqrt{[\frac{1}{2}(\text{var}(x_i) + \text{var}(y_i))]}n^{-1/6}$, where n is the number of points. The smoothed surface obtained for the susceptibles before the start of the epidemic ($t = 0$) is shown in Figure 11.2.

The spatial and temporal distance functions, $g(\cdot)$ and $h(\cdot)$, describe the contact relationships between the susceptibles and the existing infective population.

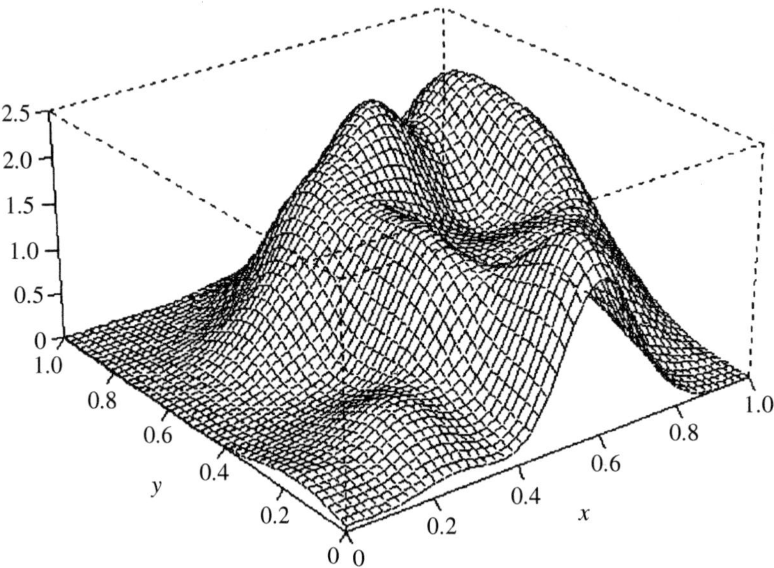

Figure 11.2 Smoothed density of susceptibles $\hat{S}(\boldsymbol{x}, 0)$. Reproduced with permission from Lawson and Leimich (2000).

11.5.2 The Spatial Distance Function *h*

For diseases easily transmitted through general contact, the spatial distance between residences can be used as a measure of exposure, and a bivariate normal function used,

$$h(\boldsymbol{x} - \boldsymbol{x}_I) = \frac{1}{2\pi\kappa} \exp\left\{ -\frac{1}{2\kappa} (\|\boldsymbol{x} - \boldsymbol{x}_I\|)^2 \right\}, \tag{11.5}$$

where $\boldsymbol{x}$ denotes the location of a susceptible, $\boldsymbol{x}_I$ the location of an infective. The one-parameter κ is a spread parameter; the larger κ, the more likely is infection across some distance. This parameter determines the spatial scale of spread.

11.5.3 The Function *g*

The function $g(\cdot)$ describes the changes of infectivity over time. Its specification is based on the infectivity pattern of measles, summarised in Table 11.1.

The times of the start of the prodrome (first symptoms), of the eruption (rash), and, if applicable, of death, are available for each infective in the data set as PRO, ERU and DEAD. Following Oesterle (1990) and Pfeilsticker (1863), we assume individuals to be equally infectious from a day before the start of the prodrome until three days after the eruption and define

$$t_I = \text{PRO} - 1, \qquad t_R = \min\{\text{ERU} + 3, \text{DEAD}\}.$$

Table 11.1 Summary of the measles infectivity pattern.

stage	susceptible	incubation		prodrome	eruption	desquamation
duration		variable	1 day	~4 days very variable	~3 days variable	
		14 days				
status	susceptible	latent	infectious			removed

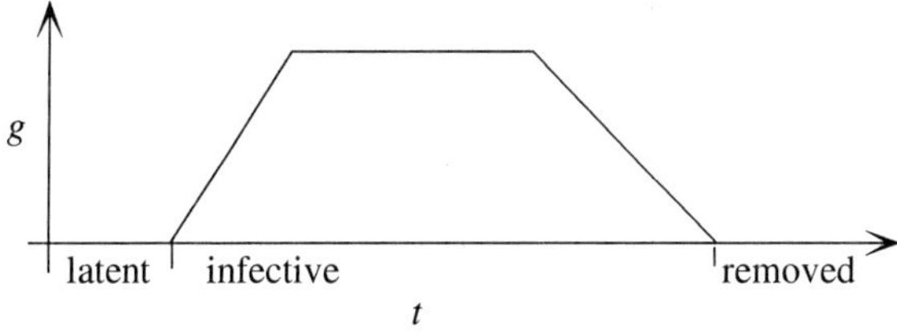

Figure 11.3 A typical function $g(\cdot)$. Reproduced with permission from Lawson and Leimich (2000).

For $g(\cdot)$, we can then use a simple uniform function

$$g(t; t_I, t_R) = \begin{cases} \gamma & \text{if } t_I < t < t_R, \\ 0 & \text{otherwise,} \end{cases} \tag{11.6}$$

rather than the more general trapezoidal function shown in Figure 11.3. The parameter γ is a constant measure of the infectivity.

11.5.4 Fitting the Model

Substituting into (11.1) and (11.3), we obtain

$$L = \prod_i \frac{\hat{S}(\boldsymbol{x}_i, t_i) \sum_{j=1}^{n(t_i)} h(\boldsymbol{x}_i - \boldsymbol{x}_{I_j}) g(t_i; t_{I_j}, t_{R_j})}{\sum_{j \in R(t_i-)} \hat{S}(\boldsymbol{x}_j, t_i) \sum_{k=1}^{n(t_i)} h(\boldsymbol{x}_j - \boldsymbol{x}_{I_k}) g(t_i; t_{I_k}, t_{R_k})}. \tag{11.7}$$

Noting that the value of $g(\cdot)$ is γ wherever it is used in (11.7), further simplification of (11.7) yields

$$L = \prod_i \frac{\hat{S}(\boldsymbol{x}_i, t_i) \sum_{j=1}^{n_{t_i}} h(\boldsymbol{x}_i - \boldsymbol{x}_{I_j})}{\sum_{j \in R(t_i-)} \hat{S}(\boldsymbol{x}_j, t_i) \sum_{k=1}^{n_{t_i}} h(\boldsymbol{x}_j - \boldsymbol{x}_{I_k})}. \tag{11.8}$$

To fit the model to the data set, the log-likelihood was maximised with respect to the single remaining parameter κ. This gave very large values for κ (see Figure 11.4(a)). The disappointing results can be explained readily by returning to the particular features of the data example. Many of the susceptibles attend the village school. The

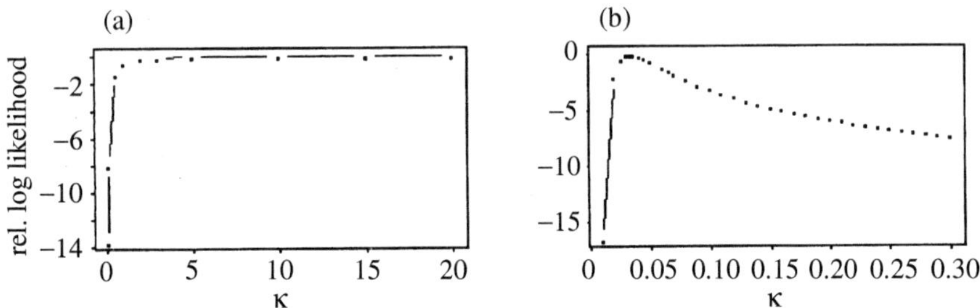

Figure 11.4 Likelihood profiles for the initial model (a) and the revised model (b). Reproduced with permission from Lawson and Leimich (2000).

spatial distance function $h(\cdot)$ currently ignores this likely place of infection, as it is based only on the distance between residences. Therefore, we would expect the model to improve, as observed, with a flattening of the distance function h, which occurs as κ increases.

11.6 REVISED MODEL

The school has two classes, one for 6–10 year olds and one for older children. The school status is known for all susceptibles. A good model should incorporate the school in the sense that infection is likely to take place at school between classmates, and to a lesser extent between children in different classes.

To implement this, the spatial distance function h is modified. There are several possible approaches, such as making κ a function of the age group, or using a non-Euclidean measure of distance. We adopt the second approach, defining the modified function h as

$$h(\mathbf{x} - \mathbf{x}_I) = \frac{1}{2\pi\kappa} \exp\left(-\frac{1}{2\kappa}(\|\mathbf{x} - \mathbf{x}_I\| \times m)^2\right), \tag{11.9}$$

where m modifies the distance according to school status:

$$m = \begin{cases} 1 & \text{if susceptible and infective not both at school,} \\ 0 & \text{if susceptible and infective in same class,} \\ \frac{1}{2} & \text{if susceptible and infective in different classes.} \end{cases}$$

Thus, being in the same class at school is associated with the same infection risk as being in the same household, while being in different classes is given a lower risk of infectivity. It is recognised that the above model might be improved by allowing the factor m to be estimable and/or using a model with different susceptible groups and separate interaction rates. However, in this example, the main concern is to provide a model which simply differentiates between type of school contact, household contact and distance based alternatives.

11.6.1 Results

Maximising the log-likelihood for the revised model yielded $\kappa_{\text{opt}} = 0.0337$ after convergence (see Figure 11.4(b)). Using the general result $2 \times (L_{\kappa_{\text{opt}}} - L_{\kappa}) \sim \chi_1^2$ to find a 95% likelihood confidence interval for κ, we obtain a CI: (0.0205, 0.0740). It is possible to compute a variance estimate from the known likelihood invoking asymptotic properties of maximum likelihood (ML) estimators. However, it is uncertain whether the asymptotic variance estimates would be valid when such asymmetry is present with a relatively small sample size. Instead we resorted to the use of an empirical approximation based on sampling the likelihood surface to provide a variance estimate for κ. Using rejection sampling from the surface, a sample of a hundred κ values was taken. The resulting standard error of κ was 0.0203. This approximation should be relatively good given a sample of such magnitude. Notice that the standard error is quite large due to the relatively flat surface, particularly above the ML estimate. This may suggest that there is some support for larger κ values in this data set.

Note that the κ parameter here solely defines the spatio-temporal aggregation of cases, and in the case of school or household contact this interaction, in the form of $1/2\pi\kappa$, can be interpreted as an instantaneous transmission rate. The fact that this rate is not confidently estimated may reflect only weak spatio-temporal interaction in this example.

11.7 CONCLUSIONS

Here, a general approach to the modelling of infectious disease behaviour has been presented, which can easily be applied to a range of data formats, whether in the form of case addresses of infectives and susceptibles, or in the form of counts of infectives within regions in fixed time periods with lower level susceptible information. Define the time period of interest as subscript $t = 1, \ldots, T$, and the region of interest as subscript $i = 1, \ldots, p$. The count in the ith area and tth time period is n_{it}. Given the conditional independence of counts in non-overlapping space-time slots under the non-homogeneous Poisson process, conditional on the susceptible field, we can assume that

$$n_{it} \sim \text{Poisson}(\Lambda_{it}),$$

$$\Lambda_{it} = \int_t \int_{A_i} S(\boldsymbol{u}, v) m\left\{ \sum_{j=1}^{I_{it}} h(\boldsymbol{u} - x_j), \sum_{j=1}^{I_{it}} g(v - t_j) \right\} \mathrm{d}\boldsymbol{u}\, \mathrm{d}v,$$

where A_i denotes the area of the ith region, $m\{\cdot\}$ is a link function, and $S(\boldsymbol{x}, t)$ is the susceptible function as before. This model generalises the earlier intensity model by allowing the introduction of a link function which can include a variety of forms.

It has been demonstrated in this example that the modelling approach is easily applied with standard statistical packages and does not require extensive programming. An advantage of the approach discussed here is that likelihood models can be developed which incorporate a variety of model assumptions applicable in different situations, but which can be analyses within the same general procedure.

Our example has been analysed using a proportional hazards type of model and we have been reasonably successful in demonstrating the importance of school and household contacts in the spatial contact process. Further work is needed in the application area and other examples to further refine the model and its components. In the example examined, only the spatio-temporal interaction of the disease has been examined, whereas in other cases it may be more important to include separate spatial and temporal components, especially if separate transmission rates are to be assessed. This extension is straightforward within the general framework.

It is also worth noting that this modelling approach assumes full knowledge of the infection process with enumeration of all infectives at the correct times and locations. In many applications, there may be considerable *under-ascertainment* of infective cases, and in that situation there could be unknown components in the cluster functions. This is equivalent to mixture models with unknown component numbers. In itself this problem does not pose significant difficulties as it is possible to invoke reversible-jump MCMC algorithms to sample the joint distribution of number and location of components. This has already been described for non-infectious clustering (see Section 6.2 and also Appendix C). In essence, the location in space-time is regarded as a parameter to be estimated (Tanner, 1996).

The above formulation and extensions to the general model have as their focus a simple conditional independence model for the infectious process. When such a model is aggregate over the population and over time, then quite complex *unconditional* dynamics can be found. This is typical of hierarchical models for stochastic systems. In general, it is possible to extend these models into a general Bayesian framework where we include prior distributions for parameters. For example, we might include random-effect terms which describe *unobserved* heterogeneities in the infection process. These could be similar to those employed in the non-infectious situation (see Section 4.3.4). This leads to relatively intractable models where the posterior distribution of the parameters must be sampled via MCMC algorithms, and likelihood methods cannot be used. Notice that this formulation is different from that of Gibson (1997), who uses a local model which leads to the immediate use of MCMC sampling because of an intractable normalising constant. Cressie and Mugglin (2000) have provided a descriptive Bayesian spatio-temporal analysis of infectious disease dynamics.

Another issue which has not been addressed within the model described here is the exact mechanism of *removal* of infectives from the population. If the focus of a study were on the removal rate for the infection, then this rate would have to be incorporated within any model. In the present development, removal is assumed to only occur after the complete infective period has been passed. This removal issue relates to that of censoring, in that if an infective recovered or otherwise changed their status with respect to infectivity within their infectivity period, then their impact on the infection spread would be reduced. This issue is addressed within models for dropout in longitudinal studies and there is likely to be considerable potential for examination of this issue within a public health context for infectious disease prediction/surveillance.

APPENDIX A

Monte Carlo Testing and Simulation Envelopes

In many applications in spatial epidemiology, large-sample (asymptotic) sampling distributions are not valid, or are unavailable due to intractable theory. The reasons for this are discussed in Section 5.4. When this occurs, resort must be made to simulation-based methods.

Before considering these simulation-based methods in detail, it is important to briefly review the role of nuisance parameters in classical inference.

A.1 NUISANCE PARAMETERS AND TEST STATISTICS

Define a statistic $T(\boldsymbol{y}; \boldsymbol{\theta})$, which is defined to be dependent on the data $\boldsymbol{y}$ and a parameter vector $\boldsymbol{\theta}$. Usually, the parameter vector is 'nuisance', in the sense that the parameters are not of primary interest in the testing situation. For example, the classical relative risk estimator, the SMR, can be used to test for $H_0 : \theta = E$ against $H_1 : \theta \neq E$, based on m regions. To test this, a suitable statistic could be based on the sum of deviations of SMRs from E, i.e. $T(\boldsymbol{n}; \boldsymbol{\theta}) = \sum_{i=1}^{m} [n_i/e_i - \theta]$. Usually, $E = 1$ and is specified. The test statistic $T(\boldsymbol{n}; \boldsymbol{\theta})$ is a non-standardised form of the score statistic (Cox and Hinkley, 1974) for a Poisson likelihood with $E(n_i) = \theta e_i$. Here, e_i is a nuisance parameter, in that it appears in the test statistic, is not of primary interest, and must be evaluated.

A variety of approaches can be adopted to the inclusion of nuisance parameters. The simplest approach is to *estimate* the nuisance parameter(s), and to make inference conditional on the estimated parameters. This is a form of *profile* inference and does not make allowance for parameter estimation uncertainty in the nuisance parameters. For $T(\boldsymbol{n}; \boldsymbol{\theta})$ above, this would represent estimation of the $\{e_i\}$ from, say, population standardised rates for regions.

An alternative is to re-express the problem so that there is no dependence on the nuisance parameter vector. It is sometimes possible to 'concentrate-out' parameters, usually via integration, so that the original model, from which the test statistic is derived, does not depend on the parameter. This approach implies that the parameter(s) arise from a distribution of values, and, in that sense, this approach is similar to the derivation of a predictive distribution in Bayesian inference. In the approach to testing described here, we examine estimation of nuisance parameters and conditional inference only.

A.2 MONTE CARLO TESTS

Monte Carlo testing is a simulation-based method for the assessment of evidence for the support of different hypotheses, in the frequentist inference paradigm. The essential ingredients of the method are the comparison of the test statistic value with a number of statistics computed from simulations of the null hypothesis. In formal terms, define t_1 to be the observed value of a statistic $T(y;\theta)$ and let t_i, $i = 2, \ldots, r$, be corresponding values generated by independent random sampling from the distribution of $T(y;\theta)$ under H_0, the null hypothesis. Let $t_{(j)}$ be the jth ranked statistic amongst the r values of t_i. Then, under H_0,

$$P_r\{t_1 = t_{(j)}\} = 1/r, \qquad j = 1, \ldots, r$$

and H_0 is rejected on the basis that t_1 ranks kth largest or higher gives an exact one-sided test of size k/r. Evidently, this probability argument can be extended to both tails as $1 - k/r$ and k/r represent equivalent quantiles in each tail. Usually, $r = 100$ or 1000 depending on the level of accuracy required (see, for example, Ripley (1987) or Cressie (1993, p. 635)).

A simple example of such a Monte Carlo test is provided by a single region count n_i and a test of whether it arose from a Poisson distribution with parameter E, where E is known. In this case there are no nuisance parameters. Formally, we examine

$$H_0 : \theta_i = E \quad \text{against} \quad H_1 : \theta_i \neq E,$$

with test statistic $T(n_i;\theta) = n_i - E$. For a given region, $n_i = 5$ and $E = 7$. For a Monte Carlo test, 99 simulations of a Poisson (7) distribution yielded a rank of 27.0 for n_i amongst the pooled sample of 100 items, and this does not reach any conventional significance level in a two-tail test. Note that in the case of discrete variates the rank ties which can result in such a simulation are usually broken by averaging. An alternative conservative rule is to assume the least extreme rank for t_1 (see, for example, Diggle (1983, p. 7)).

More complex tests arise when nuisance parameters are present, and these commonly occur in spatial epidemiology. Assume a study region consists of m regions and we wish to test whether the counts $\{n_i\}$, $i = 1, \ldots, m$, have arisen by chance, given the expected values $\{e_i\}$ in the regions. We wish to test this global criteria using $T(\boldsymbol{n};\theta) = \sum_{i=1}^{m}\{n_i/e_i - 1\}$. In this case, we have m nuisance parameters $\{e_i\}$, and we will test

$$H_0 : \theta_i = Ee_i \quad \text{against} \quad H_1 : \theta_i \neq Ee_i,$$

with $E = 1$. One approach to this problem is to estimate the $\{e_i\}$, via standardised rates (for example) and to generate samples of counts, $n^*_{i1}, \ldots, n^*_{ir}$, from an independent Poisson (e_i) distribution under H_0.

This approach leads naturally to the consideration of Monte Carlo tests for the addition of parameters and nested models. To extend the current example, consider a log-linear model as in Section 4.4, where we currently have θ_p parameters and we wish to test whether a model with θ_q $(q > p)$ should be accepted. In this case, the null hypothesis is the model with θ_p parameters, and we could compute a deviance, or other goodness-of-fit measure, for the change from θ_p to θ_q. Under H_0, θ_p parameters are estimated and regard the $\{e_i\}$ corresponding to this model as fitted values. That is, the fitted values of any null model play the role of e_is generally in $T(\boldsymbol{n}; \theta)$ above. Hence, the prescription in general is to generate count samples from the fitted model (expected) counts under H_0.

Note that all the above methods can be applied to point event (case location) data. In that case, any test statistic based on $\{\boldsymbol{x}_i\}$ can be tested for a current null model by simulating r point event realisations from the null hypothesis and computing $\{t_i\}$ from these realisations.

Difficulties can sometimes be experienced in simulation of null hypotheses for Monte Carlo tests, especially when the null is a complex spatial process. For example, if a spatially correlated prior distribution is assumed for regional rates under the null hypothesis, then r simulations of an m-variate multivariate normal distribution may be required. For large m, this could be computationally prohibitive. Ripley (1987) and Cressie (1993) discuss various methods for this simulation (e.g. Cholesky decomposition, Turning bands or spectral/harmonic methods). One possible route which could be explored, when simulations are expensive, is to resample or bootstrap the original simulation. Special methods must be used, however, which preserve the correlation structure (Hall, 1988).

Special Monte Carlo tests related to Markov chains are discussed by Besag and Clifford (1991).

A.3 SIMULATION ENVELOPES

The idea of simulation of samples from fitted values leads naturally to consideration of how model fits can be assessed over individual data points or groups of points. This area of concern is of relevance to both classical and Bayesian model fitting, in that residual diagnostics can be treated in both cases by the same methods. In classical inference, a set of fitted values $\{e_i\}$ is compared to observed values $\{n_i\}$ by computing residuals based on $r_i = n_i - e_i$. These crude residuals contain information about how the model fits at a particular observation point. Usually, the r_i are standardised to have equal variance.

As in the case of Monte Carlo testing, it is possible to generate a set of simulated counts $\{n_i^*\}$ from the model with fitted values $\{e_i\}$ and hence compute simulated residuals: $r_i^* = n_i^* - e_i$. It is possible to construct g such sets of r_i^* which can be used to construct a piecewise simulation envelope for the residuals at each observation point.

The idea of a simulation envelope can be used for residual diagnostics in Bayesian inference also. For a current parameter vector θ_P, draw a sample of θ_P from the posterior distribution, and thence simulate a data sample from $\pi(\theta_P)$, the predictive distribution of the data. The sets of simulated $\{n_i\}$ can be compared to fitted values and simulated residuals computed (Gelman *et al.*, 1995, p. 247). Simulation envelopes are useful for the pointwise analysis of residuals but are of limited use in a two-dimensional example as they cannot be displayed (or interpreted easily). Instead, it is possible to report the ranking of the data residual amongst the simulated set and thence compute a pointwise p-value for the data point considered. In this way, a p-value surface can be derived which can be displayed in two dimensions. This idea was pioneered by Kelsall and Diggle (1995b). An example of this form of residual analysis is given in Section 8.9 and a general discussion can be found in Section 5.3.

APPENDIX B

Markov Chain Monte Carlo Methods

The assessment of the absolute and relative goodness-of-fit of models relies upon the availability of methods for model estimation, or, in the Bayesian case, the ability to sample from posterior distributions of model parameters. In recent years, a range of simulation-based methods have been developed which allow posterior sampling from models of considerable complexity. Likelihood methods can be regarded as a subset of more general Bayesian models. The ability to sample from this diverse range of models is a significant facility provided by the group of methods called Markov chain Monte Carlo, or MCMC for short.

Given the generality of this approach, it is important to outline the main methods of MCMC, particularly as they are used in a variety of sections of this book.

B.1 DEFINITIONS

Denote the likelihood for data $\boldsymbol{y}$ given a parameter vector $\boldsymbol{\theta}$ as $l(\boldsymbol{y} \mid \boldsymbol{\theta})$. Prior distributions for the p components of $\boldsymbol{\theta}$ are defined as $g_i(\theta_i)$ for $i = 1, \ldots, p$. The posterior distribution of $\boldsymbol{\theta}$ and $\boldsymbol{y}$ is defined as

$$P_o(\boldsymbol{\theta} \mid \boldsymbol{y}) \propto l(\boldsymbol{y} \mid \boldsymbol{\theta}) \prod_i g_i(\theta_i). \tag{B.1}$$

The aim is to generate a sample from the posterior distribution $P_o(\boldsymbol{\theta} \mid \boldsymbol{y})$. It is often the case that $P_o(\boldsymbol{\theta} \mid \boldsymbol{y})$ can be difficult to sample from in complex models, such as those found in spatial epidemiology. It is useful to have a general method for such simulation.

Suppose we can construct a Markov chain with state space $\boldsymbol{\theta}_c$, where $\boldsymbol{\theta} \in \boldsymbol{\theta}_c \subset \mathbb{R}^k$. The chain is constructed so that the equilibrium distribution is $P_o(\boldsymbol{\theta} \mid \boldsymbol{y})$, and the chain should be easy to simulate from. If the chain is run over a long period, then it should be possible to reconstruct features of $P_o(\boldsymbol{\theta} \mid \boldsymbol{y})$ from the realised chain values. This forms the basis of the MCMC method, and algorithms are required for the construction of such chains. A selection of recent literature on this area is found in Ripley (1987), Gelman *et al.* (1995), Smith and Roberts (1993), Besag and Green

(1993), Cressie (1993), Smith and Gelfand (1992), Tanner (1996) and Robert and Casella (1999).

The basic algorithms used for this construction are

1. the Metropolis algorithm and its extension Metropolis–Hastings algorithm;
2. the Gibbs Sampler algorithm.

B.2 METROPOLIS AND METROPOLIS–HASTINGS ALGORITHMS

In all MCMC algorithms, it is important to be able to construct the correct *transition probabilities* for a chain which has $P_o(\boldsymbol{\theta} \mid \mathbf{y})$ as its equilibrium distribution. A Markov chain consisting of $\boldsymbol{\theta}^1, \boldsymbol{\theta}^2, \ldots, \boldsymbol{\theta}^t$, with state space Θ and equilibrium distribution $P_o(\boldsymbol{\theta} \mid \mathbf{y})$ has transitions defined as follows.

Define $q(\boldsymbol{\theta}, \boldsymbol{\theta}')$ as a transition probability function, such that, if $\boldsymbol{\theta}^t = \boldsymbol{\theta}$, the vector $\boldsymbol{\theta}^t$ drawn from $q(\boldsymbol{\theta}, \boldsymbol{\theta}')$ is regarded as a proposed possible value for $\boldsymbol{\theta}^{t+1}$.

B.2.1 Metropolis Algorithm

In this case choose a symmetric proposal $q(\boldsymbol{\theta}, \boldsymbol{\theta}')$ and define the transition probability as

$$p(\boldsymbol{\theta}, \boldsymbol{\theta}') = \begin{cases} \alpha(\boldsymbol{\theta}, \boldsymbol{\theta}')q(\boldsymbol{\theta}, \boldsymbol{\theta}') & \text{if } \boldsymbol{\theta}' \neq \boldsymbol{\theta}, \\ 1 - \sum_{\theta''} q(\boldsymbol{\theta}, \boldsymbol{\theta}'')\alpha(\boldsymbol{\theta}, \boldsymbol{\theta}'') & \text{if } \boldsymbol{\theta}' = \boldsymbol{\theta}, \end{cases}$$

where

$$\alpha(\boldsymbol{\theta}, \boldsymbol{\theta}') = \min\left\{1, \frac{P_o(\boldsymbol{\theta}' \mid \mathbf{y})}{P_o(\boldsymbol{\theta} \mid \mathbf{y})}\right\}.$$

In this algorithm a proposal is generated from $q(\boldsymbol{\theta}, \boldsymbol{\theta}')$ and is accepted with probability $\alpha(\boldsymbol{\theta}, \boldsymbol{\theta}')$. The acceptance probability is a simple function of the ratio of posterior distributions as a function of $\boldsymbol{\theta}$ values. The proposal function $q(\boldsymbol{\theta}, \boldsymbol{\theta}')$ can be defined to have a variety of forms but must be an irreducible and aperiodic transition function. Specific choices of $q(\boldsymbol{\theta}, \boldsymbol{\theta}')$ lead to specific algorithms.

B.2.2 Metropolis–Hastings extension

In this extension to the Metropolis algorithm the proposal function is not confined to symmetry and

$$\alpha(\boldsymbol{\theta}, \boldsymbol{\theta}') = \min\left\{1, \frac{P_o(\boldsymbol{\theta}' \mid \mathbf{y})q(\boldsymbol{\theta}', \boldsymbol{\theta})}{P_o(\boldsymbol{\theta} \mid \mathbf{y})q(\boldsymbol{\theta}, \boldsymbol{\theta}')}\right\}.$$

Some special cases of chains are found when $q(\boldsymbol{\theta}, \boldsymbol{\theta}')$ has special forms. For example, if $q(\boldsymbol{\theta}, \boldsymbol{\theta}') = q(\boldsymbol{\theta}', \boldsymbol{\theta})$, then the original Metropolis method arises and further, with

$q(\boldsymbol{\theta}, \boldsymbol{\theta}') = q(\boldsymbol{\theta}')$ (i.e. when no dependence on the previous value is assumed), then

$$\alpha(\boldsymbol{\theta}, \boldsymbol{\theta}') = \min\left\{1, \frac{w(\boldsymbol{\theta}')}{w(\boldsymbol{\theta})}\right\},$$

where $w(\boldsymbol{\theta}) = P_o(\boldsymbol{\theta} \mid \mathbf{y})/q(\boldsymbol{\theta})$ and $w(\cdot)$ are importance weights. One simple example of the method is $q(\boldsymbol{\theta}') \sim \text{Uniform}(\boldsymbol{\theta}_a, \boldsymbol{\theta}_b)$ and $g_i(\theta_i) \sim \text{Uniform}(\theta_{ia}, \theta_{ib})\ \forall\ i$, this leads to an acceptance criterion based on a likelihood ratio. Hence, the original Metropolis algorithm with uniform proposals and prior distributions leads to a stochastic exploration of a likelihood surface. This, in effect, leads to the use of prior distributions as proposals. However, in general, when the $g_i(\theta_i)$ are not uniform, this leads to inefficient sampling. The definition of $q(\boldsymbol{\theta}, \boldsymbol{\theta}')$ can be quite general in this algorithm and, in addition, the posterior distribution only appears within a ratio as a function of $\boldsymbol{\theta}$ and $\boldsymbol{\theta}'$. Hence, the distribution is only required to be known up to proportionality.

B.2.3 The Gibbs Sampler

The Gibbs Sampler has gained considerable popularity, particularly in applications in medicine, where hierarchical Bayesian models are commonly applied (Gilks *et al.*, 1993). This popularity is mirrored in the availability of software which allows its application in a variety of problems (e.g. BEAM, BUGS, CODA (see Appendix E)). This sampler is a special case of the Metropolis–Hastings algorithm where the proposal is generated from the conditional distribution of θ_i given all other $\boldsymbol{\theta}$, and the resulting proposal value is accepted with probability 1.

More formally, define

$$q(\theta_j, \theta_j') = \begin{cases} p(\theta_j^* \mid \theta_{-j}^{t-1}) & \text{if } \theta_{-j}^* = \theta_{-j}^{t-1}, \\ 0 & \text{otherwise,} \end{cases}$$

where $p(\theta_j^* \mid \theta_{-j}^{t-1})$ is the conditional distribution of θ_j given all other $\boldsymbol{\theta}$ values (θ_{-j}) at time $t-1$. Using this definition it is straightforward to show that

$$\frac{q(\boldsymbol{\theta}, \boldsymbol{\theta}')}{q(\boldsymbol{\theta}', \boldsymbol{\theta})} = \frac{P_o(\boldsymbol{\theta}' \mid \mathbf{y})}{P_o(\boldsymbol{\theta} \mid \mathbf{y})}$$

and hence $\alpha(\boldsymbol{\theta}, \boldsymbol{\theta}') = 1$.

B.2.4 M–H versus Gibbs Algorithms

There are advantages and disadvantages to M–H and Gibbs methods. The Gibbs Sampler provides a *single* new value for each $\boldsymbol{\theta}$ at each iteration, but requires the evaluation of a conditional distribution. On the other hand, the M–H step does not require evaluation of a conditional distribution but does not guarantee the acceptance of a new value. In addition, block updates of parameters are available in M–H, but not usually in Gibbs steps (unless joint conditional distributions are available). If conditional distributions are difficult to obtain or computationally expensive, then M–H can be used and is usually available.

In summary, the Gibbs Sampler may provide faster convergence of the chain if the computation of the conditional distributions at each iteration are not time-consuming. The M–H step will usually be faster at each iteration, but will not necessarily guarantee fast exploration. In straightforward hierarchical models where conditional distributions are easily obtained and simulated from, the Gibbs Sampler is likely to be favoured. In more complex problems, such as many arising in spatial statistics, resort to the M–H algorithm may be required.

B.2.5 Examples

As examples of the methods discussed above we here present some simple examples of the construction of M–H ratios for specific distributions. For the purposes of exposition, the simple case where a uniform prior distribution is assumed for any parameter. Hence, the posterior ratio reduces to a likelihood ratio.

The Poisson Distribution For the Poisson distribution it is possible to derive an M–H criteria for a simple model where only a single parameter appears. In this case the distribution can be defined as

$$P(X = x) = \begin{cases} \mathrm{e}^{-\lambda}\lambda^x/x! & x = 0, 1, 2, 3, \ldots, \\ 0 & \text{elsewhere,} \end{cases}$$

and the M–H criterion is

$$\frac{L(\lambda')}{L(\lambda)} = \left(\frac{\lambda'}{\lambda}\right)^{s_x} \mathrm{e}^{n(\lambda-\lambda')}. \tag{B.2}$$

Hence, in this rather trivial case the λ parameter would be sampled based on the likelihood ratio for λ.

Some Applied Examples

1. *Regional counts.* Assume that for m regions, the count n_i, $i = 1, \ldots, m$, is observed. In addition, the expected count in the ith region, e_i is also observed. Assume also that the counts are independently distributed and have a Poisson distribution with $E(n_i) = \theta e_i$, where θ is a constant parameter describing the relative risk over the whole study window. The likelihood in this case, bar a constant, is given by

$$L(\theta) = \exp\left(-\theta \sum_{i=1}^{m} e_i\right) \prod_{i=1}^{m} (\theta e_i)^{n_i}. \tag{B.3}$$

The maximum likelihood estimator of θ is found to be

$$\hat{\theta} = \sum_{i=1}^{m} n_i \Big/ \sum_{i=1}^{m} e_i.$$

Hence, the following M–H sampler criterion is found for the θ parameter in this case:

$$\frac{L(\theta')}{L(\theta)} = \exp\{s_e(\theta - \theta')\}\left(\frac{\theta'}{\theta}\right)^{s_n},$$

where

$$s_e = \sum_{i=1}^{m} e_i \quad \text{and} \quad s_n = \sum_{i=1}^{m} n_i.$$

2. *Case Events.* Assume that a realisation of case events occurs within a study window W of area $|W|$. In addition, it is assumed that the intensity of events relates to their distance from a fixed known point location, such as in the putative source examples of Section 7. Specifically, we assume that the events are governed by a heterogeneous Poisson process with first-order intensity given by

$$\lambda(\boldsymbol{x}, \theta) = \rho g(\boldsymbol{x})(1 + \mathrm{e}^{-\theta d(\boldsymbol{x})}), \tag{B.4}$$

where ρ is a constant rate, $g(\boldsymbol{x})$ is a function representing the local background intensity of population 'at risk' from the disease of interest, and $d(\boldsymbol{x})$ represents the distance from the point $\boldsymbol{x}$ to the fixed point. We will assume an estimate of $g(\boldsymbol{x})$, $\hat{g}(\boldsymbol{x})$ say, is available and we can make inferences conditional on the realised values of $\hat{g}(\boldsymbol{x})$ at event locations. The likelihood conditional on ρ and $\hat{g}(\boldsymbol{x})$ is then

$$\prod_{i=1}^{m}\{\rho\hat{g}(\boldsymbol{x}_i)(1 + \mathrm{e}^{-\theta d(\boldsymbol{x}_i)})\}\exp\left\{-\int_W \lambda(\theta, \boldsymbol{u})\,\mathrm{d}\boldsymbol{u}\right\}.$$

The M–H sampler criteria in this case, conditioning as noted, are

$$\frac{L(\theta')}{L(\theta)} = \prod_{i=1}^{m}\left\{\frac{1 + \exp[-\theta' d(\boldsymbol{x}_i)]}{1 + \exp[-\theta d(\boldsymbol{x}_i)]}\right\}\exp\left\{\int_W [\lambda(\theta, \boldsymbol{u}) - \lambda(\theta', \boldsymbol{u})]\,\mathrm{d}\boldsymbol{u}\right\}. \tag{B.5}$$

Clearly, in examples where greater numbers of parameters appear, more complex posterior ratios result.

APPENDIX C

Metropolis–Hastings Cluster Sampling

C.1 THE BIRTH–DEATH–DIFFUSION ALGORITHM

The basic algorithm used to sample from the posterior distribution of cluster centres and number of centres is described below. Section 6.2 provides an introduction to the relevant likelihood and Bayesian models. Define the m offspring and k related centres as

$$\{\boldsymbol{x}_i\}, i = 1, \ldots, m,$$
$$\{\boldsymbol{y}_j\}, j = 1, \ldots, k.$$

Define the likelihood conditional on m events for the Poisson process with intensity $\lambda(\boldsymbol{x} \mid \boldsymbol{y}, \theta)$ as

$$L_c = \prod_{i=1}^{m} \lambda(\boldsymbol{x}_i \mid \boldsymbol{y}, \theta) \left\{ \int_T \lambda(\boldsymbol{u} \mid \boldsymbol{y}, \theta)\, \mathrm{d}\boldsymbol{u} \right\}^{-m}. \tag{C.1}$$

This is the conditional version of the likelihood in (4.2). In general, we assume that

$$\lambda(\boldsymbol{x} \mid \boldsymbol{y}, \theta) = g(\boldsymbol{x}, \ldots) m\left(\sum_j^k h_{\phi_1}(\boldsymbol{x} - \boldsymbol{y}_j; \kappa_1); C_{\phi_2}, \ldots, C_{\phi p} \right). \tag{C.2}$$

The C_ϕ terms represent other cluster terms which could be included in the model. The first of these terms being the function of interest $C_{\phi_1} = \sum_j^k h_{\phi_1}(\boldsymbol{x} - \boldsymbol{y}_j; \kappa_1)$. The link function $m(\cdot)$ can take a variety of forms depending on the application. For example, in many epidemiological applications, an additive relative risk link of the form $1 + C_{\phi_1}$ could be appropriate. The additional cluster functions in (C.2) could represent temporal and/or space-time clusters or further multidimensional terms (Lawson and Clark, 1998).

For convenience, we rewrite (C.2) as

$$\lambda(\boldsymbol{x} \mid \boldsymbol{y}, \theta) = \hat{g} m\left(\sum_j^k h_{\phi_1}(\boldsymbol{x} - \boldsymbol{y}_j; \kappa_1); C_{\mathrm{T}} \right), \tag{C.3}$$

where $\hat{g}$ is an estimate, at $\boldsymbol{x}$, of the background modulating function, usually obtained from external data, appropriately estimated in the dimensions of the problem. The function C_{T} represents the collection of other cluster terms within the model.

C.2 PRIOR DISTRIBUTIONS

Both k and $\boldsymbol{y}$ are unknown in the problem and it is required that prior distributions be assumed for these parameters. For independent cluster models, there is a wide choice of distributions possible. One simple choice would be to assume that the centres have a uniform prior distribution over U, with the number of centres governed by a Poisson distribution. However, it has been found previously that reconstructions of cluster centres can suffer from multiple response, i.e. that centres tend to be placed close to existing centres during iterations of the algorithm. This can be combated by using an inhibition prior distribution. A simple inhibition prior distribution is the Strauss distribution (Ripley, 1988), which provides a *joint* prior distribution for centres and number of centres. The distribution $\{\boldsymbol{y}, k\} \sim \text{Strauss}(\rho, \gamma, \boldsymbol{R})$ has provided a suitable prior distribution which provides appropriate reconstructions. It is also possible to introduce hyperpriors for these parameters but these are not considered here.

C.3 METROPOLIS–HASTINGS REVERSIBLE JUMP SAMPLER

The likelihood (C.1) combined with the relevant spatial prior distributions described above provide a joint posterior distribution from which it is possible to sample. Instead of conditioning on the number of centres (k) and constructing a hierarchical model, we avoid the awkward conditioning in (C.3) by sampling from the joint posterior distribution for $(\boldsymbol{y}, k)$. This joint distribution can be sampled from by using an iterative algorithm which allows a number of different transitions to take place. These transitions represent the birth, death and shifting (diffusion) of putative cluster centres, and such transitions are iteratively evaluated using a ratio of posterior distributions.

Geyer and Møller (1994) and subsequently Green (1995) described MCMC algorithms which can have a variety of transitions. In our case, the birth, death and diffusion (shifting) of cluster centres are of interest. The type of transitions are, for the current state $\boldsymbol{y}$,

birth: addition of a randomly selected new point; the proposal is $\boldsymbol{y} \cup \{\boldsymbol{u}\}$, where $u \in T$ is a random point with probability density $b(\boldsymbol{y}, \cdot)$;

death : or deletion of an existing point; the proposal is $\boldsymbol{y} \setminus \{v_i\}$, where v_i is one of the points of $\boldsymbol{y}$ chosen with probability $d(\boldsymbol{y}, v_i)$;

diffusion: random shifting or displacement of one of the existing points; the proposal is $\boldsymbol{y} \setminus \{v_i\} \cup \{\boldsymbol{u}\}$, where v_i is one of the points of $\boldsymbol{y}$ chosen with equal probability and $u \in T$ is a random point with probability density $s(v_i, \boldsymbol{u})$.

These transitions are described for a single cluster term above, but can be defined for a series of such terms describing clusters in multidimensional problems. In those cases, the number of transitions will usually be $3d$, where d is the number of cluster terms or dimensions. For example, in space-time clustering problems there may be spatial, temporal and spatio-temporal cluster terms and hence in that case there may be nine transitions.

In the above example, we describe a basic three-transition cluster form for a single component. In that case we can define three proposal kernels which describe the probability of the different transitions. Define Q_{b}, Q_{d}, Q_{s} to describe the transition kernels for birth, death and shifting (diffusion) and assume a mixture form for the combination of these transitions, thus:

$$P(\boldsymbol{y},\cdot) = (1-p)q(\boldsymbol{y})Q_{\mathrm{b}} + (1-p)(1-q(\boldsymbol{y}))Q_{\mathrm{d}} + pQ_{\mathrm{s}},$$

where $0 \leqslant p \leqslant 1$ and $0 \leqslant q(\cdot) \leqslant 1$. That is, with probability p we propose a shift, otherwise with probability $q(\boldsymbol{y})$ we propose a birth, and otherwise propose a death. Note that for $d \succ 1$, i.e. for more than one cluster term, the $P(\boldsymbol{y},\cdot)$ will be a convex combination of d such terms with appropriate mixing probabilities.

For the single cluster case above, the Metropolis–Hastings ratios are

$$\text{birth:} \qquad M(\boldsymbol{y}, \boldsymbol{y} \cup \{u\}) = \frac{p_o(\boldsymbol{y} \cup \{u\})}{p_o(\boldsymbol{y})} \frac{1 - q(\boldsymbol{y} \cup \{u\})}{q(\boldsymbol{y})} \frac{d(\boldsymbol{y} \cup \{u\}, u)}{b(\boldsymbol{y}, u)};$$

$$\text{death:} \qquad M(\boldsymbol{y}, \boldsymbol{y} \setminus \{v_i\}) = \frac{p_o(\boldsymbol{y} \setminus \{v_i\})}{p_o(\boldsymbol{y})} \frac{q(\boldsymbol{y} \setminus \{v_i\})}{1 - q(\boldsymbol{y})} \frac{b(\boldsymbol{y} \setminus \{v_i\}, v_i)}{d(\boldsymbol{y}, v_i)};$$

$$\text{diffusion:} \quad M(\boldsymbol{y}, \boldsymbol{y} \setminus \{v_i\} \cup \{u\}) = \frac{p_o(\boldsymbol{y} \setminus \{v_i\} \cup \{u\})}{p_o(\boldsymbol{y})} \frac{s(u, v_i)}{s(v_i, u)}.$$

Convergence results for the above sampler are provided in Geyer and Møller (1994) and Lawson *et al.* (1996b).

Commonly in the above sampler some simplifying assumptions are made and the resulting ratios are considerably simplified. For example, uniform proposals can be generated from

$$R \equiv 1, \qquad q(\cdot) \equiv q, \qquad d(\boldsymbol{y}, v_i) = 1/k, \qquad b(\cdot,\cdot) = s(\cdot,\cdot) = 1/|T|,$$

but these may lead to very inefficient sampling if the likelihood is markedly peaked around a few locations. An alternative is to assume that $s(u, v) = s(u - v)$ is a symmetric kernel and

$$b(\boldsymbol{y}, u) = \frac{1}{m} \sum_{j=1}^{m} h(\boldsymbol{x}_j - u)$$

and the ratios become

$$\text{birth:} \qquad M(\boldsymbol{y}, \boldsymbol{y} \cup \{u\}) = \frac{p_o(\boldsymbol{y} \cup \{u\})}{p_o(\boldsymbol{y})} \frac{1-q}{q} \frac{m}{(k+1)\sum_{j=1}^{m} h(\boldsymbol{x}_j - u)};$$

$$\text{death:} \qquad M(\boldsymbol{y}, \boldsymbol{y} \setminus \{v_i\}) = \frac{p_o(\boldsymbol{y} \setminus \{v_i\})}{p_o(\boldsymbol{y})} \frac{q}{1-q} \frac{k \sum_{j=1}^{m} h(\boldsymbol{x}_j - v_i)}{m};$$

$$\text{diffusion:} \quad M(\boldsymbol{y}, \boldsymbol{y} \setminus \{v_i\} \cup \{u\}) = \frac{p_o(\boldsymbol{y} \setminus \{v_i\} \cup \{u\})}{p_o(\boldsymbol{y})}.$$

Note that if $q = 0.5$, which implies equal probability births and deaths, then the birth–death ratios reduce to posterior ratios modified by proposals from the cluster distribution function employed. The shift term is a simple posterior ratio.

C.4 THE POSTERIOR RATIOS FOR CLUSTER TERMS

Define the integral of the conditional intensity $\lambda(\boldsymbol{x} \mid \boldsymbol{y}, \theta)$ as $H(\boldsymbol{x} \mid \boldsymbol{y}, \theta, T) = \int_T \lambda(\boldsymbol{u} \mid \boldsymbol{y}, \theta)\, d\boldsymbol{u}$. Assuming a Strauss prior distribution for the cluster centres, the posterior ratios then become

$$\text{birth:} \quad \frac{\prod_{i=1}^{m} \lambda(\boldsymbol{x}_i \mid \boldsymbol{y} \cup u, \theta)/H(\boldsymbol{x} \mid \boldsymbol{y} \cup \boldsymbol{u}, \theta, T)^m}{\prod_{i=1}^{m} \lambda(\boldsymbol{x}_i \mid \boldsymbol{y}, \theta)/H(\boldsymbol{x} \mid \boldsymbol{y}, \theta, T)^m} \rho \gamma^{n\boldsymbol{R}(u)},$$

$$\text{death:} \quad \frac{\prod_{i=1}^{m} \lambda(\boldsymbol{x}_i \mid \boldsymbol{y} \setminus \{v_i\}, \theta)/H(\boldsymbol{x} \mid \boldsymbol{y} \setminus \{v_i\}, \theta, T)^m}{\prod_{i=1}^{m} \lambda(\boldsymbol{x}_i \mid \boldsymbol{y}, \theta)/H(\boldsymbol{x} \mid \boldsymbol{y}, \theta, T)^m} \frac{1}{\rho \gamma^{n\boldsymbol{R}(v_i)}},$$

$$\text{diffusion:} \quad \frac{\prod_{i=1}^{m} \lambda(\boldsymbol{x}_i \mid \boldsymbol{y} \setminus \{v_i\} \cup u, \theta)/H(\boldsymbol{x} \mid \boldsymbol{y} \setminus \{v_i\} \cup u, \theta, T)^m}{\prod_{i=1}^{m} \lambda(\boldsymbol{x}_i \mid \boldsymbol{y}, \theta)/H(\boldsymbol{x} \mid \boldsymbol{y}, \theta, T)^m} \gamma^{n\boldsymbol{R}(u) - n\boldsymbol{R}(v_i)},$$

where $nR(u)$ is the number of points within distance R of u.

APPENDIX D

Glossary of Estimators

In this appendix we briefly list some common estimators which have been proposed for the estimation of relative risks in disease maps. These estimators mainly arise from likelihood and EB modelling. In many cases the full Bayesian estimator is not available in closed form, and we only display closed form estimators here.

D.1 CASE EVENT ESTIMATORS

Define the relative risk of disease at location $\boldsymbol{x}$ as $R(\boldsymbol{x})$, and at the ith case location as $R(\boldsymbol{x}_i)$. Assuming that the cases are governed by a modulated Poisson process with intensity (a) $\lambda(\boldsymbol{x}) = g(\boldsymbol{x})m(\boldsymbol{x})$, or (b) $\lambda(\boldsymbol{x}) = g(\boldsymbol{x}) + m(\boldsymbol{x})$, with a study window W_t. Intensity (a) represents a multiplicative (M) model for excess risk and (b) represents an additive (A) model (Table D.1).

D.2 TRACT COUNT ESTIMATORS

The data are $\{n_i\}$, $i = 1, \ldots, m$, representing counts with small areas, and $\{\boldsymbol{x}_i\}$, $i = 1, \ldots, m$, representing the locations of cases of disease within a study window. Define the relative risk of disease in the ith small-area tract as θ_i. The following models can be specified in increasing order of complexity, based on the assumption of an independent Poisson likelihood model with $E(n_i) = e_i\theta_i$ and (if appropriate) prior distributions as specified in Table D.2.

Table D.1 Case event estimators.

Model	$R(x)$-estimator	Reference
global (M) (maximal)	$\int_{W_t} \hat{\lambda}(\boldsymbol{u})\,\mathrm{d}\boldsymbol{u} / \int_{W_t} \hat{g}(\boldsymbol{u})\,\mathrm{d}\boldsymbol{u}$	
global (A) (maximal)	$\int_{W_t} \{\hat{\lambda}(\boldsymbol{u}) - \hat{g}(\boldsymbol{u})\}\,\mathrm{d}\boldsymbol{u}$	
local (M) (minimal)	$\hat{\lambda}(x_i)/\hat{g}(x_i)$ using Dirichlet tile area information	JB, LW1
local (A) (minimal)	$\hat{\lambda}(x_i) - \hat{g}(x_i)$	
kernel (M) smoother	$\hat{\lambda}(x_i)/\hat{g}(x_i)$	JB, LW1, LW2, KD
kernel (A) smoother	$\hat{\lambda}(x_i) - \hat{g}(x_i)$	

JB, Bithell (1990); LW1, Lawson and Williams (1993); LW2, Lawson and Williams (1994); KD, Kelsall and Diggle (1995b).

Table D.2 Tract count estimators.

Model	θ_i-estimator	Ref.
1 global mean (minimal)	$\sum n_i / \sum e_i$	—
2 SMR (maximal)	n_i/e_i	—
3 simple EB	$(n_i + \alpha)/(e_i + \beta)$	CK, T
4 moment EB	$h + C(n_i/e_i - h)$, where $h = \sum n_i / \sum e_i$ and $\bar{e} = \sum e_i / m$ $C = \dfrac{\kappa - h/\bar{e}}{\kappa - h/\bar{e} + h/e_i}, \kappa = \sum_i e_i \left(\dfrac{n_i}{e_i} - h\right)^2 / \sum e_i$	Man, RM
5 moment EB (extended)	$\hat{\theta}_i^{\mathrm{EB}} = (A - W)(n_i/e_i - h)$, where A, W are weights and $\hat{\theta}_i^{\mathrm{EB}} = \{W + h(1 - W)\} n_i/e_i$ (the Manton estimator)	DL, Man
6 EB smoother	$\sum_j a_{ij} \dfrac{n_j}{e_j}$, where $a_{ij} = \begin{cases} w_i & j = i, \\ (1 - w_i)/(n_{ni} - 1) & j \neq i, \\ 0 & \text{else} \end{cases}$ and $w_i = \{1 + \overline{y_i}/(e_i v_i)\}^{-1}$ where $\overline{y_i}$, v_i are the mean and variance of the $j = 1, \ldots, n_{ni}$, neighbours	KK
7 kernel smoother	$\sum_{j=1}^{m} a_{ij} n_j / e_j$, where $a_{ij} = k_{ij} / \sum_{j=1}^{m} k_{ij}$ and k_{ij} is the kernel evaluated for the i, jth locations	BD, AL

CK, Clayton and Kaldor (1987); DL, Devine and Louis (1994); Man, Manton *et al.* (1981); RM, Marshall (1991a); T, Tsutakawa (1988); KK, Kafadar (1996); BD, Breslow and Day (1987); AL, (Lawson, 1993c).

APPENDIX E

Software

E.1 SOFTWARE

A wide variety of software is now available to provide assessment of spatial data. This ranges from modules for spatial statistical analysis in for example S-Plus, to complete Geographical Information Systems (GIS) such as MapInfo® or ArcView®, which usually do *not* have spatial statistical capabilities. However, the software available can be conveniently divided into two basic types: (1) spatial statistical tools, which are usually not integrated into a general GIS environment, and (2) general packages, which allow users to manipulate and display georeferenced data.

E.1.1 Spatial Statistical Tools

A number of packages and modules within packages now provide access to spatial statistical procedures. The most notable of these are the spatial module of S-Plus, and the SPLANCS system (University of Lancaster), which also interfaces with S-Plus. S-Plus is a widely available statistical package which is currently provided only on Unix and Windows formats, but not in other mainframe operating systems. Hence, the availability of these modules is limited by hardware configuration. The Spatial Stats module provides basic descriptive spatial analysis measures, kriging estimators and point process related methods. It does not provide a general modelling capability in applications in spatial epidemiology. The SPLANCS package, which is a set of S-Plus functions, does provide some specialist tools for the analysis of point event data in both space and space-time (e.g. kernel smoothing), and functions for analysis of putative hazard problems and other clustering problems, based on methods developed by workers at Lancaster University. The S-Plus package has a file transfer link with the GIS ArcView® also. However, none of these systems provide an integrated spatial data analysis platform, which can be used easily to carry out data manipulation and analysis.

Some packages have been developed specifically for the analysis of small-area count data and these sometimes have improved data display and management facilities. DismapWin (Schlattmann *et al.*, 1996) is a general purpose package which can display small-area count maps and provides a range of further analysis steps, including computation of SMRs, EB estimation of relative risks, mixture analysis and covariate adjustment. BEAM has also been developed to provide a platform for

Bayesian ecological analysis of mapped data, and does provide display and manipulation functions as well as statistical mapping procedures. It is also possible to use the general WinBugs MCMC software (Pascutto *et al.*, 1996) to analyse hierarchical models for mapped data, but GIS facilities are not available (as yet, although GeoBugs is promised). The MLWin software developed by the multi-level modelling project (Langford *et al.*, 1999a) can also be used to analyse hierarchical models, although based on normal approximations to distributions in the hierarchy.

For certain specific tasks, such as evaluating test statistics, some software is available, and software to provide a range of testing possibilities is currently being developed. For example, in cluster testing, *SaTScan*, software for testing spatial and spatio-temporal clustering via scan statistics is available for Windows 95/NT (Kulldorff and Nagarwalla, 1995). *Stat!* is a general package providing analysis of clustering of health events (Jacquez, 1994), which has Windows 95/NT versions in development. Other software from the same source are *gamma*, *GBAS* and *GeoMed*, which are funded by the National Cancer Institute (USA), and deal with specific aspects of spatial analysis. *GeoMed* in particular deals with general and focused clustering tests and is currently in development. The CDC (Center for Disease Control, Atlanta, USA) has also developed a program entitled *Cluster*, which can carry out a range of cluster tests. The development of cluster testing software within MapInfo® is also underway at CDC.

In addition to purpose-designed software for specific tasks, a number of general purpose statistical packages can be employed in some applications. For likelihood models of the Poisson process or Poisson-count type, packages such as GLIM, S-Plus or BMDP could be used in applications to putative health hazards or in general ecological modelling (Lawson 1992, 1993c). However, when random-effect models are employed, particularly those including correlated heterogeneity, recourse must often be made to Bayesian or multi-level software. The packages BEAM and WinBugs can provide a general hierarchical modelling framework, but do not provide any flexibility when correlation structures are to be modified, and hence emphasise the *Bayesian* rather than *spatial* aspects of the modelling process. Similar comments also apply to the MLWin software package. Approximations other than those used in the MLWin software can also be accommodated, if in simple forms, by GLIM (Aitken, 1996b).

The analysis of geostatistical data can be approached via the use of packages such as GS+® (available from Gamma Design Software: http://www.gammadesign.com). That package offers a range of facilities for the smoothing and presentation of spatially distributed data, including kriging, and variogram analysis. While these methods cannot be used directly with small-area data, it may be possible to employ these in exploratory or diagnostic analyses.

E.1.2 Geographical Information Systems

There are now a large variety of commercially available software packages which provide display and manipulation facilities for georeferenced data. These packages are usually referred to as Geographical Information Systems (GISs). The fundamental ingredient of these packages is the idea of map layers which contain different information about the mapped area. For example, in one layer might be held the tract boundaries of census small areas, while in another layer some additional information relating to the each tract can be stored and displayed: for example, census small-area labels or SMRs or crude counts. Each layer can be manipulated interactively (edited) to provide a composite map. In addition, some packages also provide facilities for selection of subareas or arbitrary transect displays. The types of display available on the most common packages is often limited to types of thematic map (choropleth, dot maps, etc.), and often contour or interpolation facilities are crude or not available in the basic package. In addition, the ability to handle (point) objects, in a reasonably sophisticated manner, has only recently become available. One *major* drawback of current systems is their lack of spatial statistical tools for analysis of spatial data.

It is widely regarded that the most common GIS packages currently in use are MapInfo®and ArcView®, and we focus here on these packages. These packages have been developing over the past 15–20 years and have different market orientations. MapInfo has as its focus, the manipulation of polygons and their associated data. Hence, small-area tract information are well suited to this format, and many business-related applications can be developed with this package. It is also possible to use MapInfo for the analysis of (point) object data via add-on software (e.g. Vertical Mapper®), which can provide interpolated surfaces and compute tessellations. On the other hand, ArcView has focused on continuous surface modelling and mapping functionality, and therefore finds considerable use in land use assessment and a wide range of environmental applications. Both packages have links to statistical software packages and to each other via data transfer facilities, and there are additional facilities which allow user programming of GIS itself. However, these packages still await the incorporation of spatial *statistical* tools.

Bibliography

Aaby, P., Oesterle, H. and Dietz, K. (1995) Severe outbreak of measles in an isolated German village, 1861. I. Mortality and secondary attack rates, epidemiology and infection. Manuscript.

Aitken, M. (1996a) Empirical Bayes shrinkage using posterior random effect means from non-parametric maximum likelihood estimation in general random effect models. In: Forcina, A., Marchetti, G.M., Hatzinger, R. and Galmacci, G. eds, *Proceedings of the 11th International Workshop on Statistical Modelling*. Graphos, Citta di Castello, pp. 87–92.

Aitken, M. (1996b) A general maximum likelihood analysis of overdispersion in generalised linear models. *Statistics and Computing* **6**, 251–262.

Alexander, F.E., Wray, N., Boyle, P., Coebergh, J.W., Draper, G., Bring, J., Levi, F., Kinney, P.A.M., Michaelis, J., Peris-Bonet, R., Petridou, E., Pukkala, E., Storm, H., Terracini, B. and Vatten, L. (1996) Clustering of childhood leukaemia: a European study in progress. *Journal of Epidemiology and Biostatistics* **1**, 13–24.

Anderson, N.H. and Titterington, D.M. (1997) Some methods for investigating spatial clustering, with epidemiological applications. *Journal of the Royal Statistical Society* **160**, 87–105.

Anderson, R.M. and May, R. (1992) *Infectious diseases of Humans: dynamics and control.* Oxford University Press, London.

Assuncao, R. and Reis, E. (1999) A new proposal to adjust Moran's I for population density. *Statistics in Medicine* **18**, 2147–2162.

Ayutha, R.S. and Böhning, D. (1995) Traffic accident mapping in Bangkok Metropolis: a case study. *Statistics in Medicine* **14**, 2445–2458.

Baddeley, A. (1993) Stereology and survey sampling theory. *Bulletin of the International Statistical Institute* (Book 2) **50**, 435–449.

Baddeley, A. and Gill, R. (1997) Kaplan–Meier estimators for interpoint distance distributions of spatial point processes. *Annals of Statistics* **25**, 263–292.

Baddeley, A. and Lieshout, M. (1993) Stochastic geometry models in high-level vision. In: Mardia, K. ed., *Statistics and Images*. Carfax, Abingdon, pp. 233–258.

Baddeley, A. and Møller, J. (1989) Nearest-neighbour Markov point processes and random sets. *International Statistical Review* **57**, 89–121.

Banfield, J.D. and Raftery, A.E. (1993) Model-based Gaussian and non-Gaussian clustering. *Biometrics* **49**, 803–821.

Barndorff-Nielsen, O.E., Kendall, W.S. and van Lieshout, M.N.M. (1999) *Stochastic Geometry: Likelihood and Computation*. Chapman and Hall, Boca Raton, FL.

Bartholomew, D.J. (1956) A sequential test of randomness for events occurring in time and space. *Biometrika* **43**, 64–78.

Becker, N.G. (1989) *Analysis of Infectious Disease Data*. Chapman and Hall, London.

Becker, N.G. (1995) Statistical challenges of epidemic data. In: Mollison, D. ed., *Epidemic Models: their Structure and Relation to Data*. Cambridge University Press, Cambridge, pp. 339–349.

Becker, N.G. and Wang, D.G. (1998) Severe outbreak of measles in an isolated German village. II. Analysis of transmission rates. Manuscript.

Berman, M. and Turner, T.R. (1992) Approximating point process likelihoods with GLIM. *Applied Statistics* **41**, 31–38.

Bernardinelli, L., Clayton, D. and Montomoli, C. (1995a) Bayesian estimates of disease maps: how important are priors? *Statistics in Medicine* **14**, 2411–2431.

Bernardinelli, L., Clayton, D., Pascutto, C., Montomoli, C., Ghislandi, M. and Songini, M. (1995b) Bayesian analysis of space-time variation in disease risk. *Statistics in Medicine* **14**, 2433–2443.

Bernardinelli, L., Pascutto, C., Best, N.G. and Gilks, W.R. (1997) Disease mapping with errors in covariates. *Statistics in Medicine* **16**, 741–752.

Bernardinelli, L., Pascutto, C., Montomoli, C., Komakec, J. and Gilks, W.R. (1999) Ecological regression with errors in covariates: an application. In: Lawson, A.B., Biggeri, A., Boehning, D., Lesaffre, E., Viel, J.-F. and Bertollini, R. eds, *Disease Mapping and Risk Assessment for Public Health*. Wiley, Chichester, ch. 26, pp. 329–348.

Bernardo, J.M. and Smith, A.F.M. (1994) *Bayesian Theory*. Wiley, New York.

Berzuini, C., Best, N., Gilks, W.R. and Larissa, C. (1997) Dynamic conditional independence models and Markov chain Monte Carlo methods. *Journal of the American Statistical Association* **92**, 1403–1412.

Besag, J. (1974) Spatial interaction and the statistical analysis of lattice systems (with discussion). *Journal of the Royal Statistical Society* B **36**, 192–236.

Besag, J. (1986) On the statistical analysis of dirty pictures (with discussion). *Journal of the Royal Statistical Society* B **48**, 259–302.

Besag, J. and Clifford, P. (1989) Generalized Monte Carlo significance tests. *Biometrika* **76**, 633–642.

Besag, J. and Clifford, P. (1991) Sequential Monte Carlo p-values. *Biometrika* **78**, 301–304.

Besag, J. and Green, P.J. (1993) Spatial statistics and Bayesian computation. *Journal of the Royal Statistical Society* B **55**, 25–37.

Besag, J. and Newell, J. (1991) The detection of clusters in rare diseases. *Journal of the Royal Statistical Society* A **154**, 143–155.

Besag, J., Newell, J. and Craft, A. (1991a) The detection of small-area anomalies in the database. In: Draper, G. ed., *The Geographical Epidemiology of Childhood Leukaemia and Non-Hodgkin Lymphoma in Great Britain, 1966–1983*. HMSO, London.

Besag, J., York, J. and A. Mollié (1991b) Bayesian image restoration with two applications in spatial statistics. *Annals of the Institute of Statistical Mathematics* **43**, 1–59.

Best, N. and Wakefield, J. (1999) Accounting for inaccuracies in population counts and case registration in cancer mapping studies. *Journal of the Royal Statistical Society* **162**, 3, 363–382.

Best, N., Arnold, R., Thomas, A., Waller, L. and Conlon, E. (1998) Bayesian models for spatially correlated disease and exposure data. In: Bernardo, J., Berger, J., Dawid, A. and Smith, A. eds, *Bayesian Statistics*. Oxford University Press, Oxford, vol. 6.

Besterfield, D.H. (1990) *Quality Control*. Prentice Hall, Englewood Cliffs, NJ, 3rd edn.

Bhopal, R., Diggle, P.J. and Rowlingson, B. (1992) Pinpointing clusters of apparently sporadic cases of legionnaires' disease. *British Medical Journal* **304**, 1022–1027.

Biggeri, A., Divino, F., Frigessi, A., Lawson, A., Böhning, D., Lesaffre, E. and Viel, J.-F. (1999) Introduction to spatial models in ecological analysis. In: Lawson, A.B., Böhning,

D., Lesaffre, E., Biggeri, A., Viel, J.-F. and Bertollini, R. eds, *Disease Mapping and Risk Assessment for Public Health*. Wiley, ch. 13, pp. 181–191.

Bithell, J. (1990) An application of density estimation to geographical epidemiology. *Statistics in Medicine* **9**, 691–701.

Bithell, J. (1995) The choice of test for detecting raised disease risk near a point source. *Statistics in Medicine* **14**, 2309–2322.

Bithell, J. and Stone, R. (1989) On statistical methods for analysing the geographical distribution of cancer cases near nuclear installations. *Journal of Epidemiology and Community Health* **43**, 79–85.

Blot, W.J. (1997) Vitamin and mineral supplementation and cancer risk: international chemoprevention trials. *Proceedings of the Society of Experimental Biology and Medicine* **216**, 291–296.

Bock, R.D. and Aitken, M. (1981) Marginal maximum likelihood estimation of item parameters: an application of an EM algorithm. *Psychometrika* **46**, 443–459.

Boehning, D., Dietz, E. and Schlattmann, P. (2000) Space-time mixture modelling of public health data. In: *Disease Mapping with Emphasis on Evaluation of Methods. Statistics in Medicine* **19**, 17/18, 2333–2344.

Bolker, B.M. and Grenfell, B. (1996) Impact of vaccination on the spatial correlation and persistence of measles dynamics. *Proceedings of the National Academy of Sciences* **93**, 12 648–12 653.

Borgefors, G. (1986) Distance transformations in digital images. *Computer Vision, Graphics and Image Processing* **34**, 344–371.

Boyle, P. and Halfacree, K. (1998) *Migration into rural areas: theories and issues*. Wiley, New York.

Breslow, N. and Clayton, D. (1993) Approximate inference in generalised linear mixed models. *Journal of the American Statistical Association* **88**, 9–25.

Breslow, N. and Day, N. (1984) *Statistical Methods in Cancer Research*. Volume 1. *The Design and Analysis of Case-Control Studies*. International Agency for Research on Cancer, Lyon.

Breslow, N. and Day, N. (1987) *Statistical Methods in Cancer Research*. Volume 2. *The Design and Analysis of Cohort Studies*. International Agency for Research on Cancer, Lyon.

Brooks, S. (1998) Markov chain Monte Carlo and its application. *The Statistician* **47**, 69–100.

Bundesamt, S. (1997) *Todesursachen*. Statistisches Bundesamt, Wiesbaden, vol. 12.

Carlin, B.P. and Louis, T.A. (1996) *Bayes and Empirical Bayes Methods for Data Analysis*. Chapman and Hall, London.

Carrat, F. and Valleron, A.J. (1992) Epidemiological mapping using the Kriging method: application to an influenza-like illness epidemic in France. *American Journal of Epidemiology* **135**, 1293–1300.

Carstairs, V. (1981) Small area analysis and health service research. *Community Medicine* **3**, 131–139.

Chen, R. (1978) A surveillance system for congenital abnormalities. *Journal of the American Statistical Association* **73**, 323–327.

Chen, R., Mantel, N. and Klingberg, M. (1984) A study of three techniques for space-time clustering in Hodgkin's disease. *Statistics in Medicine* **3**, 173–184.

Chen, R., Connelly, R. and Mantel, N. (1993) Analysing post alarm data in a monitoring system, in order to accept or reject the alarm. *Statistics in Medicine* **12**, 1807–1812.

Chen, R., Iscovich, J. and Goldbourt, U. (1997) Clustering of leukaemia cases in a city in Israel. *Statistics in Medicine* **16**, 1873–1887.

Clayton, D. and Bernardinelli, L. (1992) Bayesian methods for mapping disease risk. In: Elliott, P., Cuzick, J., English, D. and Stern, R. eds, *Geographical and Environmental Epidemiology: Methods for Small-Area Studies*. Oxford University Press, Oxford.

Clayton, D.G. (1991) A Monte Carlo method for Bayesian inference in frailty models. *Biometrics* **47**, 467–485.

Clayton, D.G. and Hills, M. (1993) *Statistical Methods in Epidemiology*. Oxford University Press, Oxford.

Clayton, D.G. and Kaldor, J. (1987) Empirical Bayes estimates of age-standardised relative risks for use in disease mapping. *Biometrics* **43**, 671–691.

Clayton, D.G., Bernardinelli, L. and Montomoli, C. (1993) Spatial correlation in ecological analysis. *International Journal of Epidemiology* **22**, 1193–1202.

Cliff, A.D. and Ord, J.K. (1981) *Spatial Processes: Models and Applications*. Pion, London.

Cliff, A., Haggett, P., Stroup, D. and Cheney, E. (1998) The changing geographical coherence of measles morbidity in the United States, 1962–1988. *Statistics in Medicine* **11**, 1409–1424.

Collings, B.J. and Margolin, B.H. (1985) Testing goodness of fit for the Poisson assumption when observations are not identically distributed. *Journal of the American Statistical Association* **80**, 411–418.

COMARE (1988) *Investigation of the Possible Increased Incidence of Leukaemia in Young People near the Dounreay Nuclear Establishment, Caithness, Scotland*. HMSO, London.

Conlon, E. and Louis, T. (1999) Addressing multiple goals in evaluating region-specific risk using Bayesian methods. In: Lawson, A., Biggeri, A., Böhning, D., Lesaffre, E., Viel, J-F. and Bertollini, R. eds, *Disease Mapping and Risk Assessment for Public Health*. Wiley, Chichester, ch. 3, pp. 31–47.

Cook, D. and Pocock, S. (1983) Multiple regression in geographical mortality studies with spatially correlated errors. *Biometrics* **39**, 361–371.

Cook-Mozaffari, P.J., Darby, S.C., Doll, R., Forman, D., Hermon, C. and Pike, M.C. (1989) Geographical variation in mortality from leukaemia and other cancers in England and Wales in relation to proximity to nuclear installations, 1969–78. *British Journal of Cancer* **59**, 476–485.

Cowles, M.K. and Carlin, B.P. (1996) Markov chain Monte Carlo convergence diagnostics: a comparative review. *Journal of the American Statistical Association* **91**, 883–904.

Cox, D.R. (1972) The statistical analysis of dependencies in point processes. In: Lewis, P.A.W. ed., *Stochastic Point Processes*. Wiley, pp. 55–66.

Cox, D.R. and Hinkley, D.V. (1974) *Theoretical Statistics*. Chapman and Hall, London.

Cox, D.R. and Isham, V. (1980) *Point Processes*. Chapman and Hall, London.

Cox, D.R. and Lewis, P.A.W. (1966) *Statistical Analysis of Series of Events*. Chapman and Hall, London.

Cressie, N. (1993) *Statistics for Spatial Data*. Wiley, New York (revised edn).

Cressie, N.A.C. (1996) Change of support and the modifiable areal unit problem. *Geographical Systems* **2**, 83–101.

Cressie, N. and Chan, N.H. (1989) Spatial modelling of regional variables. *Journal of the American Statistical Association* **84**, 393–401.

Cressie, N. and Mugglin, A. (2000) Spatio-temporal hierarchical modelling of an infectious disease from (simulated) count data. In: Bethlehem, J. and van der Heijden, P. eds, *Compstat Proceedings*. Physica Verlag, Heidelberg.

Cuzick, J. and Edwards, R. (1990) Spatial clustering for inhomogeneous populations (with discussion). *Journal of the Royal Statistical Society* B **52**, 73–104.

Cuzick, J. and Elliott, P. (1992) Small-area studies: purpose and methods. In: Elliott, P., Cuzick, J., English, D. and Stern, R. eds, *Geographical and Environmental Epidemiology: Methods for Small-Area Studies*. Oxford University Press, Oxford.

Cuzick, J. and Hills, M. (1991) Clustering and clusters-summary. In: Draper, G. ed., *Geographical Epidemiology of Childhood Leukaemia and Non-Hodgkin Lymphomas in Great Britain 1966–1983*. HMSO, London, pp. 123–125.

Daley, D. and Vere-Jones, D. (1988) *An Introduction to the Theory of Point Processes*. Springer, New York.

Dean, C.B. and Balshaw, R. (1997) Efficiency lost by analysing counts rather than event times in Poisson and overdispersed Poisson regression models. *Journal of the American Statistical Association* **92**, 1387–1398.

Devine, O. and Louis, T. (1994) A constrained empirical Bayes estimator for incidence rates in areas with small populations. *Statistics in Medicine* **13**, 1119–1133.

Diggle, P.J. (1983) *Statistical Analysis of Spatial Point Patterns*. Academic Press, London.

Diggle, P.J. (1985a) A kernel method for smoothing point process data. *Applied Statistics* **34**, 138–147.

Diggle, P.J. (1985b) A kernel method for smoothing point process data. *Journal of the Royal Statistical Society* C **34**, 138–147.

Diggle, P.J. (1989) Contribution to the 'cancer near nuclear installations' meeting. *Journal of the Royal Statistical Society* A **152**, 367–369.

Diggle, P.J. (1990) A point process modelling approach to raised incidence of a rare phenomenon in the vicinity of a prespecified point. *Journal of the Royal Statistical Society* A **153**, 349–362.

Diggle, P.J. (1993) Point process modelling in environmental epidemiology. In: Barnett, V. and Turkman, K. eds, *Statistics in the Environment SPRUCE*. Wiley, New York, vol. 1.

Diggle, P.J. and Chetwynd, A. (1991) Second-order analysis of spatial clustering for inhomogeneous populations. *Biometrics* **47**, 1155–1163.

Diggle, P.J. and Elliott, P. (1995) Statistical issues in the analysis of disease risk near point sources using individual or spatially aggregated data. *Journal of Epidemiology and Community Health* **49**, S20–S27.

Diggle, P.J. and Rowlingson, B. (1994) A conditional approach to point process modelling of elevated risk. *Journal of the Royal Statistical Society* A **157**, 433–440.

Diggle, P., Chetwynd, A., Haggvist, R. and Morris, S. (1995) Second-order analysis of space-time clustering. *Statistical Methods in Medical Research* **4**, 124–136.

Diggle, P., Morris, S., Elliott, P. and Shaddick, G. (1997) Regression modelling of disease risk in relation to point sources. *Journal of the Royal Statistical Society* A **160**, 491–505.

Diggle, P., Tawn, J. and Moyeed, R. (1998) Model-based geostatistics. *Journal of the Royal Statistical Society* C **47**, 299–350.

Diggle, P.J., Morris, S. and Wakefield, J. (2000) Point-source modelling using matched case-control data. *Biostatistics* **1**, 1–17.

Donnelly, C.A. (1995) The spatial analysis of covariates in a study of environmental epidemiology. *Statistics in Medicine* **14**, 2393–2409.

Donnelly, C.A., Ware, J.H. and Laird, N.M. (1994) Regression analysis of spatially correlated data: the Kanawha County health study. In: Patil, G.P. and Rao, C.R. eds, *Handbook of Statistics*. North Holland, Amsterdam, vol. 12, ch. 19, pp. 643–659.

Douglas, J.B. (1979) *Analysis with Standard Contagious Distributions*. International Cooperative Publishing House, Fairland.

Duncan, O.D., Cuzzort, R.P. and Duncan, B. (1961) *Statistical Geography*. The Free Press, New York.

Eberley, L. and Carlin, B. (2000) Identifiability and convergence issues for Markov chain Monte Carlo fitting of spatial models. In: *Disease Mapping with Emphasis on Evaluation of Methods. Statistics in Medicine* (Special Issue).

Elliott, P. (1995) Investigation of disease risks in small areas. *Occupational and Environmental Medicine* **52**, 785–789.

Elliott, P., Cuzick, J., English, D. and Stern, R. (eds) (1992a) *Geographical and Environmental Epidemiology: Methods for Small-Area Studies*. Oxford University Press, Oxford.

Elliott, P., Hills, M., Beresford, M., Kleinschmidt, I., Jolley, D., Pattenden, S., Rodrigues, L., Westlake, A. and Rose, G. (1992b) Incidence of cancers of the larynx and lung near incinerators of waste solvents and oils in Great Britain. *The Lancet* **339**, 854–858.

Elliott, P., Shaddick, G., Kleinschmidt, I., Jolley, D., Walls, P., Beresford, J. and Grundy, C. (1996) Cancer incidence near municipal solid waste incinerators in Great Britain. *British Journal of Cancer* **73**, 702–710.

Esman, N.A. and Marsh, G.M. (1996) Applications and limitations of air dispersion modeling in environmental epidemiology. *Journal of Exposure Analysis and Environmental Epidemiology* **6**, 339–353.

Esteve, J., Benhamou, E. and Raymond, L. (1994) *Descriptive Epidemiology*. Statistical Methods in Cancer Research, vol. IV, no. 128. International Association for Research in Cancer, Lyon.

Farrington, C.P. and Beale, A.D. (1998) The detection of outbreaks of infectious disease. In: Gierl, L., Cliff, A., Valleron, A.-J., Farrington, P. and Bull, M. eds, *Geomed '97: Proceedings of the International Workshop on Geomedical Systems*, pp. 97–117. Teubner, Leipzig.

Ferrandiz, J., Lopez, A., Llopis, A., Morales, M. and Tejerizo, M.L. (1995) Spatial interaction between neighbouring counties: cancer mortality data in Valencia (Spain). *Biometrics* **51**, 665–678.

Frisen, M. (1992) Evaluations of methods for statistical surveillance. *Statistics in Medicine* **11**, 1489–1502.

Frisen, M. and Mare, J.D. (1991) Optimal surveillance. *Biometrika* **78**, 271–280.

Gardner, M.J. (1989) Review of reported increases of childhood cancer rates in the vicinity of nuclear installations in the UK. *Journal of the Royal Statistical Society* **152**, 307–325.

Gelman, A., Carlin, J., Stern, H. and Rubin, D. (1995) *Bayesian Data Analysis*. Chapman and Hall, London.

Geyer, C. and Møller, J. (1994) Simulation procedures and likelihood inference for spatial point processes. *Scandinavian Journal of Statistics* **21**, 84–88.

Ghosh, M. and Rao, J.N.K. (1994) Small area estimation: an appraisal. *Statistical Science* **9**, 55–93.

Ghosh, M., Natarajan, K., Stroud, T. and Carlin, B. (1998) Generalized linear models for small-area estimation. *Journal of the American Statistical Association* **93**, 273–282.

Gibson, G.J. (1997) Markov chain Monte Carlo methods for fitting spatiotemporal stochastic models in plant epidemiology. *Applied Statistics* **46**, 215–233.

Gilks, W.R., Clayton, D.G., Spiegelhalter, D.J., Best, N.G., McNeil, A.J., Sharples, L.D.R and Kirby, A.J. (1993) Modelling complexity: applications of Gibbs sampling in medicine. *Journal of the Royal Statistical Society* B **55**, 39–52.

Gilks, W.R., Richardson, S. and Spiegelhalter, D.J. (eds) (1996) *Markov Chain Monte Carlo in Practice*. Chapman and Hall, London.

Glick, B.J. (1979) The spatial autocorrelation of cancer mortality. *Social Science and Medicine* **13D**, 123–130.

Green, P.J. (1995) Reversible jump MCMC computation and Bayesian model determination. *Biometrika* **82**, 711–732.

Green, P. and Sibson, R. (1978) Computing Dirichlet tessellations in the plane. *Computing Journal* **21**, 168–173.

Green, P.J. and Silverman, B.W. (1994) *Nonparametric Regression and Generalised Linear Models*. Chapman and Hall, London.

Greenberg, R.S., Daniels, S.R., Flanders, W.D., Eley, J.W. and Boring, J.R. (1996) *Medical Epidemiology*. Prentice-Hall, Englewood Cliffs, NJ, 2nd edn.

Greenland, S. (1992) Divergent biases in ecologic and individual-level studies. *Statistics in Medicine* **11**, 1209–1223.

Greenland, S. and Morgenstern, H. (1989) Ecological bias, confounding and effects modification. *International Journal of Epidemiology* **18**, 269–274.

Greenland, S. and Robins, J. (1994) Ecologic studies–biases, misconceptions and counterexamples. *American Journal of Sociology* **139**, 747–759.

Griffith, D.A. (1983) The boundary value problem in spatial statistical analysis. *Journal of Regional Science* **23**, 377–387.

Guidici, P., Knorr-Held, L. and Rasser, G. (2000) Modelling categorical covariates in Bayesian disease mapping by partition structures. In: *Disease Mapping with Emphasis on Evaluation of Methods. Statistics in Medicine* (Special Issue) **19**, 17/18, 2579–2598.

Hall, P. (1988) On confidence intervals for spatial parameters estimated from nonreplicated data. *Biometrics* **44**, 271–277.

Härdle, W. (1991) *Smoothing Techniques: with Implementation in S.* Springer, New York.

Hastie, T. and Tibshirani, R. (1990) *Generalised Additive Models.* Chapman and Hall, London.

Haybrittle, J., Yuen, P. and Machin, D. (1995) Multiple comparisons in disease mapping: letter to the editor. *Statistics in Medicine* **14**, 2503–2505.

Heisterkamp, S., Doornbos, G. and Nagelkerke, N. (2000) Assessing health impacts of environmental pollution sources using space-time models. In: *Disease Mapping with Emphasis on Evaluation of Methods. Statistics in Medicine* (Special Issue).

Henderson, R. (2000) A frailty model for spatial variation in survival data. (Manuscript.)

Hills, M. and Alexander, F. (1989) Statistical methods used in assessing the risk of disease near a source of possible environmental pollution: a review. *Journal of the Royal Statistical Society* A **152**, 353–363.

Hjort, N. (1998) Discussion of Best *et al.* paper. In: Bernardo, J., Berger, J., Dawid, A. and Smith, A. eds, *Bayesian Statistics.* Oxford University Press, Oxford, vol. 6.

Hoffmann, W. and Schlattmann, P. (1999) An analysis of the geographical distribution of leukaemia incidence in the vicinity of a suspected point source: a case study. In: Lawson, A.B., Biggeri, A., Boehning, D., Lesaffre, E., Viel, J.-F. and Bertollini, R. eds, *Disease Mapping and Risk Assessment for Public Health.* Wiley, New York, ch. 30, pp. 395–409.

Howe, G.M. (1963) *National Atlas of Disease Mortality in the United Kingdom.* Nelson, London.

Inskip, H., Beral, V., Fraser, P. and Haskey, P. (1983) Methods for age-adjustment of rates. *Statistics in Medicine* **2**, 483–493.

Jacquez, G. (1994) STATL: *statistical software for the clustering of health events.* Biomedware, Ann Arbor, MI.

Jacquez, G.M. (1996) Disease cluster statistics for imprecise space-time locations. *Statistics in Medicine* **15**, 873–886.

Jarpe, E. (1998) Surveillance of spatial patterns. Technical report 3, Department of Statistics, Goteborg University, Sweden.

Kafadar, K. (1996) Smoothing geographical data, particularly rates of disease. *Statistics in Medicine* **15**, 2539–2560.

Katsouyanni, K. and Pershagen, G. (1997) Ambient air pollution exposure and cancer. *Cancer Causes and Control* **8**, 284–291.

Keeling, M.J., Rand, D.A. and Morris, A.J. (1997) Correlation models for childhood epidemics. *Proceedings of the Royal Society of London* B **264**, 1149–1156.

Kelsall, J. and Diggle, P.J. (1995a) Kernel estimation of relative risk. *Bernoulli* **1**, 3–16.

Kelsall, J. and Diggle, P.J. (1995b) Non-parametric estimation of spatial variation in relative risk. *Statistics in Medicine* **14**, 2335–2342.

Kelsall, J. and Diggle, P.J. (1998) Spatial variation in risk of disease: a nonparametric binary regression approach. *Applied Statistics* **47**, 559–573.

Kinlen, L.J. (1995) Epidemiological evidence for an infective basis in childhood leukaemia. *British Journal of Cancer* **71**, 1–5.

Knorr-Held, L. (2000) Bayesian modelling of inseparable space-time variation in disease risk. In: *Disease Mapping with Emphasis on Evaluation of Methods. Statistics in Medicine* (Special Issue) 19, 17/18, 2555–2568.

Knorr-Held, L. and Besag, J. (1998) Modelling risk from disease in time and space. *Statistics in Medicine* **17**, 2045–2060.

Knorr-Held, L. and Rasser, G. (2000) Bayesian detection of clusters and discontinuities in disease maps. *Biometrics* **56**, 13–21.

Knox, E.G. (1964) The detection of space-time interactions. *Applied Statistics* **13**, 25–29.

Knox, E.G. (1989) Detection of clusters. In: Elliott, P. ed., *Methodology of Enquiries into Disease Clustering*. Small Area Health Statistics Unit, London, pp. 17–20.

Kong, A., Lai, J. and Wong, W. (1994) Sequential imputations and Bayesian missing data problems. *Journal of the American Statistical Association* **89**, 278–288.

Kulldorff, M. and Hjalmars, U. (1999) The Knox method and other tests for space-time interaction. *Biometrics* **55**, 544–552.

Kulldorff, M. and Nagarwalla, N. (1995) Spatial disease clusters: detection and inference. *Statistics in Medicine* **14**, 799–810.

Kulldorff, M., Athas, W., Feuer, E., Miller, B. and Key, C. (1998) Evaluating cluster alarms: a space-time scan statistic and brain cancer in Los Alamos. *American Journal of Public Health* **88**, 1377–1380.

Kunsch, H. (1987) Intrinsic autoregressions and related models on the two-dimensional lattice. *Biometrika* **74**, 517–524.

Lai, T.L. (1995) Sequential changepoint detection in quality control and dynamical systems. *Journal of the Royal Statistical Society* **57**, 613–658.

Lancaster, P. and Salkauskas, K. (1986) *Curve and Surface Fitting: an Introduction*. Academic Press, London.

Langford, I., Leyland, A.H., Rashbash, J., Goldstein, H., McDonald, A.-L. and Bentham, G. (1999a) Multilevel modelling of area-based health data. In: Lawson, A.B., Biggeri, A., Boehning, D., Lesaffre, E., Viel, J.-F. and Bertollini, R. eds, *Disease Mapping and Risk Assessment for Public Health Decision Making*. Wiley, ch. 16, pp. 217–227.

Langford, I.H., Leyland, A.H., Rashbash, J. and Goldstein, H. (1999b) Multilevel modelling of the geographical distributions of diseases. *Applied Statistics* **48**, 253–268.

Lawson, A.B. (1989) Contribution to the 'cancer near nuclear installations' meeting. *Journal of the Royal Statistical Society* A **152**, 374–375.

Lawson, A.B. (1992) GLIM and normalising constant models in spatial and directional data analysis. *Computational Statistics and Data Analysis* **13**, 331–348.

Lawson, A.B. (1993a) A deviance residual for heterogeneous spatial Poisson processes. *Biometrics* **49**, 889–897.

Lawson, A.B. (1993b) On composite intensity score tests. *Communications in Statistics – Theory and Methods* **22**, 3223–3235.

Lawson, A.B. (1993c) On the analysis of mortality events around a prespecified fixed point. *Journal of the Royal Statistical Society* A **156**, 363–377.

Lawson, A.B. (1994a) On bivariate Cramer–von Mises types of test for spatial randomness. *Journal of the Royal Statistical Society* C **43**, 259–260.

Lawson, A.B. (1994b) On using spatial Gaussian priors to model heterogeneity in environmental epidemiology. In *Proceedings of the Practical Bayesian Statistics Conference. The Statistician* **43**, 69–76.

Lawson, A.B. (1995) Markov chain Monte Carlo methods for putative pollution source problems in environmental epidemiology. *Statistics in Medicine* **14**, 2473–2486.

Lawson, A.B. (1996a) Markov chain Monte Carlo methods for spatial cluster processes. *Computer Science and Statistics: Proceedings of the Interface* **27**, 314–319.

Lawson, A.B. (1996b) Use of deprivation indices in small area studies: letter. *Journal of Epidemiology and Community Health* **50**, 689–690.

Lawson, A.B. (1997) Some spatial statistical tools for pattern recognition. In: Stein, A., de Vries, F.W.T.P. and Schut, J. eds, *Quantitative Approaches in Systems Analysis*. C.T. de Wit Graduate School for Production Ecology, Wageningen, vol. 7, pp. 43–58.

Lawson, A.B. (2000) Cluster modelling of disease incidence via RJMCMC methods: comparative evaluation. *Statistics in Medicine* **19**, 17/18, 2361–2376.

Lawson, A.B. and Clark, A.B. (1998) Space-time cluster modelling of small area data via MCMC methods. In: *Proceedings of the Biometrics Section of the ASA*. American Statistical Association, Washington, pp. 1–9.

Lawson, A.B. and Clark, A. (1999a) Markov chain Monte Carlo methods for clustering in case event and count data in spatial epidemiology. In: Halloran, M.E. and Berry, D. eds, *Statistics and Epidemiology: Environment and Clinical Trials*. Springer, New York, pp. 193–218.

Lawson, A.B. and Clark, A. (1999b) Markov chain Monte Carlo methods for putative sources of hazard and general clustering. In: Lawson, A.B., Böhning, D., Lesaffre, E., Biggeri, A., Viel, J.-F. and Bertollini, R. eds, *Disease Mapping and Risk Assessment for Public Health*. Wiley, ch. 9, pp. 119–141.

Lawson, A.B. and Clark, A.B. (1999c) Small area cluster modelling via RJMCMC methods. *Journal of the National Institute of Public Health* **48**(2), 113–120.

Lawson, A.B. and Cressie, N. (2000) Spatial statistical methods for environmental epidemiology. In: Rao, C.R. and Sen, P.K. eds, *Handbook of Statistics: Bio-Environmental and Public Health Statistics*. Elsevier, Amsterdam, vol. 18, pp. 357–396.

Lawson, A.B. and Harrington, N.W. (1996) The analysis of putative environmental pollution gradients in spatially correlated epidemiological data. In: Jeffers, J. ed., *Statistics in the Environment. Journal of Applied Statistics* (Special Issue) **23**, 301–310.

Lawson, A.B. and Leimich, P. (2000) Approaches to space-time modelling of infectious disease behaviour. *IMA Journal of Mathematics Applied to Medicine and Biology* **17**, 1–13.

Lawson, A.B. and Viel, J.-F. (1995) Tests for directional space-time interaction in epidemiological data. *Statistics in Medicine* **14**, 2383–2392.

Lawson, A.B. and Waller, L. (1996) A review of point pattern methods for spatial modelling of events around sources of pollution. *Environmetrics* **7**, 471–488.

Lawson, A.B. and Williams, F. (1993) Applications of extraction mapping in environmental epidemiology. *Statistics in Medicine* **12**, 1249–1258.

Lawson, A.B. and Williams, F. (1994) Armadale: a case study in environmental epidemiology. *Journal of the Royal Statistical Society* A **157**, 285–298.

Lawson, A.B. and Williams, F. (2000) Spatial competing risk models in disease mapping. *Statistics in Medicine* (Special Issue) **19**, 17/18, 2451–2468.

Lawson, A.B., Biggeri, A. and Lagazio, C. (1996a) Modelling heterogeneity in discrete spatial data models via MAP and MCMC methods. In: Forcina, A., Marchetti, G., Hatzinger, R. and Galmacci, G. eds, *Proceedings of the 11th International Workshop on Statistical Modelling*. Graphos, Citta di Castello, pp. 240–250.

Lawson, A.B., van Lieshout, M. and Baddeley, A. (1996b) Markov chain Monte Carlo inference for spatial cluster processes. Manuscript.

Lawson, A., Biggeri, A. and Williams, F.L.R. (1999a) A review of modelling approaches in health risk assessment around putative sources. In: Lawson, A.B., Böhning, D., Lesaffre, E., Biggeri, A., Viel, J.-F. and Bertollini, R. eds, *Disease Mapping and Risk Assessment for Public Health*. Wiley, ch. 17, pp. 231–245.

Lawson, A.B., Biggeri, A. and Dreassi, E. (1999b) Edge effects in disease mapping. In: Lawson, A.B., Böhning, D., Lesaffre, E., Biggeri, A., Viel, J.-F. and Bertollini, R. eds, *Disease Mapping and Risk Assessment for Public Health*. Wiley, ch. 6, pp. 85–97.

Lawson, A.B., Biggeri, A., Boehning, D., Lesaffre, E., Viel, J.-F., Clark, A., Schlattmann, P. and Divino, F. (2000a) Disease mapping models: an empirical evaluation. In: *Disease Mapping with Emphasis on Evaluation of Methods. Statistics in Medicine* (Special Issue) **19**, 17/18, 2217–2242.

Lawson, A.B., Simeon, S., Kulldorff, M., Biggeri, A. and Magnani, C. (2000b) Spatial cluster modelling: a comparison of object models with flexible forms. (Submitted.)

Lawson, D.H. and Wilson, G.M. (1974) Detecting adverse drug reactions. *British Journal of Hospital Medicine* **12**, 790–798.

Lee, D.T. and Schacter, B.J. (1980) Two algoritms for constructing a Delauney triangulation. *International Journal of Computer and Information Science* **9**, 219–242.

Lenihan, J. (1985) *Bonnybridge/Denny Morbidity Review*. Scottish Home and Health Department, HMSO, Edinburgh.

Lewandowsky, S., Herrmann, D., Behrens, J., Li, S.-C., Pickle, L. and Jobe, J. (1993) Perception of clusters in statistical maps. *Applied Cognitive Psychology* **7**, 533–551.

Lloyd, O. (1982) Mortality in a small industrial town. In: Gardner, A. ed., *Current Approaches to Occupational Health*. Wright, London, vol. 2, pp. 283–309.

Loizeaux, M. and McKeague, I. (2000) Bayesian inference for spatial point processes via perfect sampling. (Submitted.)

Lucas, J.M. (1985) Counted data cusums. *Technometrics* **27**, 129–144.

McCullagh, P. and Nelder, J. (1989) *Generalised Linear Models*. Chapman and Hall, London, 2nd edn.

MacEachren, A.M. (1995) *How Maps Work: Representation, Visualisation, and Design*. Guildford Press, New York.

McNab, Y. and Dean, C. (2000) Parametric bootstrap and penalised quasi-likelihood inference in conditional autoregressive models. In: *Disease Mapping with Emphasis on Evaluation of Methods. Statistics in Medicine* (Special Issue) **19**, 17/18, 2421–2436.

Mantel, N. (1967) The detection of disease clustering and a generalised regression approach. *Cancer Research* **27**, 209–220.

Manton, K., Woodbury, M. and Stallard, E. (1981) A variance components approach to categorical data models with heterogeneous mortality rates in North Carolina counties. *Biometrics* **37**, 259–269.

Marshall, R. (1991a) Mapping disease and mortality rates using empirical Bayes estimators. *Applied Statistics* **40**, 283–294.

Marshall, R. (1991b) A review of methods for the statistical analysis of spatial patterns of disease. *Journal of the Royal Statistical Society* A **154**, 421–441.

Matérn, B. (1986) *Spatial Variation*. Lecture Notes in Statistics, no. 36. Springer, New York.

Miles, R.E. (1974) On the elimination of edge effects in planar sampling. In: Harding, E. and Kendall, D.G. eds, *Stochastic Geometry*. Wiley, New York, pp. 228–247.

Møller, J., Syversveen, A. and Waagepetersen, R.P. (1998) Log Gaussian Cox processes. *Scandinavian Journal of Statistics* **25**, 451–482.

Mollie, A. 1999 Bayesian and empirical Bayes approaches to disease mapping. In: Lawson, A.B., Biggeri, A., Boehning, D., Lesaffre, E., Viel, J.-F. and Bertollini, R. eds, *Disease Mapping and Risk Assessment for Public Health*. Wiley, New York, ch. 2, pp. 15–29.

Mollison, D. ed. (1995) *Epidemic Models: Their Structure and Relation to Data*. Cambridge University Press, Cambridge.

Monmonier, M. (1996) *How to Lie with Maps*. University of Chicago Press, London, 2nd edn.

Montgomery, D.C. (1991) *Introduction to Statistical Quality Control*. Wiley, New York, 2nd edn.

Mugglin, A. and Carlin, B. (1998) Hierarchical modeling in geographic information systems: population interpolation over incompatible zones. *Journal of Agricultural, Biological and Environmental Statistics* **3**, 111–130.

Mulmuley, K. (1993) *Computational Geometry*. Prentice-Hall, New York.

Mungiole, M., Pickle, L. and Simonson, K. (1999) Application of a weighted head-banging algorithm to mortality maps. *Statistics in Medicine* **18**, 3201–3209.

Nejjari, C., Tessier, J.F., Dartigues, J., Barberger-Gateau, P., Letenneur, L. and Salamon, R. (1993) The relationship between dyspnoea and main lifetime occupation in the elderly. *International Journal of Epidemiology* **22**, 848–854.

Neutra, R.R. (1990) Counterpoint from a cluster buster. *American Journal of Epidemiology* (Supplement) **132**, 1–8.

Oden, N. (1995) Adjusting Moran's I for population density. *Statistics in Medicine* **14**, 17–26.

Oesterle, H. (1990) *Statistische Reanalyse einer Masernepidemie 1861 in Hagelloch*. PhD thesis, Eberhard–Karls Universität, Tübingen.

Ogata, Y. (1988) Statistical models for earthquake occurences and residual analayis for point processes. *Journal of the American Statistical Association* **83**, 9–27.

Openshaw, S., Charlton, M., Wymer, C. and Craft, A. (1987) A mark I geographical analysis machine for the automated analysis of point data sets. *International Journal of Geographical Information Systems* **1**, 335–358.

Panopsky, M.A. and Dutton, J.A. (1984) *Atmospheric Turbulence*. Wiley, New York.

Pascutto, C., Bernardinelli, L., Best, N.G. and Gilks, W.R. (1996) Ecological regression with errors in covariates: an application. In: Forcina, A., Marchetti, G.M., Hatzinger, R. and Galmacci, G. eds, *Statistical Modelling: Proceedings of the 11th International Workshop on Statistical Modelling*. Graphos, Citta di Castello, pp. 299–307.

Pascutto, C., Wakefield, J., Best, N., Bernardinelli, L., Elliott, P., Richardson, S., and Staines, A. (2000) Statistical issues in the analysis of disease mapping data. In: *Disease Mapping with Emphasis on Evaluation of Methods. Statistics in Medicine* (Special Issue).

Pfeilsticker, A. (1863) *Beiträge zur Pathologie der Masern mit besonderer Berücksichtgung der Statistischen Verhältnisse*. PhD thesis, Eberhard–Karls Universität, Tübingen.

Pickle, L. (2000) Exploring spatio-temporal patterns of mortality using mixed effects models. In: *Disease Mapping with Emphasis on Evaluation of Methods. Statistics in Medicine* (Special Issue) **19**, 17/18, 2251–2264.

Pickle, L.W. and Hermann, D.J. (1995) Cognitive aspects of statistical mapping. Technical report 18, NCHS Office of Research and Methodology, Washington, DC.

Pickle, L., Mungiole, M., Jones, G. and White, A. (1999) Exploring spatial patterns of mortality: the new atlas of United States mortality. *Statistics in Medicine* **18**, 3211–3220.

Plummer, M. and Clayton, D.G. (1996) Estimation of population exposure in ecological studies. *Journal of the Royal Statistical Society* B **58**, 113–126.

Potthoff, R.F. and Whittinghill, M. (1966) Testing for homogeneity. I. The binomial and multinomial distributions. *Biometrika* **53**, 167–182.

Prentice, R. and Sheppard, L. (1995) Aggregate data studies of disease risk factors. *Biometrika* **82**, 113–125.

Preparata, F. and Shamos, M. (1985) *Computational Geometry*. Springer, New York.

Press, S.J. (1989) *Bayesian Statistics*. Wiley, New York.

Quian, W. and Titterington, D. (1991) Estimation of parameters in hidden Markov models. *Philosophical Transactions of the Royal Society of London* A **337**, 407–428.

Rao, C.R. (1973) *Linear Statistical Inference*. Wiley, New York, 2nd edn.

Raubertas, R.F. (1988) Spatial and temporal analysis of disease occurence for detection of clustering. *Biometrics* **44**, 1121–1129.

Rhodes, C.J. and Anderson, R.M. (1996) Power laws governing epidemics in isolated populations. *Nature* **381**, 600–602.

Richardson, S. (1992) Statistical methods for geographical correlation studies. In: Elliott, P., Cuzick, J., English, D. and Stern, R. eds, *Geographical and Environmental Epidemiology: Methods for Small Area Studies.* Oxford University Press, Oxford, pp. 181–204.

Richardson, S., Guihenneuc, C. and Laserre, V. (1992) Spatial linear models with autocorrelated error structure. *The Statistician* **41**, 539–557.

Ripley, B.D. (1981) *Spatial Statistics.* Wiley, New York.

Ripley, B.D. (1987) *Stochastic Simulation.* Wiley, New York.

Ripley, B.D. (1988) *Statistical Inference for Spatial Processes.* Cambridge University Press, Cambridge.

Robert, C.P. and Casella, G. (1999) *Monte Carlo Statistical Methods.* Springer, New York.

Robinson, W.S. (1950) Ecological correlation and the behaviour of individuals. *American Sociological Review* **15**, 351–357.

Rogerson, P.A. (1997) Surveillance systems for monitoring the development of spatial patterns. *Statitistics in Medicine* **16**, 2081–2093.

Rosenfeld, A., Klette, R. and Sloboda, F. (1998) *Advances in Digital and Computational Geometry.* Springer, New York.

Ross, A. and Davis, S. (1990) Point pattern analysis of the spatial proximity of residences prior to diagnosis of persons with Hodgkin's disease. *American Journal of Epidemiology* (Supplement) **132**, 53–62.

Rothman, K.J. (1986) *Modern Epidemiology.* Little, Brown and Co., Boston, MA.

Rothman, K.J. (1990) A sobering start to the cluster busters' conference. *American Journal of Epidemiology* (Supplement) **132**, S6–S13.

Sans, S., Elliott, P., Kleinschmidt, I., Shaddick, G., Pattenden, S., Walls, P., Grundy, C. and Dolk, H. (1995) Cancer incidence and mortality near the Baglan Bay petrochemical works, south Wales. *Occupational and Environmental Medicine* **52**, 217–224.

Schlattman, P. and Böhning, D. (1993) Mixture models and disease mapping. *Statistics in Medicine* **12**, 1943–1950.

Schlattmann, P., Dietz, E. and Böhning, D. (1996) Covariate adjusted mixture models with the program DismapWin. *Statistics in Medicine* **15**, 919–929.

Schulman, J., Selvin, S. and Merrill, D.W. (1988) Density equalised map projections: a method for analysing clusters around a fixed point. *Statistics in Medicine* **7**, 491–505.

Schumm, S.A. and Lichty, R.W. (1965) Time, space and causality in geomorphology. *American Journal of Science* **263**, 110–119.

Schweder, T. and Spjotwoll, E. (1982) Plots of p-values to evaluate many tests simultaneously. *Biometrika* **69**, 493–502.

Searle, S., Cassella, G. and McCulloch, C. (1992) *Variance Components.* Wiley, New York.

Sibson, R. (1980) The Dirichlet tessellation as an aid in data analysis. *Scandinavian Journal of Statistics* **7**, 14–20.

Siegmund, D. (1985) *Sequential Analysis.* Springer, New York.

Silverman, B.W. (1986) *Density Estimation for Statistics and Data Analysis.* Chapman and Hall, London.

Smith, A.F.M. and Gelfand, A.E. (1992) Bayesian statistics without tears: a sampling–resampling perspective. *American Statistician* **46**, 84–88.

Smith, A.F.M. and Roberts, G. (1993) Bayesian computation via the Gibbs sampler and related Markov chain Monte Carlo methods. *Journal of the Royal Statistical Society* **55**, 3–23.

Snow, J. (1854) *On the Mode of Communication of Cholera*. Churchill Livingstone, London, 2nd edn.

Snyder, D.L. (1975) *Random Point Processes*. Wiley, New York.

Spiegelhalter, D., Best, N., Gilks, W.R. and Inskip, H. (1996) Hepatitis B: a case study in MCMC methods. In: Gilks, W.R., Richardson, S. and Spiegelhalter, D. eds, *Markov Chain Monte Carlo in Practice*. Chapman and Hall, London.

Steel, D.G. and Holt, D. (1996) Analysing and adjusting aggregation effects: the ecological fallacy revisited. *International Statistical Review* **64**, 39–60.

Stern, H. and Cressie, N.A. (1999) Inference for extremes in disease mapping. In: Lawson, A.B., Biggeri, A., Boehning, D., Lesaffre, E., Viel, J.-F. and Bertollini, R. eds, *Disease Mapping and Risk Assessment for Public Health*. Wiley, New York, ch. 5.

Stern, H. and Cressie, N. (2000) Posterior predictive model checks for disease mapping models. In: *Disease Mapping with Emphasis on Evaluation of Methods. Statistics in Medicine* (Special Issue) **19**, 17/18, 2377–2398.

Stone, R. (1988) Investigations of excess environmental risks around putative sources: statistical problems and a proposed test. *Statistics in Medicine* **7**, 649–660.

Stoyan, D., Kendall, W. and Mecke, J. (1987) *Stochastic geometry and its applications*. Akademie, Berlin.

Sun, D., Tsutakawa, R. and Kim, H. (2000) Spatio-temporal interaction with disease mapping. *Statistics in Medicine* **19**(15), 2015–2035.

Tango, T. (1995) A class of tests for detecting 'general' and 'focussed' clustering of rare diseases. *Statistics in Medicine* **14**, 2323–2334.

Tango, T. (1999) Comparison of general tests for spatial clustering. In: Lawson, A.B., Biggeri, A., Boehning, D., Lesaffre, E., Viel, J.-F. and Bertollini, R. eds, *Disease Mapping and Risk Assessment for Public Health*. Wiley, New York, ch. 8.

Tanner, M.A. (1996) *Tools for Statistical Inference*. Springer, New York, 3rd edn.

Thacker, S. (1994) Historical development. In: Teusch, S. and Churchill, R. eds, *Principles and Practice of Public Health Surveillance*. Oxford University Press, New York, pp. 3–17.

Thacker, S. and Berkelman, R. (1992) History of public health surveillance. In: Halperin, W., Baker, L. and Monson, R. eds, *Public Health Surveillance*. Van Nostrand Rheinhold, New York, pp. 1–15.

Thomas, D.C. (1985) The problem of multiple inference in identifying point-source environmental hazards. *Environmental Health Perspectives* **62**, 407–414.

Thomson, S. (1992) *Sampling*. Wiley, New York.

Tomatis, L., Aitio, A., Heseltine, E., Kaldor, J., Mier, A.B., Parkin, D.M. and Riboli, E. (1990) *Cancer: Causes, Occurence and Control*. IARC, Lyon.

Tsutakawa, R. (1988) Mixed model for analysing geographic variability in mortality rates. *Journal of the American Statistical Association* **83**, 37–42.

Turnbull, B., Iwano, E., Burnett, W., Howe, H. and Clark, L. (1990) Monitoring for clusters of disease: application to leukaemia incidence in upstate New York. *American Journal of Epidemiology* (Supplement) **132**, 136–143.

Wackernagel, H. (1995) *Multivariate Geostatistics*. Springer, New York.

Waller, L. and Lawson, A.B. (1995) The power of focussed tests to detect disease clustering. *Statistics in Medicine* **14**, 2291–2308.

Waller, L., Turnbull, B., Clark, L. and Nasca, P. (1993) Chronic disease surveillance and testing of clustering of disease and exposure: application to leukaemia incidence and TCE-contaminated dumpsites in upstate New York. *Environmetrics* **3**, 281–300.

Waller, L., Carlin, B., Xia, H. and Gelfand, A. (1997) Hierarchical spatio-temporal mapping of disease rates. *Journal of the American Statistical Association* **92**, 607–617.

Walter, S.D. (1993) Visual and statistical assessment of spatial clustering in mapped data. *Statistics in Medicine* **12**, 1275–1291.

Walter, S. and Birnie, S. (1991) Mapping mortality and morbidity patterns: an international comparison. *International Journal of Epidemiology* **20**, 678–689.

Watson, D.F. (1981) Computing the n-dimensional Delauney triangulation with application to Voronoi polytopes. *The Computer Journal* **24**, 167–172.

Webster, R., Oliver, M.A., Muir, K.R. and Mann, J.R. (1994) Kriging the local risk of a rare disease from a register of diagnoses. *Geographical Analysis* **26**, 168–185.

Whittemore, A., Friend, N., Brown, B. and Holly, E. (1987) A test to detect clusters of disease. *Biometrika* **74**, 631–635.

Wolpert, R.L. and Ickstadt, K. (1998) Poisson/gamma random field models for spatial statistics. *Biometrika* **85**, 251–267.

Xia, H. and Carlin, B. (1998) Spatio-temporal models with errors in covariates: mapping Ohio lung cancer mortality. *Statistics in Medicine* **17**, 2025–2043.

Yasui, Y. and Lele, S. (1997) A regression method for spatial disease rates: an estimating function approach. *Journal of the American Statistical Association* **92**, 21–33.

Yasui, Y., Liu, H., Benach, J. and Winger, M. (2000) An empirical evaluation of various priors in empirical Bayes estimation of small-area disease risks. In: *Disease Mapping with Emphasis on Evaluation of Methods. Statistics in Medicine* (Special Issue).

Zelterman, D. (1987) Goodness-of-fit tests for large sparse multinomial distributions. *Journal of the American Statistical Association* **82**, 624–629.

Zhu, L. and Carlin, B. (2000) Comparing hierarchical models for spatio-temporally misaligned data using the DIC criterion. In: *Disease Mapping with Emphasis on Evaluation of Methods. Statistics in Medicine* (Special Issue) **19**, 17/18, 2265–2278.

Zidek, J., White, R. and Le, N.D. (1999) Using spatial data in assessing the association between air pollution episodes and respiratory morbidity. In: Barnett, V., Stein, A. and Turkman, K.F. eds, *Statistics for the Environment SPRUCE.* Wiley, New York, vol. 4, ch. 7, pp. 117–135.

Index

WILEY SERIES IN PROBABILITY AND STATISTICS
ESTABLISHED BY WALTER A. SHEWHART AND SAMUEL S. WILKS

Probability and Statistics Section

*ANDERSON · The Statistical Analysis of Time Series
ARNOLD, BALAKRISHNAN, and NAGARAJA · A First Course in Order Statistics
ARNOLD, BALAKRISHNAN, and NAGARAJA · Records
BACCELLI, COHEN, OLSDER, and QUADRAT · Synchronization and Linearity: An Algebra for Discrete Event Systems
BARNETT · Comparative Statistical Inference, *Third Edition*
BASILEVSKY · Statistical Factor Analysis and Related Methods: Theory and Applications
BERNARDO and SMITH · Bayesian Theory
BILLINGSLEY · Convergence of Probability Measures, *Second Edition*
BOROVKOV · Asymptotic Methods in Queuing Theory
BOROVKOV · Ergodicity and Stability of Stochastic Processes
BRANDT, FRANKEN, and LISEK · Stationary Stochastic Models
CAINES · Linear Stochastic Systems
CAIROLI and DALANG · Sequential Stochastic Optimization
CONSTANTINE · Combinatorial Theory and Statistical Design
COOK · Regression Graphics
COVER and THOMAS · Elements of Information Theory
CSÖRGŐ and HORVÁTH · Weighted Approximations in Probability Statistics
CSÖRGŐ and HORVÁTH · Limit Theorems in Change Point Analysis
*DANIEL · Fitting Equations to Data: Computer Analysis of Multifactor Data, *Second Edition*
DETTE and STUDDEN · The Theory of Canonical Moments with Applications in Statistics, Probability, and Analysis
DEY and MUKERJEE · Fractional Factional Plans
*DOOB · Stochastic Processes
DRYDEN and MARDIA · Statistical Shape Analysis
DUPUIS and ELLIS · A Weak Convergence Approach to the Theory of Large Deviations
ETHIER and KURTZ · Markov Processes: Characterization and Convergence
FELLER · An Introduction to Probability Theory and Its Applications, Volume 1, *Third Edition*, Revised; Volume II, *Second Edition*
FULLER · Introduction to Statistical Time Series, *Second Edition*

---

*Now available in a lower priced paperback edition in the Wiley Classics Library.

Probability and Statistics Section (Continued)

FULLER · Measurement Error Models
GHOSH, MUKHOPADHYAY, and SEN · Sequential Estimation
GIFI · Nonlinear Multivariate Analysis
GUTTORP · Statistical Inference for Branching Processes
HALL · Introduction to the Theory of Coverage Processes
HAMPEL · Robust Statistics: The Approach Based on Influence Functions
HANNAN and DEISTLER · The Statistical Theory of Linear Systems
HUBER · Robust Statistics
HUŠKOVÁ, BERAN, and DUPAČ · Collected Works of Jaroslav Hájek—With Commentary
IMAN and CONOVER · A Modern Approach to Statistics
JUREK and MASON · Operator-Limit Distributions in Probability Theory
KASS and VOS · The Geometrical Foundations of Asymptotic Inference
KAUFMAN and ROUSSEEUW · Finding Groups in Data: An Introduction to Cluster Analysis
KELLY · Probability, Statistics, and Optimization
KENDALL, BARDEN, CARNE, and LE · Shape and Shape Theory
LINDVALL · Lectures on the Coupling Method
McFADDEN · Management of Data in Clinical Trials
MANTON, WOODBURY, and TOLLEY · Statistical Applications Using Fuzzy Sets
MARDIA and JUPP · Directional Statistics
MORGENTHALER and TUKEY · Configural Polysampling: A Route to Practical Robustness
MUIRHEAD · Aspects of Multivariate Statistical Theory
OLIVER and SMITH · Influence Diagrams, Belief Nets, and Decision Analysis
*PARZEN · Modern Probability Theory and Its Applications
PEÑA, TIAO, and TSAY · A Course in Time Series Analysis
PRESS · Bayesian Statistics: Principles, Models, and Applications
PUKELSHEIM · Optimal Experimental Design
RAO · Asymptotic Theory of Statistical Inference
RAO · Linear Statistical Inference and Its Applications, *Second Edition*
RAO and SHANBHAG · Choquet-Deny Type Functional Equations with Applications to Stochastic Models
ROBERTSON, WRIGHT, and DYKSTRA · Order Restricted Statistical Inference
ROGERS and WILLIAMS · Diffusions, Markov Processes, and Martingales, Volume I: Foundations, *Second Edition*, Volume II: Itô Calculus
RUBINSTEIN and SHAPIRO · Discrete Event Systems: Sensitivity Analysis and Stochastic Optimization by the Score Function Method
RUZSA and SZEKELEY · Algebraic Probability Theory
SALTELLI, CHAN and SCOTT · Sensitivity Analysis
SCHEFFÉ · The Analysis of Variance
SEBER · Linear Regression Analysis
SEBER · Multivariate Observations
SEBER and WILD · Nonlinear Regression
SERFLING · Approximation Theorems of Mathematical Statistics
SHORACK and WELLNER · Empirical Processes with Applications to Statistics
SMALL and McLEISH · Hilbert Space Methods in Probability and Statistical Inference
STAPLETON · Linear Statistical Models
STAUDTE and SHEATHER · Robust Estimation and Testing
STOYANOV · Counterexamples in Probability
TANAKA · Time Series Analysis: Nonstationary and Noninvertible Distribution Theory

---

*Now available in a lower priced paperback edition in the Wiley Classics Library.

Probability and Statistics Section (Continued)

THOMPSON and SEBER · Adaptive Sampling
WELSH · Aspects of Statistical Inference
WHITTAKER · Graphical Models in Applied Multivariate Statistics
YANG · The Construction Theory of Denumerable Markov Processes

Applied Probability and Statistics Section

ABRAHAM and LEDOLTER · Statistical Methods for Forecasting
AGRESTI · Analysis of Ordinal Categorical Data
AGRESTI · Categorical Data Analysis
ANDERSON, AUQUIER, HAUCK, OAKES, VANDAELE, and WEISBERG Statistical Methods for Comparative Studies
ARMITAGE and DAVID (editors) · Advances in Biometry
*ARTHANARI and DODGE · Mathematical Programming in Statistics
ASMUSSEN · Applied Probability and Queues
*BAILEY · The Elements of Stochastic Processes with Applications to the Natural Sciences
BARNETT and LEWIS · Outliers in Statistical Data, *Third Edition*
BARTHOLOMEW, FORBES, and McLEAN · Statistical Techniques for Manpower Planning, *Second Edition*
BATES and WATTS · Nonlinear Regression Analysis and Its Applications
BECHHOFER, SANTNER, and GOLDSMAN · Design and Analysis of Experiments for Statistical Selection, Screening, and Multiple Comparisons
BELSLEY · Conditioning Diagnostics: Collinearity and Weak Data in Regression
BELSLEY, KUH, and WELSCH · Regression Diagnostics: Identifying Influential Data and Sources of Collinearity
BHAT · Elements of Applied Stochastic Processes, *Second Edition*
BHATTACHARYA and WAYMIRE · Stochastic Processes with Applications
BIRKES and DODGE · Alternative Methods of Regression
BLISCHKE and PRABHAKAR MURTHY · Reliability: Modeling, Prediction, and Optimization
BLOOMFIELD · Fourier Analysis of Time Series: An Introduction, *Second Edition*
BOLLEN · Structural Equations with Latent Variables
BOULEAU · Numerical Methods for Stochastic Processes
BOX · Bayesian Inference in Statistical Analysis
BOX and DRAPER · Empirical Model-Building and Response Surfaces
*BOX and DRAPER · Evolutionary Operation: A Statistical Method for Process Improvement
BUCKLEW · Large Deviation Techniques in Decision, Simulation, and Estimation
BUNKE and BUNKE · Nonlinear Regression, Functional Relations, and Robust Methods: Statistical Methods of Model Building
CHATTERJEE and HADI · Sensitivity Analysis in Linear Regression
CHERNICK · Bootstrap Methods: A Practitioner's Guide
CHILÈS and DELFINER · Geostatistics: Modeling Spatial Uncertainty
CHOW and LIU · Design and Analysis of Clinical Trials: Concepts and Methodologies
CLARKE and DISNEY · Probability and Random Processes: A First Course with Applications, *Second Edition*
*COCHRAN and COX · Experimental Designs, *Second Edition*
CONOVER · Practical Nonparametric Statistics, *Second Edition*

---

*Now available in a lower priced paperback edition in the Wiley Classics Library.

Applied Probability and Statistics (Continued)

CORNELL · Experiments with Mixtures, Designs, Models, and the Analysis of Mixture Data, *Second Edition*
*COX · Planning of Experiments
CRESSIE · Statistics for Spatial Data, *Revised Edition*
DANIEL · Applications of Statistics to Industrial Experimentation
DANIEL · Biostatistics: A Foundation for Analysis in the Health Sciences, *Sixth Edition*
DAVID · Order Statistics, *Second Edition*
*DEGROOT, FIENBERG, and KADANE · Statistics and the Law
DODGE · Alternative Methods of Regression
DOWDY and WEARDEN · Statistics for Research, *Second Edition*
DUNN and CLARK · Applied Statistics: Analysis of Variance and Regression, *Second Edition*
*ELANDT-JOHNSON and JOHNSON · Survival Models and Data Analysis
*FLEISS · The Design and Analysis of Clinical Experiments
FLEISS · Statistical Methods for Rates and Proportions, *Second Edition*
FLEMING and HARRINGTON · Counting Processes and Survival Analysis
GALLANT · Nonlinear Statistical Models
GLASSERMAN and YAO · Monotone Structure in Discrete-Event Systems
GNANADESIKAN · Methods for Statistical Data Analysis of Multivariate Observations. *Second Edition*
GOLDSTEIN and LEWIS · Assessment: Problems, Development, and Statistical Issues
GREENWOOD and NIKULIN · A Guide to Chi-squared Testing
*HAHN · Statistical Models in Engineering
HAHN and MEEKER · Statistical Intervals: A Guide for Practitioners
HAND · Construction and Assessment of Classification Rules
HAND · Discrimination and Classification
HEDAYAT and SINHA · Design and Inference in Finite Population Sampling
HEIBERGER · Computation for the Analysis of Designed Experiments
HINKELMAN and KEMPTHORNE · Design and Analysis of Experiments, Volume 1: Introduction to Experimental Design
HOAGLIN, MOSTELLER, and TUKEY · Exploratory Approach to Analysis of Variance
HOAGLIN, MOSTELLER, and TUKEY · Exploring Data Tables, Trends and Shapes
HOAGLIN, MOSTELLER, and TUKEY · Understanding Robust and Exploratory Data Analysis
HOCHBERG and TAMHANE · Multiple Comparison Procedures
HOCKING · Methods and Applications of Linear Models: Regression and the Analysis of Variables
HOGG and KLUGMAN · Loss Distributions
HOSMER and LEMESHOW · Applied Logistic Regression
HØYLAND and RAUSAND · System Reliability Theory: Models and Statistical Methods
HUBERTY · Applied Discriminant Analysis
HUNT and KENNEDY · Financial Derivatives in Theory and Practice
JACKSON · A User's Guide to Principal Components
JOHN · Statistical Methods in Engineering and Quality Assurance
JOHNSON · Multivariate Statistical Simulation
JOHNSON & KOTZ · Distributions in Statistics
JOHNSON, KOTZ, and BALAKRISHNAN · Continuous Univariate Distributions, Volume 1, *Second Edition*
JOHNSON, KOTZ, and BALAKRISHNAN · Continuous Univariate Distributions, Volume 2, *Second Edition*

*Now available in a lower priced paperback edition in the Wiley Classics Library.

Applied Probability and Statistics (Continued)

JOHNSON, KOTZ, and BALAKRISHNAN · Discrete Multivariate Distributions
JOHNSON, KOTZ, and KEMP · Univariate Discrete Distributions, *Second Edition*
JUREČKOVÁ and SEN · Robust Statistical Procedures: Asymptotics and Interrelations
KADANE · Bayesian Methods and Ethics in a Clinical Trial Design
KADANE and SCHUM · A Probabilistic Analysis of the Sacco and Vanzetti Evidence
KALBFLEISCH and PRENTICE · The Statistical Analysis of Failure Time Data
KELLY · Reversibility and Stochastic Networks
KHURI, MATHEW, and SINHA · Statistical Tests for Mixed Linear Models
KLUGMAN, PANJER, and WILLMOT · Loss Models: From Data to Decisions
KLUGMAN, PANJER, and WILLMOT · Solutions Manual to Accompany Loss Models: From Data to Decisions
KOTZ, BALAKRISHNAN and JOHNSON · Continuous Multivariate Distributions, Volume 1, *Second Edition*
KOVALENKO, KUZNETZOV, and PEGG · Mathematical Theory of Reliability of Time-Dependent Systems with Practical Applications
LACHIN · Biostatistical Methods: The Assessment of Relative Risks
LAD · Operational Subjective Statistical Methods: A Mathematical, Philosophical, and Historical Introduction
LANGE, RYAN, BILLARD, BRILLINGER, CONQUEST, and GREENHOUSE · Case Studies in Biometry
LAWLESS · Statistical Models and Methods for Lifetime Data
LAWSON · Statistical Methods for Spatial Epidemiology
LEE · Statistical Methods for Survival Data Analysis, *Second Edition*
LEPAGE and BILLARD · Exploring the Limits of Bootstrap
LEYLAND and GOLDSTEIN · Multilevel Modelling of Health Statistics
LINHART and ZUCCHINI · Model Selection
LITTLE and RUBIN · Statistical Analysis with Missing Data
LLOYD · The Statistical Analysis of Categorical Data
MAGNUS and NEUDECKER · Matrix Differential Calculus with Applications in Statistics and Econometrics, *Revised Edition*
MALLER and ZHOU · Survival Analysis with Long Term Survivors
MANN, SCHAFER, and SINGPURWALLA · Methods for Statistical Analysis of Reliability and Life Data
McLACHLAN and KRISHNAN · The EM Algorithm and Extensions
McLACHLAN · Discriminant Analysis and Statistical Pattern Recognition
McNEIL · Epidemiological Research Methods
MEEKER and ESCOBAR · Statistical Methods for Reliability Data
*MILLER · Survival Analysis, *Second Edition*
MONTGOMERY and PECK · Introduction to Linear Regression Analysis, *Second Edition*
MYERS and MONTGOMERY · Response Surface Methodology: Process and Product in Optimization Using Designed Experiments
NELSON · Accelerated Testing, Statistical Models, Test Plans, and Data Analyses
NELSON · Applied Life Data Analysis
OCHI · Applied Probability and Stochastic Processes in Engineering and Physical Sciences
OKABE, BOOTS, CHUI, and SUGIHARA · Spatial Tesselations: Concepts and Applications of Voronoi diagrams, *Second Edition*
PANKRATZ · Forecasting with Dynamic Regression Models
PANKRATZ · Forecasting with Univariate Box–Jenkins Models: Concepts and Cases
PIANTADOSI · Clinical Trials: A Methodologic Perspective

*Now available in a lower priced paperback edition in the Wiley Classics Library.

Applied Probability and Statistics (Continued)

PORT · Theoretical Probability for Applications
PUTERMAN · Markov Decision Processes: Discrete Stochastic Dynamic Programming
RACHEV · Probability Metrics and the Stability of Stochastic Models
RÉNYI · A Diary on Information Theory
RIGDON and BASU · Statistical Methods for the Reliability of Repairable Systems
RIPLEY · Spatial Statistics
RIPLEY · Stochastic Simulation
ROLSKI, SCHMIDLI, SCHMIDT, and TEUGELS · Stochastic Processes for Insurance and Finance
ROUSSEEUW and LEROY · Robust Regression and Outlier Detection
RUBIN · Multiple Imputation for Nonresponse in Surveys
RUBINSTEIN · Simulation and the Monte Carlo Method
RUBINSTEIN and MELAMED · Modern Simulation and Modeling
RYAN · Statistical Methods for Quality Improvement, *Second Edition*
SCHIMEK · Smoothing and Regression: Approaches, Computation and Applications
SCHUSS · Theory and Applications of Stochastic Differential Equations
SCOTT · Multivariate Density Estimation: Theory, Practice, and Visualization
*SEARLE · Linear Models
SEARLE · Linear Models for Unbalanced Data
SEARLE, CASELLA, and McCULLOCH · Variance Components
SENNOT · Stochastic Dynamic Programming and the Control of Queuing Systems
STOYAN, KENDALL, and MECKE · Stochastic Geometry and Its Applications, *Second Edition*
STOYAN and STOYAN · Fractals, Random Shapes, and Point Fields: Methods of Geometrical Statistics
SUTTON, ABRAMS, JONES, SHELDON and SONG · Methods for Meta-analysis in Medical Research
THOMPSON · Empirical Model Building
THOMPSON · Sampling
THOMPSON · Simulation: A Modeler's Approach
TIJMS · Stochastic Modeling and Analysis: A Computational Approach
TIJMS · Stochastic Models: An Algorithmic Approach
TITTERINGTON, SMITH, and MARKOV · Statistical Analysis of Finite Mixture Distributions
UPTON and FINGLETON · Spatial Data Analysis by Example, Volume 1: Point Pattern and Quantitative Data
UPTON and FINGLETON · Spatial Data Analysis by Example, Volume II: Categorical and Directional Data
VAN RIJCKEVORSEL and DE LEEUW · Component and Correspondence Analysis
VIDAKOVIC · Statistical Modeling by Wavelets
WEISBERG · Applied Linear Regression, *Second Edition*
WESTFALL and YOUNG · Resampling-Based Multiple Testing: Examples and Methods for p-Value Adjustment
WHITTLE · Systems in Stochastic Equilibrium
WINKER · Optimization Heuristics in Econometrics: Applications of Threshold Accepting
WOODING · Planning Pharmaceutical Clinical Trials: Basic Statistical Principles
WOOLSON · Statistical Methods for the Analysis of Biomedical Data
*ZELLNER · An Introduction to Bayesian Inference in Econometrics

---

*Now available in a lower priced paperback edition in the Wiley Classics Library.

Texts and References Section

AGRESTI · An Introduction to Categorical Data Analysis
ANDERSON · An Introduction to Multivariate Statistical Analysis, *Second Edition*
ANDERSON and LOYNES · The Teaching of Practical Statistics
ARMITAGE and COLTON · Encyclopedia of Biostatistics. 6 Volume set
BARTOSZYNSKI and NIEWIADOMSKA-BUGAJ · Probability and Statistical Inference
BENDAT and PIERSOL · Random Data: Analysis and Measurement Procedures, *Third Edition*
BERRY, CHALONER, and GEWEKE · Bayesian Analysis in Statistics and Econometrics: Essays in Honor of Arnold Zellner
BHATTACHARYA and JOHNSON · Statistical Concepts and Methods
BILLINGSLEY · Probability and Measure, *Second Edition*
BOX · R. A. Fisher, the Life of a Scientist
BOX, HUNTER, and HUNTER · Statistics for Experimenters: An Introduction to Design, Data Analysis, and Model Building
BOX and LUCEÑO · Statistical Control by Monitoring and Feedback Adjustment
BROWN and HOLLANDER · Statistics: A Biomedical Introduction
CHATTERJEE and PRICE · Regression Analysis by Example, *Third Edition*
COOK and WEISBERG · An Introduction to Regression Graphics
COOK and WEISBERG · Applied Regression Including Computing and Graphics
COX · A Handbook of Introductory Statistical Methods
DILLON and GOLDSTEIN · Multivariate Analysis: Methods and Applications
*DODGE and ROMIG · Sampling Inspection Tables, *Second Edition*
DRAPER and SMITH · Applied Regression Analysis, *Third Edition*
DUDEWICZ and MISHRA · Modern Mathematical Statistics
DUNN · Basic Statistics: A Primer for the Biomedical Sciences, *Second Edition*
EVANS, HASTINGS and PEACOCK · Statistical Distributions, *Third Edition*
FISHER and VAN BELLE · Biostatistics: A Methodology for the Health Sciences
FREEMAN and SMITH · Aspects of Uncertainty: A Tribute to D. V. Lindley
GROSS and HARRIS · Fundamentals of Queueing Theory, *Third Edition*
HALD · A History of Probability and Statistics and their Applications Before 1750
HALD · A History of Mathematical Statistics from 1750 to 1930
HELLER · MACSYMA for Statisticians
HOEL · Introduction to Mathematical Statistics, *Fifth Edition*
HOLLANDER and WOLFE · Nonparametric Statistical Methods, *Second Edition*
HOSMER and LEMESHOW · Applied Logistic Recession, *Second Edition*
HOSMER and LEMESHOW · Applied Survival Analysis: Regression Modeling of Time to Event Data
JOHNSON and BALAKRISHNAN · Advances in the Theory and Practice of Statistics: A Volume in Honor of Samuel Kotz
JOHNSON and KOTZ (editors) · Leading Personalities in Statistical Sciences: From the Seventeenth Century to the Present
JUDGE, GRIFFITHS, HILL, LÜTKEPOHL, and LEE · The Theory and Practice of Econometrics, *Second Edition*
KHURI · Advanced Calculus with Applications in Statistics
KOTZ and JOHNSON (editors) · Encyclopedia of Statistical Sciences. Volumes 1 to 9 with Index
KOTZ and JOHNSON (editors) · Encyclopedia of Statistical Sciences: Supplement Volume

---

*Now available in a lower priced paperback edition in the Wiley Classics Library.

Texts and References Section (Continued)

KOTZ, REED, and BANKS (editors) · Encyclopedia of Statistical Sciences: Update Volume 1
KOTZ, REED, and BANKS (editors) · Encyclopedia of Statistical Sciences: Update Volume 2
LAMPERTI · Probability: A Survey of the Mathematical Theory, *Second Edition*
LARSON · Introduction to Probability Theory and Statistical Inference, *Third Edition*
LE · Applied Categorical Data Analysis
LE · Applied Survival Analysis
MALLOWS · Design, Data, and Analysis by Some Friends of Cuthbert Daniel
MARDIA · The Art of Statistical Science: A Tribute to G. S. Watson
MASON, GUNST, and HESS · Statistical Design and Analysis of Experiments with Applications to Engineering and Science
MURRAY · X-STAT 2.0 Statistical Experimentation, Design Data Analysis, and Nonlinear Optimization
PURI, VILAPLANA, and WERTZ · New Perspectives in Theoretical and Applied Statistics
RENCHER · Methods of Multivariate Analysis
RENCHER · Linear Models in Statistics
RENCHER · Multivariate Statistical Inference with Applications
ROBINSON · Practical Strategies for Experimenting
ROSS · Introduction to Probability and Statistics for Engineers and Scientists
ROHATGI · An Introduction to Probability Theory and Mathematical Statistics
ROHATGI and SALEH · An Introduction to Probability and Statistics, *Second Edition*
RYAN · Modern Regression Methods
SCHOTT · Matrix Analysis for Statistics
SEARLE · Matrix Algebra Useful for Statistics
STYAN · The Collected Papers of T. W. Anderson: 1943–1985
TIAO, BISGAARD, HILL, PEÑA, and STIGLER (editors) · Box on Quality and Discovery: with Design, Control, and Robustness
TIERNEY · LISP-STAT: An Object-Oriented Environment for Statistical Computing and Dynamic Graphics
WONNACOTT and WONNACOTT · Econometrics, *Second Edition*
WU and HAMADA · Experiments: Planning, Analysis, and Parameter Design Optimization

WILEY SERIES IN PROBABILITY AND STATISTICS

ESTABLISHED BY WALTER A. SHEWHART AND SAMUEL S. WILKS

Editors
Robert M. Groves, Graham Kalton, J. N. K. Rao, Norbert Schwarz, Christopher Skinner

Survey Methodology Section

BIEMER, GROVES, LYBERG, MATHIOWETZ, and SUDMAN · Measurement Errors in Surveys

---

*Now available in a lower priced paperback edition in the Wiley Classics Library.

COCHRAN · Sampling Techniques, *Third Edition*
COUPER, BAKER, BETHLEHEM, CLARK, MARTIN, NICHOLLS and O'REILLY (editors) · Computer Assisted Survey Information Collection
COX, BINDER, CHINNAPPA, CHRISTIANSON, COLLEDGE, and KOTT (editors) · Business Survey Methods
*DEMING · Sample Design in Business Research
DILLMAN · Mail and Telephone Surveys: The Total Design Method
GROVES · Survey Errors and Survey Costs
GROVES and COUPER · Nonresponse in Household Interview Surveys
GROVES, BIEMER, LYBERG, MASSEY, NICHOLLS, and WAKSBERG · Telephone Survey Methodology
*HANSEN, HURWITZ, and MADOW · Sample Survey Methods and Theory, Volume I: Methods and Applications
*HANSEN, HURWITZ, and MADOW · Sample Survey Methods and Theory, Volume II: Theory
KISH · Statistical Design for Research
*KISH · Survey Sampling
KORN and GRAUBARD · Analysis of Health Surveys
LESSLER and KALSBEEK · Nonsampling Error in Surveys
LEVY and LEMESHOW · Sampling of Populations: Methods and Applications
LYBERG, BIEMER, COLLINS, de LEEUW, DIPPO, SCHWARZ, TREWIN (editors) · Survey Measurement and Process Quality
SIRKEN, HERRMANN, SCHECHTER, SCHWARZ, TANUR and TOURNANGEAU (editors) · Cognition and Survey Research
VALLIANT, DORFMAN, and ROYALL · Finite Population Sampling and Inference: A Prediction Approach

---

*Now available in a lower priced paperback edition in the Wiley Classics Library.